THE VARIETIES OF ORTHOGRAPHIC KNOWLEDGE

NEUROPSYCHOLOGY AND COGNITION

VOLUME 8

The purpose of the Neuropsychology and Cognition series is to bring out volumes that promote understanding in topics relating brain and behavior. It is intended for use by both clinicians and research scientists in the fields of neuropsychology, cognitive psychology, psycholinguistics, speech and hearing, as well as education. Examples of topics to be covered in the series would relate to memory, language acquisition and breakdown, reading, attention, developing and aging brain. By addressing the theoretical, empirical, and applied aspects of brain-behavior relationships, this series will try to present the information in the fields of neuropsychology and cognition in a coherent manner.

The titles published in this series are listed at the end of this volume.

THE VARIETIES OF ORTHOGRAPHIC KNOWLEDGE

I: Theoretical and Developmental Issues

Edited by

VIRGINIA WISE BERNINGER
University of Washington, Seattle, U.S.A.

KLUWER ACADEMIC PUBLISHERS
DORDRECHT / BOSTON / LONDON

Library of Congress Cataloging-in-Publication Data

The varieties of orthographic knowledge / edited by Virginia Wise Berninger.
p. cm.
Contents: 1. Theoretical and developmental issues.
ISBN 0-7923-3081-1 (set). -- ISBN 0-7923-3080-3 (v. 1)
1. Language and languages--Orthography and spelling. 2. Language acquisition. 3. Literacy. I. Berninger, Virginia Wise.
P240.2.V37 1994
411--dc20 94-30307

ISBN 0-7923-3080-3 (Volume 1)
ISBN 0-7923-3081-1 (Set of 2 volumes)

Published by Kluwer Academic Publishers,
P.O. Box 17, 3300 AA Dordrecht, The Netherlands.

Kluwer Academic Publishers incorporates
the publishing programmes of
D. Reidel, Martinus Nijhoff, Dr W. Junk and MTP Press.

Sold and distributed in the U.S.A. and Canada
by Kluwer Academic Publishers,
101 Philip Drive, Norwell, MA 02061, U.S.A.

In all other countries, sold and distributed
by Kluwer Academic Publishers Group,
P.O. Box 322, 3300 AH Dordrecht, The Netherlands.

Printed on acid-free paper

Printed in the Netherlands

This 2-volume series on orthography is dedicated to ongoing dialogue and scientific investigation about the varieties of orthography knowledge and their role in reading and writing acquisition.

TABLE OF CONTENTS - VOLUME I

Commentaries on Volume I

Acknowledgements

I thank R. Malatesha Joshi, Editor of the Neuropsychology and Cognition Series published by Kluwer, for his encouragement in bringing these two edited volumes on orthography to fruition. He has believed for a long time that orthography has not been given sufficient attention by reading acquisition researchers, who have tended to emphasize the role of phonology in learning to read. It was at his invitation that this project was initiated. I also thank Sylvia Mirsepassi at the University of Washington who converted all the contributions to these volumes into camera-ready copy. Without her computer expertise this project would not have been possible. I am also grateful to all the contributors to these volumes whose enthusiasm inspired me to pursue this project and whose cooperation in meeting deadlines made it possible to complete this project in a timely manner. Finally, I thank Barbara Foorman, Esther Geva, and Dale Willows for their thoughtful commentaries at the end of each volume.

Virginia W. Berninger,
Editor

The role of orthography in reading and writing is not a new topic of inquiry. For example, in 1970 Venezky made a seminal contribution with *The Structure of English Orthography* in which he showed how both sequential redundancy (probable and permissible letter sequences) and rules of letter-sound correspondence contribute to orthographic structure. In 1980 Ehri introduced the concept of orthographic images, that is, the representation of written words in memory, and proposed that the image is created by an amalgamation of the word's orthographic and phonological properties. In 1981 Taylor described the evolution of orthographies in writing systems—from the earliest *logographies* for pictorial representation of ideas to *syllabaries* for phonetic representation of sounds to *alphabets* for phonemic representation of sounds. In 1985 Frith proposed a stage model for the role of orthographic knowledge in development of word recognition: Initially in the logographic stage a few words can be recognized on the basis of partial spelling information; in the alphabetic stage words are recognized on the basis of grapheme-phoneme correspondence; in the orthographic stage spelling units are recognized automatically without phonological mediation. For an historical overview of research on visual processing of written language spanning the earliest records of writing to the early work in experimental psychology, see Venezky (1993).

During the past two decades, however, the role of orthography has not received as much attention as has the role of phonology in reading and writing acquisition. This lack of attention to orthography is ironic because during the same two decades substantial converging evidence has verified that in normal readers visual information in printed words is processed fully and not merely sampled to test top-down hypotheses (Rayner & Pollatsek, 1989). What might account for this lack of attention to orthography?

One contributing factor proposed by Willows and her co-editors in their recent book, *Visual Processes in Reading and Reading Disabilities*, is that research on the visual processes in reading is widely scattered throughout diverse literatures. Thus there is need for volumes like theirs and this 2-volume series to provide a common forum for research on orthography from diverse perspectives.

Another contributing factor has been the lack of clarity about the distinction between non-orthographic visual processes and orthographic processes (Berninger, 1990, 1991, 1994). Not all visual processing is orthographic processing, which is visual processing specific to written words. Much of the early research on the role of visual perception and visual memory in reading disabilities used non-linguistic visual stimuli such as geometric figures and line drawings. Thus, whenVellutino argued that linguistic factors rather than visual perception and visual memory were causal mechanisms in dyslexia (Vellutino, 1979a), he was not ruling out orthographic factors (Vellutino, 1979b). This 2-volume series will focus exclusively on orthographic knowledge specific to written words and will not deal with the relationship between the physiology of vision and the acquisition of orthographic knowledge (see Willows et al., 1993, especially chapters 4, 5, and 14).

Yet another contributing factor was the paradigm shift in the early 1980's from research on the visual perceptual deficit hypothesis to the linguistic deficit hypothesis of dyslexia. This shift was due in large part to the pioneering efforts of Liberman and Shankweiler and their colleagues at the Haskins Laboratory (e.g., their 1974 article in the *Journal of Experimental Child Psychology)* regarding the role of phonology in beginning reading andVellutino's persuasive demonstration of the linguistic nature of reading disabilities in his influential 1979 book, *Dyslexia: Theory and Research.* This paradigm shift was maintained, in large part, by the considerable number of subsequent studies confirming the role of phonology and other linguistic factors in reading (e.g., Brady & Shankweiler, 1991). A consequence of this paradigm shift was that research on orthography was less fashionable although it did not come to a standstill (e.g., Aaron & Joshi, 1987; Henderson, 1984; Templeton & Bear, 1992).

Still another contributing factor is theoretical. We lack a well established theory of orthography and its role in reading and writing acquisition. In contrast, a well established theory of phonology developed by Liberman, Cooper, Shankweiler, and Studdert-Kennedy (1967) predated research on the role of phonology in reading acquisition and this clearly articulated theory may have facilitated the progress we have made in understanding the role of phonology in learning to read. A major purpose of Volume I of this 2-volume series is therefore to integrate existing work on orthography to stimulate thinking about a theoretical framework to guide future research and to use in evaluating existing research. Such theory must take into account changes in orthographic knowledge over skill development as reading and writing are developmental processes. Also, as Wagner and Barker (chapter 7) conclude, such theory should integrate orthographic and phonological processing in a comprehensive model.

A final contributing factor is methodological. Orthography and phonology are probably confounded in the normal reading and writing process, rendering it difficult to design tasks that measure orthography independently of phonology or phonology independently of orthography. Volume II of this 2-volume series will therefore consider alternative methodological approaches (experimental, electrophysiological, and statistical) for dissecting analytically processes that are functionally integrated.

Despite these five factors contributing to the relative neglect of orthography, a paradigm shift may be looming in which attention is switching from a relatively exclusive focus on phonology to increasing attention to the relationship between orthography and phonology (e.g., Gough, Ehri, & Treiman, 1993). Orthographic-phonological relationships are therefore examined in both volumes. Yet each volume has a unique focus.

Volume I explores a number of theoretical issues, often from a developmental perspective. What are the different kinds of orthographic knowledge that have been investigated and discussed in the literature? Which kinds of orthographic knowledge are most relevant at various stages of literacy acquisition? Which tasks tap each of these kinds of knowledge? Is orthographic knowledge constrained by genetic inheritance? Is orthographic knowledge constrained by linguistic universals common to all languages or is it unique to specific languages? What role does oral language, for example, naming skills, play in acquiring knowledge of orthographic structure? What role does knowledge of letter-sound relationships play in acquiring phonological awareness, which in turn plays an important role in learning to read and spell? How early in development is orthographic awareness acquired? Do orthographic measures account for unique variance in reading or writing over and beyond that accounted for by phonological measures alone? Is orthographic processing important only in word recognition in isolation or also in context? What are the implications of the alternative theories such as dual route theory or connectionism for the study of orthographic knowledge?

Volume II focuses on orthographic-phonological, orthographic-spelling, and orthographic-reading relationships. An overview of the basic principles of orthographic-sound relationships is provided. A theoretical model of the multiple sources of orthographic and orthographic-phonological knowledge contributing to skilled, fluent reading is proposed. New approaches to the study of spelling are discussed: investigation of developmental and individual differences in strategy use and of retention of spelling knowledge over time. The importance of orthography in normal and disabled reading and in reading isolated words versus connected text is explored. Three methodologies for analytically teasing apart the independent contribution of orthography and phonology are presented: experimental manipulations of a novel alphabet with orthographic but not phonological properties; electrophysiological techniques for detecting differences in brain response on orthographic and phonological tasks; and statistical techniques such as analysis of covariance structures in structural equation modeling for assessing the relative contribution of correlated factors to explaining the variance in reading or writing skills.

As pointed out by Wagner and Barker in Volume I, at present there is no consensus about which tasks are most appropriate for measuring orthographic skills or even if orthographic skills are important in understanding literacy acquisition. Contributors to this 2-volume series offer a diversity of perspectives on orthography, but support the position that orthography is relevant to literacy. They differ in their theoretical orientation and measurement approach. Our goal is to promote constructive dialogue about the theoretical and measurement issues. Ultimately, the most appropriate measures of orthography will probably depend on the research question at hand; and the perceived importance of orthography will depend on a conceptual framework that recognizes that orthography is both separate from and functionally intertwined with phonology.

References

Aaron, P.G., & Joshi, R.M. (Eds.) (1987). *Reading and writing disorders in different orthographic systems. Proceedings of the NATO Advanced Study Institute on Developmental and Acquired Disorders of Reading and Writing Systems in Different Languages: A cognitive neuropsychological perspective.* Dordrecht, The Netherlands: Kluwer Academic Publishers.

Berninger, V. (1991). Overview of "Bridging the gap between development, cognitive, and neuropsychological approaches to reading." *Learning and Individual Differences, 3,* 163-179.

Berninger, V. (1990). Multiple orthographic codes: Key to alternative instructional methodologies for developing orthographic-phonological connections underlying word identification. *School Psychology Review, 19,* 518-533.

Berninger, V. (1994). *Reading and writing acquisition. A developmental neuropsychological perspective.* Madison, WI: WCB Brown & Benchmark.

Brady, S.A., & Shankweiler, D.P. (Eds.) (1991). *Phonological processes in literacy.* Hillsdale, NJ: Lawrence Erlbaum Associates.

Ehri, L. (1980). The development of orthographic images. In U. Frith (Ed.), *Cognitive processes in spelling* (pp. 311-338). London: Academic Press.

Frith, U. (1985). Beneath the surface of developmental dyslexia. In K.E. Patterson, J.C. Marshall, & M. Coltheart (Eds.), *Surface dyslexia* (pp. 301-330). London: Lawrence Erlbaum Associates.

Gough, P., Ehri, L., & Treiman, R. (Eds.) (1993). *Reading acquisition.* Hillsdale, NJ: Erlbaum.

Henderson, L. (1984). *Orthographies and reading. Perspectives from Cognitive Psychology, Neuropsychology, and Linguistics.* Hillsdale, NJ: Lawrence Erlbaum Associates.

Liberman, A.M., Cooper, F.S., Shankweiler, D.P., & Studdert-Kennedy, M. (1967). Perception of the speech code. *Psychological Review, 74,* 431-461.

Liberman, I., Shankweiler, D., Fischer, F., & Carter, B. (1974). Explicit syllable and phoneme segmentation in the young child. *Journal of Experimental Child Psychology, 18,* 201-212.

Rayner, K., & Pollatsek, A. (1989). *The psychology of reading.* Englewood Cliffs, NJ: Prentice-Hall.

Taylor, I. (1981). Writing systems and reading. In *Reading research: Advances in theory and practice* (Vol. 2, pp. 1-51). New York: Academic Press.

Templeton, S., & Bear, D. (1992). *Development of orthographic knowledge and the foundations of literacy.* Hillsdale, NJ: Lawrence Erlbaum Associates.

Vellutino, F. (1979a). *Dyslexia: Theory and research.* Cambridge, MA: The MIT Press.

Vellutino, F. (1979b). The validity of perceptual deficit explanations of reading disability: A reply to Fletcher and Saby. *Journal of Learning Disabilities, 12,* 27-34.

Venezky, R. (1970). *The structure of English orthography.* The Hague: Mouton.

Venezky, R. (1993). History of interest in the visual component of reading. In D. Willows, R. Kruk, & E. Corcos (Eds.), *Visual processes in reading and reading disabilities.* Hillsdale, NJ: Lawrence Erlbaum Associates.

Wagner, R., & Barker, T. (1994). The development of orthographic processing ability. In V. Berninger (Ed.), *The varieties of orthographic knowledge I: Theoretical and developmental issues* (pp. 181-206). Dordrecht, The Netherlands: Kluwer Academic Publishers.

Willows, D., Kruk, R., & Corcos, E. (1993). *Visual processes in reading and reading disabilities.* Hillsdale, NJ: Lawrence Erlbaum.

VIRGINIA W. BERNINGER

INTRODUCTION TO THE VARIETIES OF ORTHOGRAPHIC KNOWLEDGE I: THEORETICAL AND DEVELOPMENTAL ISSUES

Visual processes in reading have been studied for over a century by experimental psychologists and neuropsychologists (Venezky, 1993). However, advances in psycholinguistics over the past two decades led to a relative focus on the linguistic aspects of reading, particularly the phonological processes involved, and a relative neglect of the visual processes. Recently interest in the visual processes involved in reading and writing the orthography of the language has reappeared (Willows, Kruk, & Corcos, 1993), but the lack of consensus on how to define orthographic processes and measure them has impeded progress.

DEFINITIONAL ISSUES

One reason for the lack of consensus on how to measure orthographic processing (see Table 1 in chapter 7 by Wagner & Barker) is that orthographic processing involves multiple kinds of orthographic knowledge and different investigators are focusing on different kinds of orthographic knowledge. The schema in Table 1 summarizes the kinds of orthographic knowledge discussed in the literature and proposes whether their representation in memory is declarative or procedural. Declarative representations contain knowledge about the writing system. The content or structure of a visible word is represented and can be accessed; or relationships between spoken and written forms of words are stored that can be accessed in translating written words into spoken words or spoken words into written words; or linguistic awareness of properties and functions of written words is represented. Procedural representations, on the other hand, contain procedures of mind (Kolers & Roediger, 1984) for acting upon representations of written words in the mind's eye. These procedures play a role in creating declarative representations of

V.W. Berninger (ed.), The varieties of orthographic knowledge I: Theoretical and developmental issues, 1-25.

Table 1

Varieties of Orthographic Knowledge	Declarative Knowledge	Procedural Knowledge
Orthographic Structure	X	
spatial redundancy		
sequential redundancy (based on statistical probability or orthographic structure rules)		
Orthographic Coding (accuracy and speed)		X
whole word (its constituent letters)		
letter in a word		
letter cluster in a word		
Orthographic-Linguistic Mapping (bidirectional)		
Orthographic Code Connections to		X
phonological codes		
name code (whole word)		
syllable		
onsets and rimes		
phoneme(s)		
semantic/morphemic /syntactic codes		
Spelling-Sound Knowledge	X	
Spelling-Semantic/Syntactic Knowledge	X	
Internal Lexicon (Storage)	X	
partial orthographic images		
complete orthographic images		
interconnections with phonological, semantic, and syntactic representations		
rules ± exceptions		
Metacognitive Knowledge about the Writing System		
Concepts of Print	X	
Concepts of Processing Print		X
Strategies		X

words in memory and in accessing those declarative representations. Procedural representations may also underlie strategies for utilizing orthographic knowledge. The various kinds of orthographic knowledge most likely come from exposure to and interaction with reading materials and from experience in writing. After providing a brief overview of each of the various kinds of orthographic knowledge, I discuss which of these kinds of knowledge is the focus of each contributor to Volume I.

Orthographic Structure. Mason (1975) studied sixth graders and showed that good readers and poor readers differed in utilization of *spatial redundancy* information, which arises from the relationship among distinctive visual features and certain letters occurring more often in certain positions than others, but not from utilization of distinctive visual features (like curves, angles, and lines in words) per se. She also showed that good readers processed highly spatially redundant nonwords faster than common real words which were not as spatially redundant but were composed of the same letters.

Venezky (1979) and Venezky and Massaro (1979), on the other hand, discussed *sequential redundancy* based on letter sequences. Sequential redundancy contributes to orthographic structure which can be defined in two contrasting ways. One approach uses frequency of occurrence data, based upon types or tokens, to define a goodness of fit or probability of occurrence. The other approach uses rules or patterns based upon structural analyses. The former approach, which yields letter probabilities, positional frequencies, and sequential redundancy patterns, will always assign a low score to a non-occurring pattern. The latter approach, in contrast, will evaluate all patterns—occurring or non-occurring—according to rules or templates and assign a conformity index. Venezky and Massaro proposed that automatic word recognition depends on having abstracted knowledge of *orthographic regularity*, based on statistical probability or rules, through repeated exposure to the orthographic structure in text. They emphasized that orthographic regularity is not the same as letter-sound regularity. Phonically irregular words may be orthographically regular (e.g., eighth), and orthographically irregular strings may be pronounceable by applying phonics rules (e.g., ssilf). For example, even if the rime of a syllable contains irregular grapheme-phoneme correspondences, the rime as unit is probably orthographically regular (Berninger, 1990).

Orthographic Coding. Johnson (1978) reviewed the concept of codes as used in cognitive psychology. Codes are procedures for transforming stimulus information into unitary mental representations. They should not be confused with the information they represent; the content of a code only becomes available when the decoding process is complete. Written words can be coded into whole word units, single letters in words, or letter clusters in words (Barron, 1986; Berninger, 1987; Shallice, Warrington, & McCarthy, 1983) in memory. Whole word unit does not imply that letters are not processed or that only configuration is processed; rather letters are processed in parallel within a word, that is, the orthographic structure for the whole word is processed. The coding operations refer to the size of the unit chunked in the unitary mental representation—the whole word, a single element, or a series of elements smaller than the whole. Orthographic structure probably plays a role in orthographic coding.

Orthographic-Linguistic Mapping. Procedural operations create interconnections among orthographic codes and other linguistic codes. Spelling-sound knowledge results from and may influence these operations.

Orthographic Code Connections. Orthographic codes map onto phonological codes of corresponding size (Van Orden, Pennington, & Stone, 1990). For example, whole written words map onto name codes for whole spoken words, single letters map onto phonemes, letter clusters map onto syllables, rimes, or phonemes (Berninger, 1994). Orthographic codes can also map onto semantic codes for lexical items as in the direct route in Dual Route Theory (Coltheart, 1978) or onto morphemic codes for sublexical affixes to lexical items. Code connections may form inductively through repeated exposure to words (Seidenberg & McClelland, 1989; Van Orden et al., 1990) or deductively through explicit instruction in rules of letter-sound relationship and structural analysis (Adams, 1990; Foorman, Francis, Novy, & Liberman, 1991; Venezky, 1970). Code connections may be formed in the other direction as well, with phonological codes (or other linguistic codes) mapping onto orthographic codes of corresponding unit size.

Spelling-Sound Knowledge. In contrast to code connections, which are procedural operations for transforming stimulus words into mental representations, spelling-sound knowledge is based on the content that becomes available when the decoding process is complete. This content may consist of automatic sight words, phonics rules, phonograms (word families), or structural analysis rules (for syllabication, accent patterns, or modification of roots with affixes). Spelling-sound knowledge may be more complex than relationships between single graphemes and phonemes; it also involves relationships between letter sequences and phonemes, rimes, or syllables *and* the positioning of single letters or letter sequences within a word. (See Venezky, in press, Volume II, for model of five (0-4) orders or levels of spelling-sound knowledge in reading.) Sound-spelling knowledge is also represented (see Barron, chapter 6) and is reflected in the content of encoded written productions.

Internal Lexicon (Storage). Ehri (1980a, 1980b) introduced the concept of an orthographic image, which is a word-specific representation stored in memory. Creating orthographic images in memory requires knowledge of letter-sound relations, written syllable-spoken syllable relationships, and spelling patterns associated with rhyming words (Ehri, 1980a), that is, knowledge based on orthographic-phonological connections. When children learn to read, the orthographic representation of a word amalgamates with the phonological, syntactic, and semantic representations of a word already in the lexicon and forms an integrated unit that can be partial or complete, depending on whether all the letters in a word's spelling are completely represented and linked with a complete phonological representation of spoken and silent sounds (Ehri, 1992a). These orthographic images are accessed in reading and in spelling words, but spelling may be more adversely affected by partial orthographic images than is reading. The issue of how orthographic knowledge is stored requires further research. Venezky (personal communication, June 1, 1994) has suggested that it might be (a) regenerated when needed from stored lexical images, (b) stored as rules with exceptions, or (c) represented by some combination of these. The first possibility suggests that procedural knowledge might also be involved in storage.

Metacognitive Knowledge of the Writing System. Clay's (1979) Concepts of Print assesses both declarative knowledge about orthography (e.g., sentences begin with a capital letter and end with a period, question mark, or exclamation point) and procedural knowledge about processing print (e.g., reading proceeds left to right). Strategies might operate on any of the kinds of orthographic knowledge. For example, for spelling-sound mapping, strategies might include scan left to right; try placing the stress on the next to the last syllable and see if the word is familiar; or try thinking of a word with the same spelling pattern and pronounce the unknown word the same way (i.e., the analogy strategy, Glushko, 1979; Goswami, 1988). Other strategies reviewed by Varnhagen (in press) include retrieve spelling sequence and perform phonological check; analyze unknown word into morphemic components; segment word into syllable, subsyllable, onset and rime, or individual phonemes; apply idiosyncratic mnemonics for exception words; or access external consultant (dictionary or another writer). Formal assessment tools are lacking for metacognitive knowledge about orthography in developing and skilled readers and writers.

KINDS OF ORTHOGRAPHIC KNOWLEDGE DISCUSSED IN VOLUME I

Olson, Forsberg, and Wise (chapter 1) use three measures of orthographic coding: word-pseudohomophone choice, homophone choice, and PIAT spelling. The first task requires choosing the real word in a pair of words that also contains a nonword pronounced exactly the same as the real word. Even if readers code the words orthographically and rely on orthographic-phonological connections to decode the words, the task cannot be solved correctly without accessing an orthographic image of the real word in the memory. The second task requires choosing one of two homonyms that correctly answers a question. Again, a correct response requires more than coding and decoding; it requires accessing an amalgamation of a word's spelling and its associated semantic representation. The last task requires selection of the correct written spelling for a spoken word from a set of four orthographically similar alternatives. Taken together, these three tasks provide operational measures of *orthographic images* in the lexicon (see Table 1).

Jackson, Lu, and Ju (chapter 2) review literature showing that Chinese cannot be read solely in terms of orthographic coding. Rather, it, like English, involves orthographic connections to phonological codes and orthographic connections to semantic codes. However, unlike an alphabet system such as English, which maps letters onto phonemes, Chinese maps strokes within characters onto phonetic radicals, which most often provide clues to pronunciation of the rime part of the syllable. Also, unlike English, which marks written word boundaries, Chinese maps strokes within characters onto semantic radicals that are morphemes, which convey meaning at the subword level. In their empirical work Jackson et al. compared two approaches to teaching Chinese to English-speaking ninth graders. One approach involved direct connections between characters and meaning of single-syllable Chinese words. The other approach used a non-Roman alphabetic system to teach letter-sound correspondence. Two of Olson's orthographic tasks were given but did not predict performance in learning the character-meaning associations. This finding makes sense in that these orthographic tasks measure orthographic images or word-specific representations already acquired rather than coding procedures for creating new representations during the learning process. Taken together, findings in this chapter add to our understanding of orthographic code connections to phonological and semantic codes (see Table 1).

Assink and Kattenberg (chapter 3) use measures that tap two kinds of orthographic knowledge in Table 1. Their "word-image skill" measure, which requires rejection of illegal letter combinations, is an operational measure of orthographic structure (sequential redundancy). Their spelling tasks are designed to assess two basic types of orthographic problems in Dutch: spelling homophones that make syntactic distinctions not present in oral language; and non-homophones that express simple sound-spelling correspondences. According to the authors, correct spelling of the latter requires memory of word-specific representations; thus, these spelling tasks are operational measures of word images in the lexicon.

Wolf, Pfeil, Lotz, and Biddle (chapter 4) discuss the intriguing finding that incidence of reading disability is relatively constant across languages that vary considerably in regularity of letter-sound correspondence or type of orthography (alphabetic or non-alphabetic). They question whether phonological core deficits are the only source of reading disabilities. They note that pseudoword accuracy, which is widely accepted as the best discriminator of poor reading in English, is not a good discriminator of poor reading in German, which is more regular than English. Naming speed on rapid automatized naming tasks (RAN) is a good predictor of reading differences in both German and English dyslexics. However, they point out that RAN tasks tap more than phonological processes. They also tap orthographic processes, also a theme in chapter 5, and thus serve as a marker of disruption in automatic processes underlying abstraction of orthographic regularity and rapid access to lexical codes.

Bowers, Golden, Kennedy, and Young (chapter 5) review literature demonstrating that rapid automatized naming (RAN) tasks tap speed of accessing names of highly automatized printed symbols. They then demonstrate significant relationships between RAN scores and both letter cluster coding and reading skills in primary grade children. They hypothesize that if a child is slow in identifying single letters, then single letters will not be activated in close temporal proximity allowing the child to abstract patterns of coocurrence among letters. They refer to this hypothesis as the orthographic redundancy interpretation of naming speed's relationship to letter cluster knowledge. Thus, they are integrating the constructs of orthographic coding, letter-cluster name connections, and orthographic structure (sequential redundancy) in their conceptual framework. (see Table 1). Like Venezky and Massaro (1979), they emphasize the link between automatization and orthographic structure; however, they introduce the automatized naming side of the link whereas Venezky and Massaro introduced the orthographic structure side of the link (orthographic regularity). Further research is needed to evaluate whether bidirectional influences may be operating between orthographic structure and automatized naming in creating orthographic-phonological connections. Olson et al. (chapter 1) report modest correlations, at best, between their rapid naming and orthographic factors, leading them to dismiss Bower and Wolf's (1993a, 1993b) proposal that orthographic deficits and rapid naming are related. However, Olson et al.'s orthographic factor is based on orthographic images rather than orthographic structure, which is more relevant to the Bower and Wolf hypothesis.

Barron (chapter 6) reviews a sizeable literature documenting auditory-orthographic effects in prereaders, beginning and developing readers, skilled readers, and dyslexics. This effect is attributed to connections between letter clusters and sounds in the rime part of the syllable and to letter-phoneme connections as well as emerging letter-sound knowledge; thus, his theoretical framework is relevant to both the code connections and spelling-sound knowledge in Table 1.

Wagner and Barker (chapter 7) use four different tasks to operationalize orthographic processing, two of which tap orthographic-phonological mappings and letter-sound knowledge (letter name knowledge and invented spellings), one of which taps orthographic images (homophone choice, see discussion of Olson et al.'s tasks), and one of which taps metacognitive knowledge (concepts of print) (see Table 1).

Berninger and Abbott (chapter 8) focus on receptive orthographic coding and orthographic-phonological code connections in their primary grade sample, when the primary research question was how word-specific representations get created in memory. However, in their intermediate grade sample, when the primary research questions were about the role of existing word-specific representations in memory and automatization of coding processes, they focus on orthographic images as well as expressive orthographic coding and speeded orthographic coding (see Table 1).

Collectively, the chapters in this volume deal with all the kinds of orthographic knowledge summarized in Table 1, but individual investigators do not. Thus, conclusions about orthographic processing in regard to dyslexics or poor readers (see chapters by Olson et al., Assink & Kattenberg, Wolf et al., Bowers et al., Barron, and Berninger & Abbott, Volume I, and Lennox & Siegel, Volume II) will depend on what measures were used and which kind of orthographic knowledge was assessed. It is unlikely that any one task will suffice to measure orthographic processing for all purposes considering that any one task cannot measure all kinds of orthographic knowledge and no one task is likely to be a pure measure of orthographic processes independent of other cognitive processes (see Geva & Willows' Commentary, Volume I). Selecting the most appropriate task(s) will depend on the specific aims of a particular research study.

Conclusions may also depend on characteristics of the sample studied. Wolf et al. (chapter 4), Bowers and Wolf (1993) and Bowers et al. (chapter 5) propose the Double Deficit hypothesis—that severe dyslexics have deficits in both phonemic skills and rapid naming whereas milder dyslexics may have deficits only in phonemic skills. If the Bower and Wolf hypothesis of a relationship between rapid automatized naming and orthographic structure is correct (see chapter 5), then deficits in orthographic regularity may only be found if the sample contains enough children with deficits in rapid automatized naming. Thus, the fact that Olson et al. (Volume I) and Lennox and Siegel (Volume II) did not find evidence that dyslexics have difficulty with orthographic structure (permissible letter sequences) but Assink and Kattenberg (Volume I) did, may reflect differences in the incidence of automatized naming deficits in their samples.

THEORETICAL ISSUES

Real or Artifactual Phenomenon. Wagner and Barker (chapter 7) acknowledge that orthography as a topic of research has been controversial, with some investigators questioning whether orthographic processing really exists. One argument against its existence is that phonological processing alone is sufficient to explain reading and writing acquisition. A common defense to this position is to demonstrate the statistical independence of orthographic and phonological skills, that is, that orthographic skills contribute unique variance, over and beyond that contributed by phonological skills, in explaining reading or writing achievement (see Olson et al., chapter 1; Wagner & Barker, chapter 7; and Berninger & Abbott, chapter 8). Another argument against its existence is that orthographic processing tasks merely measure word-recognition or spelling ability (Vellutino, Scanlon, & Tanzman, 1994). Indeed, Olson et al. initially conceptualized their orthographic measures as tapping the direct route of Dual Route Theory in word recognition (see chapter 1). Evidence against the argument that orthographic measures merely tap word recognition or spelling ability is the causal modeling of Wagner and Barker (chapter 7), who found that orthographic measures accounted for variance in word recognition independent of the auto-regressive effects of word recognition, phonological processing, and verbal ability. Additional evidence against this argument is the low to modest correlations between orthographic measures and word recognition and spelling skills in a large-scale psychometric study that included a battery of multiple orthographic measures, including those used by Olson et al. (see Berninger & Abbott, chapter 8).

Multiple Code Activation. One of the difficulties in studying orthographic processes is that it is impossible to design pure measures of orthographic processing that do not also tap phonological processing to some degree. Likewise, it is impossible to design pure measures of phonological processing that do not tap orthographic processing to some degree (see Wagner & Barker, chapter 7). The reason is that phonological codes activate orthographic codes and orthographic codes activate phonological codes in adult skilled readers (e.g., Tanenhaus, Flanigan, & Seidenberg, 1980), in novice readers who have acquired some letter-sound knowledge but cannot yet pronounce or spell words, and in beginning readers (Barron, chapter 6). Although many investigators consider pseudoword (nonword) reading to be a pure measure of phonological processing, both orthographic codes and phonological codes contribute to reading pseudowords in primary grade and intermediate grade children (see Berninger & Abbott, chapter 8). Thus pseudoword reading is probably a measure of orthographic-phonological code connections.

Orchestration of Mind. Some researchers have investigated orthographic processing from the perspective of Dual Route Theory (e.g., Olson et al., chapter 1; and Bowers et al., chapter 5). Others have investigated it from the perspective of connectionism (Berninger & Abbott, chapter 8). Yet others have not adopted any theoretical framework regarding the role orthographic processing plays in word recognition (Wagner & Barker, chapter 7). Whereas Dual Route Theory assumes independence of an orthographic route and phonological route to word recognition, connectionism assumes interaction between orthographic and phonological processing; however, see chapter 8 and Foorman's Commentary for discussion of differences among connectionist models. Given evidence for multiple code activation, a pure orthographic module and a pure phonological module seem unlikely. Although Olson et al. (chapter 1) showed that orthographic and phonological skills are statistically independent in regression analyses, they also found that word recognition loads on both the phonological and orthographic factors and that phonological coding and orthographic coding have very similar patterns of genetic and shared environmental effects. They concluded that phonological and orthographic factors are distinct yet substantially related. Although they began with a dual route perspective, they end by adopting Ehri's (1992a) integrative view. This integrative view is consistent with the metaphor of orchestration of mind introduced by Posner, Petersen, Fox, and

Raichle (1988). As in the orchestra in which separate musicians function together in concert, neuroanatomically separate orthographic and phonological codes can function together during word recognition (for further discussion, see Berninger, 1994, chapters 1 and 2).

Bidirectionality of Connections. In contrast to much literacy research that has focused on the print-to-sound connections, Barron (chapter 6) calls attention to the sound-to-print connections. The challenge for the beginning reader and writer, as well as researchers who study the literacy acquisition process, is that these bidirectional connections are asymmetric. (See Venezky, 1970, in press, for further discussion of the lack of symmetry in the spelling-sound system.) As Snowling (1987) pointed out, there are more phoneme-grapheme correspondences to learn (44 phoneme to 102 functional spelling units) than grapheme-phoneme correspondences (26 graphemes–44 phonemes).

Genetic Determinism versus Genetic Constraints. Are our brains prewired to process orthographic information in predetermined ways? Results of twin studies by Olson and colleagues (chapter 1) support the conclusion that genetic inheritance may constrain the brain architecture underlying both orthographic and phonological processing to some extent, but that genes do not completely determine orthographic and phonological processing abilities. Environmental influences such as experience with reading material and quality of instruction also play a role. The results reported in Chapter 1 are of particular interest because they differ from trends reported previously when the sample size was smaller—that phonological but not orthographic skills are heritable. Now that sample size and power have increased, both orthographic skills (using measures tapping orthographic images) and phonological skills (requiring decoding of printed nonwords) are shown to be heritable. The fact that Olson et al. are modifying their theoretical position from a dual route view (orthographic or phonological access to the lexicon) to an integrated view (orthographic and phonological processes are interrelated) suggests an alternative interpretation for these findings. Not only integration at the whole word level (tapped by the orthographic tasks) but also integration at subword level (tapped by the phonological tasks) is influenced by genes.

Nevertheless it is important to keep in mind that Olson et al. found both shared variance and independent variance between orthographic and phonological coding deficits. So orthographic and phonological processes may have shared (integrated) as well as independent (separate) genetic pathways.

Olson et al. make the important point that just because orthographic skills are genetically constrained it does not mean that they cannot be remediated to some degree. The two remedial case studies discussed by Assink and Kattenberg (chapter 3) illustrate this point. Their observation that spelling deficits related to lack of knowledge of spelling rules are more easily remediable than spelling deficits related to lack of knowledge of orthographic structure warrants further research. Results of treatment studies cited by Berninger and Abbott (chapter 8) also support the conclusion that orthographic skills can be remediated.

Role of Experience. Several of the contributors (Olson et al.; Jackson et al.; Barron; and Wagner & Barker) used or discussed measures of print exposure (e.g., Stanovich, West, & Cunningham, 1992), which are an operational measure of reading experience. Measures of orthographic processing explain independent variance in reading over and beyond that explained by reading experience (see Wagner & Barker, chapter 7). Bowers et al. (chapter 5) reviewed research that shows good readers benefit more from practice than do poor readers (also see Assink & Kattenberg, 1991, for additional evidence). It may well be that deficits or delays in orthographic processing skills may be responsible for poor readers not benefitting from practice in the same way that normal readers do. It also follows that not all children will acquire orthographic skills simply from print exposure, especially if genetic constraints are operating.

Universal versus Language-Specific Characteristics. On the one hand, reading any orthography probably requires orthographic-phonological connections, although specific orthographies may differ in the units of orthography and units of phonology involved in forging connections. For example, Jackson, Lu, and Ju's review of the literature supports the conclusion reached by Leong (1987) that Chinese does not bypass phonology. However, it maps characters onto phonetic radicals rather than on phonemes as an alphabetic language such as English does. Other evidence for commonalities across languages is the fact that reading and spelling disabilities occur in all orthographies (Arabic, Chinese, Danish, Dutch, English, French, German, Greek, Hebrew, Italian, Japanese, Kannada—a South Indian language, Spanish, and Turkish, see Aaron & Joshi, 1987)—even in those with almost perfect orthographic-phonological correspondence. On the other hand, some aspects of the orthography may be specific to a given language. For example, Assink and Kattenberg discussed the analogy principle in Dutch spelling by which homophones make *syntactic* distinctions (about grammatical person, tense, active/passive voice, number, etc.), whereas in English homophone spelling makes *lexical* distinctions. Unlike English or German, Dutch orthography contains syntactic information not represented in the oral language. Wolf et al. (chapter 4) argue that differences across languages with differing orthographies may help sort out the contribution of orthographic processing to reading disability.

Visual and orthographic processes. Although the visual and the orthographic systems in the brain are not identical (Berninger, 1994; Carr & Posner, in press), they most likely share subprocesses (see Geva & Willows Commentary this volume). Of the kinds of orthographic knowledge in Table 1, orthographic structure (particularly spatial redundancy) and orthographic coding are most likely to draw upon visual subprocesses. The relationship between the psychophysiology of visual processes (see Willows et al., 1993) and orthographic structure and orthographic coding warrants further research.

DEVELOPMENTAL ISSUES

Emergent literacy. The orthographic system undergoes considerable development, independent of the developing phonological system, before a child can read, that is, pronounce printed words and attach meaning to them (Berninger, 1994). Beginning with the "fundamental graphic act" when the young child discovers that scribbling with a crayon or pencil leaves a graphic trace, orthographic production follows a predictable developmental pattern: random scribbling; zig-zag lines; variation in elements without segmentation into units; linear, word-like arrangement of elements; true letters; words; sequences of related words; and finally sentences (Gibson &

Levin, 1975). Lavine (1972) investigated preschoolers' perception of the orthographic system and reported a number of intriguing findings. Not only do nonreading three year olds' graphic productions resemble writing that can be differentiated from pictures but also they are able to distinguish pictures from writing on formal sorting tasks. Although four and five year olds use global features of the string such as linear arrangement, nonrepetetiveness of units, and presence of multiple units to sort graphic displays into writing or nonwriting categories, the most important criteria they use are the features of the letters. By age five, nonreaders exposed to printed English categorized 100% of the displays with Roman or Hebrew letters as writing, but only 73% of the displays with artificial characters (composed of distinctive features of Roman letters) and only 20% of the displays with Chinese characters (not composed of distinctive features of Roman letters).

Thus, the notion that literacy is equated with pronouncing and spelling words needs to be reexamined, as Barron (chapter 6) argues. Considerable protoliterate knowledge (Barron, 1991) is acquired during the preschool years (also see Adams, 1990) before children show conventional signs of literacy. That is, receptive knowledge precedes expressive knowledge of phonological-orthographic connections. Evidence of this protoliterate knowledge is the auditory-orthographic effect in novice readers who have letter-sound knowledge but are not able to pronounce or spell words (Barron, chapter 6). Presumably letter-sound knowledge allows novice readers to detect the phonemes in the rime unit of word pairs and react differently to word pairs that are spelled and pronounced the same than to those that are spelled the same but pronounced differently. Thus, as confirmed by causal modeling (Wagner, Torgesen, & Rashotte, 1994), letter-sound knowledge (sounds associated with letters) may promote development of phonological awareness, which then promotes further development of application of letter-sound knowledge (decoding).

Development of Various Kinds of Orthographic Knowledge (see Table 1). Little is known about the development of *orthographic structure,* but some research evidence suggests that the reading disabled do not differ from normal readers in their knowledge of orthographic structure (see Lennox & Siegel, in press). For example, Siegel, Geva, and Share (1990) showed that learning disabled children and normal grade-matched readers did not differ on a task with pairs of pronounceable pseudowords in which one contained a bigram that never occurs in a particular position in English (e.g., fily) and the other contained a bigram that does occur in a particular position in English (e.g., filk). However, research has not yet addressed whether the reading disabled and normal readers may have differed in knowledge of orthographic structure in the earliest stages of reading acquisition.

Although no one has examined developmental patterns in acquiring spatial or sequential redundancy, there are suggestions in the literature that abstraction of orthographic regularity begins early. Pick (1978) reported that first graders rejected orthographically illegal letter strings as not being real words. Berninger (1988) found that first graders consistently at the beginning, middle, and end of the year rejected letter strings, which violate orthographic regularity, more accurately than pronounceable nonwords, which do not violate orthographic regularity, as not being real words. Apparently these first graders had the concept that a real word must conform to allowable letter sequences but did not yet have the concept that a real word must not only be pronounceable but also activate meaning. However, early knowledge of orthographic structure probably undergoes significant development before sufficient knowledge of orthographic regularity is acquired to support automatization of word recognition (see Venezky & Massaro, 1979).

The development of *orthographic coding* from kindergarten (nonreaders) to first grade (beginning readers) (Berninger, 1987) and from first to second to third grade (Berninger, Yates, & Lester, 1991) has been investigated. Developmental trends were noted in that proficiency in coding a whole word unit seems to develop earlier than proficiency in coding a letter in a word, which seems to develop earlier than proficiency in coding a letter cluster in a word. However, by the end of first grade, most children had some proficiency with all codes, suggesting that they had sufficient orthographic coding skill to learn sight words (spelling sequence of whole word), beginning phonics (single letters in words), and word families or analogies (letter clusters in words). Whole word coding was more related to component reading and writing skills early in literacy acquisition, and letter cluster coding was more related to component reading and writing skills by third grade (also see

Bowers, chapter 5).

Although Frith (1985) did not propose her developmental model of word recognition—from logographic to alphabetic to orthographic stages—within a connectionist framework, it could be modified to fit such a framework (see Multiple Connections Model discussed in chapter 8). With this modification, the model makes predictions about the development of *orthographic-phonological code connections*. The logographic (sight word) stage involves whole written word-whole spoken word (name code) connections. The alphabetic stage involves letter-phoneme connections. The orthographic stage involves letter cluster-syllable/rime/or phoneme connections, in keeping with Ehri's (1992b) claim that even complex spelling regularities depend on sound. Presumably letter cluster-rime connections underlie end analogies that Goswami (1989) has shown to be effective in beginning reading. Although children may not proceed through these stages in a rigid sequence (Vellutino, 1992), this stage model captures the alternative strategies children may use to learn to read and spell their orthography (also see Firth, 1972).

The importance of distinguishing between orthographic structure and spelling-sound knowledge is supported by neuropsychological evidence (McCarthy & Warrington, 1990). Dissociations occur between visual word-form dyslexias (analogous to orthographic structure of the coded or stored word) and central dyslexias (analogous to spelling-sound or sound-spelling transformations). Thus, it makes sense that development of spelling-sound knowledge may occur independent of development of orthographic structure knowledge in some cases.

Development of *spelling-sound knowle*dge has been investigated. Barron (chapter 6) and Wagner et al. (1994) showed that this knowledge begins to develop before children can pronounce words. Likewise, Berninger (1988) found that first graders were consistently better at the beginning, middle, and end of the year in making receptive judgments about which stimuli were real words than they were in pronouncing words or pseudowords, that is, in applying orthographic-phonological knowledge productively. Rosinsky and Wheeler (1972) showed children pairs of nonsense words (one was pronounceable, one was not) and asked them to point to one that was more like a real word. First graders performed only at chance level, but third and fifth graders averaged 70% to 80% correct responses, respectively. Apparently older children judge a word as real not only on the basis of having a permissible orthographic structure but also on the basis of being able to translate that orthographic structure into sound.

Orthographic structure knowledge must be integrated not only with phonological knowledge but also with semantic/syntactic knowledge. Biemiller (1970) demonstrated that beginning readers' errors first reflect a reliance on contextual (semantic/syntactic) information, next reflect a greater reliance on orthographic information in text, and finally reflect a co-reliance on both orthographic and contextual information. However, Barr (1972) demonstrated that this developmental sequence may be modified by the nature of the instructional program—phonics instruction draws children's attention to orthographic (letter) information more than does the sight word method.

The development of *orthographic images* or word-specific representations in memory plays an important role in reading and spelling development. Still, word-specific representations are not perfectly related to reading and writing achievement (see chapter 8) and are probably but one source of knowledge in reading words orally or silently or spelling words in writing (see Venezky, Volume II). (For a different perspective, see Vellutino et al., 1994). Measures of orthographic images may be related more to some components of reading than to others. Wagner and Barker (chapter 7) reviewed their work showing that the homophone choice task accounted for more variance in reading connected text than in reading isolated words and in timed than untimed measures. The relationship between speed of orthographic processing (see chapters by Wolf et al. and Bowers et al.) and acquisition of orthographic images requires further research. Future research should also address how the internal organization of the lexicon (relationship of orthographic representations and other linguistic representations) may change over the course of development.

The development of metacognitive knowledge about orthography has probably received less attention than has the development of other kinds of orthographic knowledge. What research exists has focused primarily on the emerging literacy stage (e.g., Clay, 1979) or adult, skilled reading (see Venezky Volume II).

The different kinds of orthographic knowledge in Table 1 are conceptually distinct but not orthogonal components of orthographic processing. In the course of development one kind of orthographic knowledge may influence acquisition of another kind of orthographic knowledge. For example, orthographic coding affects development of orthographic-phonological code connections (see chapter 8) and spelling-sound knowledge affects acquisition of orthographic images (Ehri, 1992a).

Summary

The definitional, theoretical, developmental, and measurement issues discussed in this introduction, subsequent chapters, and two commentaries at the end are far from resolved. Hopefully this series will stimulate dialogue and research to resolve these issues eventually. Clearly much more research is needed to understand fully the development of the various kinds of orthographic knowledge and their role in literacy acquisition.

Acknowledgements

I thank Richard Venezky and Richard Wagner for thoughtful comments on an earlier version of the introduction.

REFERENCES

Aaron, P.G., & Joshi, R.M. (Eds.) (1987). *Reading and writing disorders in different orthographic systems.* Dordrecht, The Netherlands: Kluwer Academic Publishers.

Adams, M. (1990). *Beginning to read: Thinking and learning about print.* Cambridge, MA: MIT Press.

Assink, E., & Kattenberg, G. (1991, April). *The use of orthographic structure in normal and poor readers.* American Educational Research Association, Chicago.

Assink, E., & Kattenberg, G. (1994). Higher-order linguistic influences on development of orthographic knowledge: Illustrations from spelling problems in Dutch and assessment tools. In V.W. Berninger (Ed), *The varieties of orthographic knowledge I: Theoretical and developmental issues* (pp. 111-136). Dordrecht, The Netherlands: Kluwer Academic Publishers.

Barr, R. (1972). The influence of instructional conditions on word recognition errors. *Reading Research Quarterly, 7*, 509-529.

Barron, R.W. (1986). Word recognition in early reading: A review of the direct and indirect access hypotheses. *Cognition, 24,* 93-119.

Barron, R. (1991). Proto-literacy, literacy, and the acquisition of phonological awareness. *Learning and Individual Differences, 3,* 243-255.

Barron, R. (1994). The sound-to-spelling connections: Orthographic-activation in auditory word recognition and its implications for the acquisition of phonological awareness and literacy skills. In V.W. Berninger (Ed), *The varieties of orthographic knowledge I: Theoretical and developmental issues* (pp. 219-242). Dordrecht, The Netherlands: Kluwer Academic Publishers.

Berninger, V. (1987). Global, component, and serial procedures for printed words in beginning reading. *Journal of Experimental Child Psychology, 43,* 387-418.

Berninger, V. (1988). Acquisition of linguistic procedures for printed words: Neuropsychological implications for learning. *International Journal of Neuroscience, 42,* 267-281.

Berninger, V. (1990). Multiple orthographic codes: Key to instructional interventions for developing orthographic-phonological connections underlying word identification. *School Psychology Review, 19,* 518-533.

Berninger, V. (1994). *Reading and writing acquisition. A developmental neuropsychological perspective.* Dubuque, IA: Brown & Benchmark.

Berninger, V., & Abbott, R. (1994). Multiple orthographic and phonological codes in literacy acquisition: An evolving research program. In V.W. Berninger (Ed), *The varieties of orthographic knowledge I: Theoretical and developmental issues* (pp. 277-317). Dordrecht, The Netherlands: Kluwer Academic Publishers.

Berninger, V., Yates, C., & Lester, K. (1991). Multiple orthographic codes in reading and writing acquisition. *Reading and Writing: An Interdisciplinary Journal, 3,* 115-149.

Biemiller, A. (1970). The development of the use of graphic and contextual information as children learn to read. *Reading Research Quarterly, 6,* 75-96.

Bowers, P., Golden, J., Kennedy, A., & Young, A (1994). Limits upon orthographic knowledge due to processes indexed by naming speed. In V.W. Berninger (Ed), *The varieties of orthographic knowledge I: Theoretical and developmental issues* (pp. 173-218). Dordrecht, The Netherlands: Kluwer Academic Publishers.

Bowers, P., & Wolf, M. (1993a, March). *A double-deficit hypothesis for developmental reading disorders*. New Orleans: Society for Research in Child Development.

Bowers, P.G., & Wolf, M. (1993b). Theoretical links among naming speed, precise timing mechanisms, and orthographic skill in dyslexia. *Reading and Writing, 5*, 69-85.

Carr, T. H., & Posner, M. I. (in press). The impact of learning to read on the functional anatomy of language processing. In B. de Gelder & J. Morais (Eds.), *Language and literacy: Comparative approaches*. Cambridge, MA: MIT Press.

Clay, M.M. (1979). *Reading: The patterning of complex behavior*. Auckland, New Zealand: Heinemann.

Coltheart, M. (1978). Lexical access in simple reading tasks. In G. Underwood (Ed.), *Strategies of information processing* (pp. 151-216). London: Academic Press.

Ehri, L.C. (1980a). The development of orthographic images. In U. Frith (Ed.), *Cognitive processes in spelling* (pp. 311-338). London, England: Academic Press.

Ehri, L. (1980b). The role of orthographic images in learning printed words. In J.F. Kavanagh & R.L. Venezky (Eds.), *Orthography, reading, and dyslexia* (pp. 155-170). Baltimore: University Park Press.

Ehri, L.C. (1992a). Reconceptualizing the development of sight word reading and its relationship to recoding (pp. 107-144). In P. Gough, L. Ehri, & R. Treiman (Eds.), *Reading acquisition*. Hillsdale, NJ: Lawrence Erlbaum Associates.

Ehri, L. (1992b). Review and commentary: Stages of spelling development. In S. Templeton & D. Bear (Eds.), *Development of orthographic knowledge and the foundations of literacy* (pp. 307-332). Hillsdale, NJ: Lawrence Erlbaum Associates.

Firth, I. (1972). *Components of reading disability*. Unpublished doctoral dissertation, University of New South Wales, Australia.

Foorman, B. (1994). Phonological and orthographic processing: Separate but equal? In V.W. Berninger (Ed.), *Varieties of orthographic knowledge I: Theoretical and developmental issues* (pp. 241-266). Dordrecht, The Netherlands: Kluwer Academic Publishers.

Foorman, B., Francis, D., Novy, D., & Liberman, D. (1991). How letter-sound instruction mediates progress in first-grade reading and spelling. *Journal of Educational Psychology, 83,* 456-469.

Frith, U. (1985). Beneath the surface of developmental dyslexia. In K. Patterson, J. Marshall, & M. Coltheart (Eds.), *Surface dyslexia* (pp. 301-330). London: Erlbaum.

Geva, E., & Willows, D. (1994). Orthographic knowledge is orthographic knowledge is orthographic knowledge. In V. W. Berninger (Ed.), *The varieties of orthographic knowledge I: Theoretical and developmental issues* (pp. 357-378). Dordrecht, The Netherlands: Kluwer Academic Publishers.

Gibson, E., & Levin, H. (1975). *The psychology of reading.* Cambridge, MA: MIT Press.

Glushko, R. (1979). The organization and activation of orthographic knowledge in reading aloud. *Journal of Experimental Psychology: Human Perception and Performance, 5,* 674-691.

Goswami, U. (1988). Orthographic analogies and reading development. *Quarterly Journal of Experimental Psychology, 40A,* 239-268.

Goswami, U. (1989, March). *Orthographic units and transfer in reading.* San Francisco: American Educational Research Association.

Jackson, N., Lu, W-H., Ju, D. (1994). Reading Chinese and reading English: Similarities, differences, and second-language learning. In V.W. Berninger (Ed), *The varieties of orthographic knowledge I: Theoretical and developmental issues* (pp. 73-109). Dordrecht, The Netherlands: Kluwer Academic Publishers.

Johnson, N.F. (1978). Coding processes in memory. In W.K. Estes (Ed.), *Handbook of learning and cognitive processes* (Vol. 6, pp. 87-129). Hillsdale, NJ: Erlbaum.

Kolers, P., & Roediger, H. (1984). Procedures of mind. *Journal of Verbal Learning and Verbal Behavior, 23,* 425-449.

Lavine, L.O. (1972). The development of perception of writing in pre-reading children: A cross-cultural study. Unpublished doctoral dissertation, Department of Human Development, Cornell University.

Lennox, C., & Siegel, L. (in press). Development of orthographic and phonological processes in normal and disabled reading. In V.W. Berninger (Ed.), *The varieties of orthographic knowledge II: Relationships to phonology, reading, and writing*. Dordrecht, The Netherlands: Kluwer Academic Publishers.

Leong, C.K. (1987). Reading and reading difficulties in a morphemic script. Chinese does not bypass phonology. In P.G. Aaron & R. Malatesha Joshi (Eds.), *Reading and writing disorders in difference orthographic systems* (pp. 267-282). Dordrecht, The Netherlands: Kluwer Academic Press.

Mason, M. (1975). Reading ability and letter search times: Effects of orthographic structure defined by single-letter positional frequency. *Journal of Experimental Psychology: General, 104,* 146-166.

McCarthy, R., & Warrington, E. (1990). *Cognitive neuropsychology. A clinical introduction.* New York: Academic Press.

Olson, R., Forsberg, H., & Wise, B. (1994). Genes, environment, and the development of orthographic skills. In V.W. Berninger (Ed), *The varieties of orthographic knowledge I: Theoretical and developmental issues* (pp. 27-71). Dordrecht, The Netherlands: Kluwer Academic Publishers.

Pick, A. (1978). Perception in the acquisition of reading. In F. Murray, H. Sharp, & J. Pikulski, (Eds.), *The acquisition of reading: Cognitive, linguistic, and perceptual prerequisites* (pp. 99-122). Baltimore: University Park Press.

Posner, M., Petersen, S., Fox, P., & Raichle, M. (1988). Localization of cognitive operations in the human brain. *Science, 240,* 1627-1631.

Rosinsky, R.R., & Wheeler, K.E. (1972). Children's use of orthographic structure in word discrimination. *Psychonomic Science, 26,* 97-98.

Seidenberg, M., & McClelland, J. (1989). A distributed, developmental model of word recognition and naming. *Psychological Review, 96,* 523-568.

Shallice, T., Warrington, E., & McCarthy, R. (1983). Reading without semantics. *Quarterly Journal of Experimental Psychology, 35A,* 111-138.

Siegel, L.S., Geva, E., & Share, D. (1990). *The development of orthographic skills in normal and disabled readers*. Unpublished manuscript.

Snowling, M. (1987). Developmental dyslexia: A cognitive developmental perspective. In P.G. Aaron & R.M. Joshi (Eds.), *Reading and writing disorders in different orthographic systems* (pp. 1-23). Dordrecht, The Netherlands: Kluwer Academic Publishers.

Stanovich, K.E., West, R.F., & Cunningham, A.E. (1992). Beyond phonological processes: Print exposure and orthographic processing. In S.A. Brady & D. Shankweiler (Eds.), *Phonological processes in literacy* (pp. 219-235). Hillsdale, NJ: Lawrence Erlbaum Associates.

Tanenhaus, M.K., Flanigan, H.P., & Seidenberg, M.K. (1980). Orthographic and phonological activation in auditory and visual word recognition. *Memory and Cognition, 8*, 513-520.

Van Orden, G., Pennington, B., & Stone, G. (1990). Word identification in reading and the promise of subsymbolic psycholinguistics. *Psychology Review, 97*, 1-35.

Varnhagen, C.K. (in press). Children's spelling strategies. In V.W. Berninger (Ed.), *The varieties of orthographic knowledge II: Their relationships to phonology, reading, and writing*. Dordrecht, The Netherlands: Kluwer Academic Press.

Vellutino, F. (1992). Afterword. In S. Templeton & D. Bear (Eds.), *Development of orthographic knowledge and foundations of literacy* (pp. 353-357). Hillsdale, NJ: Lawrence Erlbaum Associates.

Vellutino, F.R., Scanlon, D.M., & Tanzman, M.S. (1994). Components of reading ability: Issues and problems in operationalizing word identification, phonological coding, and orthographic coding. In G.R. Lyon (Ed.), *Frames of reference for the assessment of learning disabilities: New views on measurement issues* (pp. 279-332). Baltimore, MD: Paul Brookes Publishing.

Venezky, R. (1970). *The structure of English orthography*. The Hague: Mouton.

Venezky, R. (1979). Orthographic regularities in English words. In P. Kolers, M. Wrolstad, & H. Bouma (Eds.), *Processing of visible language* (pp. 283-293). New York: Plenum Press.

Venezky, R. (1993). History of interest in the visual component of reading. In D. Willows, R. Kruk, & E. Corcos (Eds.), *Visual processes in reading and reading disabilities*. Hillsdale, NJ: Lawrence Erlbaum.

Venezky, R. (in press). From orthography to reading to psychology. In V.W. Berninger (Ed.), *The varieties of orthographic knowledge II: Their relationships to phonology, reading, and writing.* Dordrecht, The Netherlands: Kluwer Academic Publishers.

Venezky, R., & Massaro, D. (1979). The role of orthographic regularity in word recognition. In L. Resnick, & P. Weaver (Eds.), *Theory and practice of early reading* (Vol. 1, pp. 85-108). Hillsdale, NJ: Erlbaum.

Wagner, R., & Barker, T. (1994). The development of orthographic processing ability. In V.W. Berninger (Ed), *The varieties of orthographic knowledge I: Theoretical and developmental issues* (pp. 243-276). Dordrecht, The Netherlands: Kluwer Academic Publishers.

Wagner, R.K., Torgesen, J.K., & Rashotte, C.A. (1994). The development of reading-related phonological processing abilities: New evidence of bi-directional causality from a latent variable longitudinal study. *Development Psychology, 30,* 73-87.

Willows, D., Kruk, R., & Corcos, E. (Eds.) (1993). *Visual processes in reading and reading disabilities.* Hillsdale, NJ: Lawrence Erlbaum.

Wolf, M., Pfeil, C., Lotz, R., & Biddle, K. (1994). Towards a more universal understanding of the developmental dyslexias: The contribution of orthographic factors. In V.W. Berninger (Ed), *The varieties of orthographic knowledge I: Theoretical and developmental issues* (pp. 137-171). Dordrecht, The Netherlands: Kluwer Academic Publishers.

Address correspondence to:

Virginia W. Berninger, Ph.D.
University of Washington
Miller Hall DQ-12
Seattle, WA 98195
U.S.A.

RICHARD K. OLSON, HELEN FORSBERG, & BARBARA WISE

GENES, ENVIRONMENT, AND THE DEVELOPMENT OF ORTHOGRAPHIC SKILLS

1. INTRODUCTION

Researchers have taken two somewhat different views regarding the nature and development of orthographic and phonological knowledge in spelling and reading. A strongly integrative view holds that development in both areas depends on a common underlying knowledge base. For example, Ehri (1989, 1992) has argued that alphabetic "orthographic images" involved in both reading and spelling are amalgamated with the phonological information pertaining to the word (see also, Barron, 1986; Goswami & Bryant, 1990; Stuart & Coltheart, 1988). A more separatist view is represented in "dual-route" theories that emphasize the independence of two routes to the lexicon; an indirect phonological-decoding route operating through the reader's knowledge of grapheme-phoneme correspondences, and a direct "visual" route that uses orthographic knowledge to access the lexicon without phonological mediation (Coltheart, 1978; Morton, 1969). The "dual-route" view has been very influential in attempts to account for individual differences in acquired and developmental reading disorders (Boder, 1973; Castles & Coltheart, 1993; Coltheart, Curtis, Atkins, & Haller, 1993; Mitterer, 1982; Patterson, Marshal, & Coltheart, 1985; Seymour, 1986), as well as individual differences across the normal continuum of reading ability (Baron, 1979; Baron & Strawson, 1976; Freebody & Byrne, 1988; Treiman, 1984). In this chapter we selectively review earlier research and present new behavioral-genetic evidence on the degree of developmental independence between disabled readers' skills in the indirect (phonological) and direct (orthographic) routes for the identification of printed words.

V.W. Berninger (ed.), The varieties of orthographic knowledge I: Theoretical and developmental issues, 27-71.

In the Colorado Learning Disabilities Research Center (CLDRC),[1] we are examining the genetic and environmental etiology of disabled readers' deficits in component reading, language, and perceptual skills (DeFries, Olson, Pennington, & Smith, 1991; Olson, Wise, Conners, Rack, & Fulker, 1989). Because deficits in printed word recognition and spelling are fundamental to most reading disabilities (Perfetti, 1985), we began our research with an attempt to assess separately subjects' skills in the direct and indirect pathways for word recognition posited by "dual-route" theory (Olson, Kliegl, Davidson, & Foltz, 1985). Our assessment of skill in the indirect phonological-decoding route followed the long-standing tradition of having subjects read pronounceable nonwords. Measures of skill in the direct orthographic route were based on the homophonic nature of English words and nonwords: Identical sounding words and nonwords can be produced by different spelling patterns. Based on earlier research by Baron and Strawson (1976) with normal college students, we developed a computer-based measure of orthographic coding that required a speeded forced-choice between a word and a phonologically identical "pseudohomophonic" nonword (e.g., rain rane) (Olson et al., 1985). The task was called an "orthographic-coding" measure because subjects had to recognize the correct orthographic pattern for the word independent from its phonology. Although subjects may automatically engage phonological decoding processes when presented with the word and its pseudohomophone (Van Orden, 1987; Perfetti & Bell, 1991), their phonological decoding of the two choices in this task would not yield the correct answer. Therefore, it was assumed that performance on the orthographic task yielded a measure of processing in the direct lexical route of "dual-route" theory.

The present reassessment of independence between orthographic and phonological coding skills is based first on the question of statistical independence, second, on the question of differential deficits in disabled readers' orthographic and phonological coding, and third, on differences in the genetic and environmental etiology of those deficits. In the next section (2) of this chapter we review the results of several studies that have shown independent but also overlapping contributions of orthographic and phonological coding skills to variance in word recognition. Results from recent factor analyses in the Colorado Reading Project will reveal the unique relations between orthographic and phonological coding and other variables related to reading and spelling.

In the third chapter section, we summarize results from studies of older reading-disabled and younger reading-level-matched normal groups. The evidence is strong for a unique deficit in most disabled readers' phonological coding, but the disabled and normal groups' relative performance in orthographic coding apparently depends on the type of orthographic task. Some orthographic tasks have yielded a deficit for reading-disabled groups that is similar to that for phonological coding. Other orthographic tasks result in performance that is consistent with or even superior to the disabled group's level of word recognition.

In the fourth section of the chapter, genetic and environmental influences on group deficits in phonological and orthographic coding are evaluated by comparing similarities within identical and same-sex fraternal twin pairs. Contrary to earlier reports of twin data suggesting low heritability for orthographic coding and high heritability for phonological coding (Olson et al., 1989; Stevenson, 1991), new data from a much larger twin sample and new orthographic tasks indicates substantial heritability for deficits in *both* skills. Bivariate genetic analyses show that the correlated variance between orthographic and phonological coding deficits is largely due to the same genes, and deficits in both skills are genetically linked to deficits in phonological awareness. However, there is some preliminary evidence that the reliable uncorrelated variance in both orthographic and phonological coding is also significantly heritable.

In a concluding section, the new behavioral-genetic evidence leads to a re-evaluation of our earlier views about the etiological independence of orthographic and phonological skills in disabled readers. We conclude that Ehri's (1989, 1992) integrative view provides a better fit to the data, although we also support Stanovich and West's (1989) view that print exposure may play a special role in the development of orthographic knowledge.

2. ORTHOGRAPHIC AND PHONOLOGICAL CONTRIBUTIONS TO WORD RECOGNITION

Conners and Olson (1990) reported the results of path analyses that found independent contributions from orthographic and phonological coding to variance in word recognition within groups of older disabled and younger reading-level-matched normal subjects. In this section, the question of independent contributions to individual differences in word recognition is reevaluated in a new sample and with new measures of phonological and orthographic coding. We discuss a factor analysis that confirms the existence of separate orthographic and phonological coding factors and clarifies the nature of these factors through their relations to other variables. First, the subject sample and measures will be described.

2.1 Subjects in the Colorado Learning Disabilities Research Center (CLDRC)

Subjects in the CLDRC include identical and fraternal twin pairs who are identified from school records in 27 Colorado school districts. Permission is then sought from the parents to examine the twins' files for any evidence of a reading problem. This evidence variously includes comments from teachers, referrals to resource rooms or remedial reading programs, and/or low standardized achievement test scores. Twin pairs containing at least one member with any evidence of a reading problem are invited to the University of Colorado for laboratory testing. A smaller comparison sample of normal twins with no school record of reading problems is also invited to the laboratory for testing.

From 1983 to 1993, the ongoing CLDRC twin study has completed laboratory testing for 459 twin pairs with at least one twin having some sort of school-record evidence of a reading problem. In addition, 297 twin pairs have been tested who had no school-record evidence of reading problems. The behavioral-genetic analyses reported in Section 4 are based on this large sample. However, the factor and regression analyses reported in the present section included only the twins tested since 1989 when the test battery was modified to include some important new measures.

The twins under 17 years of age are given the Wechsler Intelligence Scale for Children-Revised (WISC-R). Those over 17 are given the Weschler Adult Intelligence Scale-Revised (WAIS-R) (Wechsler, 1974). For the analyses reported in this chapter, all subjects had Verbal or Performance IQ scores of at least 85, no evidence of neurological or severe emotional problems, and no uncorrected auditory or visual acuity deficits.

The 296 subjects included in the present factor and regression analyses were all members of identical and fraternal twin pairs referred for having at least one member with a reading problem. The mean age was 11.1 years (range = 8 to 18.6). All of the subjects' scores on the various measures described below were standardized against those of the normally distributed comparison sample, which included some poor readers, in spite of the absence of such evidence in their school records. The reading disabled sample included a wide range of reading deficits for the affected twins. Some individual members of the twin pairs had normal or above normal levels of reading skill. Occasionally both members had normal reading skills in spite of evidence of a deficit in their school records. The group's word recognition scores were normally distributed around a mean that was -1.77 (range = -6.48 to +2.37) standard deviation units below the mean for the normal comparison group. The present factor and regression analyses were performed on this relatively deviant group because we are most interested in the variance associated with different degrees of reading deficit.

2.2. *Measures Used in the Factor and Regression Analyses*

Groups of measures were related to hypothesized skill areas that included orthographic coding, phonological coding, phonological awareness, rapid verbal and perceptual processing, verbal and perceptual IQ, and word recognition. Print exposure was included as an environmental variable. The measures are described below in each of the categories.

2.2.1. *Orthographic Coding.* The three tasks hypothesized to be measures of orthographic coding all required the recognition of the correct spelling of a target word with phonologically similar background foils. Our *Word-Pseudohomophone Choice* (WPC) task described earlier (rain rane; sammon salmon) contained 80 trials with a wide range of target-word frequencies and orthographic regularity (Olson et al., 1985, 1989). Subjects pressed a left or right button to designate the correct orthographic pattern as quickly as possible after a pair appeared on the computer screen. Feedback was given for latency and accuracy after each trial (see Olson, Forsberg, Wise, & Rack, 1994, for a detailed description of this task). A similar procedure was used for the *Homophone Choice* (HC) task wherein subjects heard a sentence such as "Which is a fruit?"

and subsequently were shown a pair of homophones on the computer (pair pear) for forced choice (see Barker, Torgesen, & Wagner, 1992; Stanovich & West, 1989, for similar tasks). A final variable was created for each of the above tasks by adding the *z* scores for subjects' percent correct and their median latency on correct responses. The third forced-choice task was the *Peabody Individual Achievement Test* (PIAT) for spelling (Dunn & Markwardt, 1970). The PIAT test involves the oral presentation of a target word, then the word in a sentence, and finally the isolated word. Subjects then make an untimed forced choice among four orthographically and often phonologically similar alternatives printed on a card (e.g., "cloudy": clowdy cloady cloudey cloudy). As can be seen in this example, the choices are not all strictly homophonic, so phonological coding might make a greater contribution to performance in this task than it would for the other two forced-choice tasks. The 84 target words were arranged in increasing order of difficulty and the test was halted if subjects made 5 errors in any 7 consecutive responses.

The *Wide Range Achievement Test* (WRAT) (Jastak & Jastak, 1978) spelling production test was also given. We hypothesized that this measure would load more strongly on a phonological factor because on many trials a correct response could be produced by the application of common phoneme-grapheme correspondence rules. Form 1 of the test (45 items) was used for children under 12 years and form 2 (46 items) was used with older children. The items were presented orally in isolation, then in a sentence, then in isolation again, in increasing order of difficulty, and subjects wrote down the target word. Testing was halted after subjects made ten consecutive errors.

2.2.2. Phonological Decoding. Two measures of phonological decoding included an oral nonword reading task and a silent nonword reading task. In the *Oral Nonword Reading* (ONR) task (Olson et al., 1989; 1994), the nonwords are presented on the computer one at a time and response latency is measured with a voice key. All responses are recorded for off-line analyses of errors. The first section of the test includes 45 one-syllable nonwords, ranging from vcv to cccvcv structure (e.g., ter, strale). The second section contains forty two-syllable nonwords (e.g., hodfen, lobsel, strempick). Accuracy scores and median correct reaction times are standardized for each of the two sections of the tasks. Composite scores used in the present analyses are created by combining each subject's standard scores for accuracy and median correct latency. In the *Silent Nonword Reading* (SNR) task (Olson et al., 1985, 1994), three pronounceable letter strings are presented side by side on the computer (e.g., coam - baim - goam; dysical - fotograph - barmacy). Subjects push one of three buttons as quickly as possible to designate the letter string that would sound like a common word if read aloud. Subjects receive 65 trials. Great care was taken to balance the targets and distractors in terms of their visual similarity to real words. Thus, subjects could not respond by simply picking the most visually familiar letter-string. The task requires first that the subject generate the internal sound codes for the nonwords. (Because there is no oral response, variability in articulatory skills should not have any direct influence on performance in this task.) Second, the task also requires the subject to match the phonetic code for the nonword (e.g., coam) to a word (e.g., comb) in his/her lexicon. Z scores for percent correct and median latency on correct responses were added to form a composite measure for the present analyses.

2.2.3. *Phonological Awareness.* Three measures of phonological awareness, broadly defined as the ability to be aware of and manipulate the phonemic segments of speech, included a "pig-latin" game, a phoneme deletion task, and the Lindamood Auditory Conceptualization test (Lindamood & Lindamood, 1979). In our *Phoneme Segmentation and Transposition* (PST) task (Olson et al., 1989), subjects take the first sound off the front of a word, put it at the end, and add the sound /ay/. For example, "rope" would become "ope-ray." The test consists of 9 practice and 45 test items. All words are within the listening vocabulary of elementary school aged children. There is no time constraint. The *Phoneme Deletion* (PD) task is based on the Bruce (1964) phoneme deletion task and the Rosner and Simon (1971) auditory analysis task. The phoneme deletion task consists of 6 practice and 40 test trials. First, subjects hear a nonword which they are asked to repeat. They are then asked to remove a specified phoneme from the nonword and if done correctly, the result is a word (e.g., "say prot," "now say prot without the /r/ sound"—"pot"). The task is presented via a tape player. Two seconds are allowed for the subjects to repeat the initial stimulus, 4 seconds are allowed for the subjects to give their response to the deletion instructions. The end of each response period is signalled by a tone and then the next instruction is given. In the *Lindamood Auditory Conceptualization* (LAC) test, colored blocks are used to represent phonemes and the subjects are required to add, remove or transpose blocks to reflect changes in nonwords or sequences of sounds spoken by the tester (Lindamood & Lindamood, 1979). For example the subject might be shown three different colored blocks in a row and told: "if that says aps, show me asp"; the subject should therefore exchange the positions of the second and third blocks. This task has the major advantage that subjects are not required to give spoken responses; thus it assesses segmentation skills that are independent of subjects' phonemic blending abilities. Subjects' scores on all of the three phonological awareness tasks were based on percent correct responses.

2.2.4. Rapid Naming and Visual Search. Two measures of rapid naming were derived from the *Rapid Automatic Naming* (RAN) test (Denkla & Rudel, 1974). Subjects in this task are asked to name from left to right, as rapidly as possible, separate sets of randomly ordered letters (a, d, o, p, and s), numbers (2, 4, 6, 7, and 9), colors (red, blue, green, and yellow circles), or picture (familiar line drawings) items distributed in rows across a card. The number of items for each category that are named correctly in 15 seconds is the subject's score for that category. Based on the results of a prior factor analysis, naming speed for numbers and letters was combined for one variable *(RAN NL)* and colors and pictures were combined for another variable *(RAN CP)*.

A third test in this group required speeded visual matching without naming. In the Educational Testing Service *Identical Pictures Test* (IPT) (French, Ekstrom, & Price, 1963), subjects attempt to match, as quickly as possible, an abstract line drawing at the beginning of each row with an identical picture among four minimally different distractors distributed across the page to the left. The test is administered in two parts with 1.5 minutes for each part. The subject's score is the total number of correct responses minus the number of wrong responses.

2.2.5. IQ. Verbal and Perceptual IQ scores were constructed based on Kaufman's (1975) factor analysis of the WISC-R. Subjects' *z* scores on the Information, Vocabulary, Comprehension, and Similarities subscales were averaged for a Verbal score. Scores on the Picture Completion, Picture

Arrangement, Block Design, and Object Assembly subscales were combined for a Perceptual score.

2.2.6. *Word Recognition.* Two measures of word recognition were combined for this variable. The first measure was the *Peabody Individual Achievement Test* (PIAT) for word recognition (Dunn & Markwardt, 1970). The PIAT contains 66 words of increasing difficulty in rows across a page. The subject reads the words aloud in sequence until 5 of the last 7 items are missed, or the end of the list is reached. Grade-level assignments are standardized for the 1st to 12th grades. The second test was our experimental *Timed Word Recognition Test* (TWRT) (Olson et al., 1989; 1994). This test assessed word-recognition accuracy and latency when single words were presented on the computer screen. The response to a word was counted correct only if the correct response was initiated and detected by a voice key within two seconds. Our goal was to assess level of word-recognition accuracy while also requiring a minimal level of speed or fluency. To begin the test, a short screener list of 14 words was presented to all subjects. They were instructed to read each word aloud as quickly and as accurately as possible. Pronunciation accuracy was scored on-line by the experimenter. Performance on the 14 item screener list was used to determine initial placement into a difficulty-scaled list of 182 words. Presentation of the words continued until the subject made 10 errors out of the last 20 words or until the end of the list was reached. Pronunciation errors and voice-onset times longer than two seconds were both errors for list placement purposes. The z scores for the PIAT and TWRT tests were combined for a single measure of subjects' word recognition.

2.2.7. *Print Exposure.* Stanovich and West (1989) have developed measures of print exposure to explore its effects on a variety of reading and language skills. Their measures require subjects to identify age-appropriate book titles, magazine titles, or authors and distinguish them from foil items. The particular measure used here was a book *Title Recognition Test* (TRT) containing 40 items, with 25 actual titles of popular children's books (Cunningham & Stanovich, 1991). The subjects' score was the number of real titles chosen minus the number of foils chosen.

2.2.8. Summary of General Testing Procedure. The above tests were presented in a fixed order as part of a larger test battery during two 2.5 hour sessions. The IQ, PIAT, RAN, and IPT tests were administered in one session in John DeFries' laboratory at the Institute for Behavioral Genetics. The orthographic tasks (WPC & HC), phonological decoding tasks (ONR & SNR), phonological awareness tasks (PST, PD, LAC), word recognition (TWRT), and print exposure (TRT) tasks were administered in a different session on the same day in Richard Olson's laboratory at the Department of Psychology.

2.3. Exploratory Factor Analysis

Subjects' scores on the above measures were adjusted for the linear and quadratic effects of age. Then the distributions for each variable were examined for their normality. Natural log transformations of the median latency scores and the truncation of a few outlier scores were needed to normalize the distributions. The scores were then entered in a Principal-Components factor analysis. The rotation was oblique because we expected at least some of the factors to be correlated. (A varimax rotation yielded essentially the same factor structure but the factors were not correlated.) The unique patterns of variable loadings on the individual factors are described below.

2.3.1. Phonological Factor. The factor structure matrix and factor correlation matrix are presented in Table 1. The loadings in the structure matrix represent the correlations between the individual variables and the specific factors. The first factor, accounting for 41% of the variance, is distinguished by uniquely high loadings for word recognition, phonological decoding (ONR & SNR), and phonological awareness (PST, PD, & LAC), and WRAT spelling. This factor is identified as the phonological factor. The existence of a common factor for word recognition, phonological decoding, and phonological awareness is entirely consistent with a vast body of research relating these variables (c.f., Adams, 1990; Catts, 1989; Liberman, Shankweiler, & Liberman, 1989; Morais, 1991; Stanovich, 1986; Vellutino & Scanlon, 1987; Wagner, Torgesen, & Rashotte, 1994).

The WRAT spelling production task also loads strongly on the phonological factor. This may be due to the presence of mostly regular words in the lower range of this test where subjects could use their knowledge of phoneme-grapheme correspondence rules to produce the correct spelling even when they were not familiar with the printed word.

2.3.2. *Orthographic Factor.* The third factor, accounting for 10% of the variance, is the only other factor that also shows a high loading with word recognition. It is distinguished from the phonological factor by high loadings with the orthographic tasks (WPC, HC, PIAT), and the Title Recognition Test. The hypothesized greater involvement of phonological skills in the PIAT spelling task, compared to the other orthographic tasks, was supported by its relatively high loading on the phonological factor.

The uniquely high loading of the Title Recognition Test on the orthographic factor is consistent with the task demands. Previous print exposure for the specific target words in the orthographic tasks (e.g., rain rane; salmon sammon) is a logical necessity for accurate performance, regardless of how good subjects' phonological decoding skills might be (Gough, Juel, & Griffith, 1992). In several previous studies, correlations between print exposure, word recognition, and orthographic coding have been significant, but correlations between print exposure and phonological decoding or phoneme awareness are usually lower and often not significant (Cipielewski & Stanovich, 1992; Cunningham & Stanovich, 1991, 1993; Stanovich & West, 1989). These previous studies and the present results suggest that print exposure contributes to the development of word recognition primarily through its influence on the development of accurate orthographic codes. The fact that print exposure did not also show a high loading on the phonological factor suggests that variance in this factor may be more due to biological constraints and/or the effects of specific training in phonological coding (see Section 4).

2.3.3. *IQ Factor.* The second factor, accounting for 10% of the variance, is distinguished by high loadings on the Kaufman Verbal and Perceptual IQ measures as well as the Identical Pictures Test. Therefore, the second factor is given the "IQ" label. The Verbal measure also loads at a moderate level and about equally on the phonological and orthographic factors. In contrast, the Perceptual measure and the Identical Pictures Test showed very low loadings on these factors. The latter result seems to contradict the idea that deficits in orthographic coding

Table 1

FACTOR STRUCTURE MATRIX

	Phonological Factor 1	IQ Factor 2	Orthographic Factor 3	Rapid Naming Factor 4
Word Recognition	.79	-.06	.76	.27
Oral Nonwords	.80	-.18	.57	.28
Silent Nonwords	.74	-.02	.52	.18
Phoneme Segmentation	.72	.18	.32	.31
Phoneme Deletion	.87	.15	.20	.15
Lindamood (LAC)	.77	.28	.28	.05
WRAT Spelling Prod.	.84	.00	.65	.29
Word-Pseudohomophone	.42	-.01	.81	.38
Homophone Choice	.26	.07	.84	.27
PIAT Spelling Choice	.54	-.07	.74	.34
Title Recognition	.29	.15	.67	.08
RAN Letters & Numbers	.36	-.04	.32	.83
RAN Pictures & Colors	.17	.11	.25	.79
Identical Pictures	.04	.63	.18	.57
Kaufman Verbal IQ	.43	.62	.39	-.06
Kaufman Perceptual IQ	.16	.89	.03	.10

FACTOR CORRELATION MATRIX

	FACTOR 1	FACTOR 2	FACTOR 3
FACTOR 2	.09		
FACTOR 3	.43	.04	
FACTOR 4	.18	.05	.25

are uniquely associated with deficits in visual-perceptual skills (Corcos & Willows, 1993; Seymour & Evans, 1993). With the possible exception of a few case studies (c.f., Goulandris & Snowling, 1991), we are not aware of any visual processing deficits that have been specifically linked to deficits in orthographic coding but not to phonological coding. However, it is possible that the visual processing involved in orthographic coding is quite different from that involved in the present perceptual tasks (Seymour & Evans, 1993). Carr and Posner (in press) reviewed PET scan evidence suggesting that the left medial prestriate visual cortex is a primary location for some stage of orthographic processing. This cortical region is nearby and strongly connected to the primary visual cortex. In contrast, the processing of pictorial information tends to be more dominant in parietal and temporal areas of the right hemisphere.

2.3.4. *Rapid Naming Factor.* Finally, the fourth factor, accounting for 7% of the variance, is uniquely specified by high loadings on the Rapid Automatic Naming (RAN) tasks and to a smaller degree on the Identical Pictures Test (IPT). Although the IPT test did not involve naming, it did emphasize processing speed. There has been much interest of late in the relation between rapid naming, general processing speed, and reading disabilities. Felton and Wood (1992) have noted that the prognosis is particularly bad for young disabled readers with deficits in both phonological decoding and rapid naming. However, within the present sample, the rapid naming tasks exhibit only modest and similar correlations with the phonological and orthographic factors. The latter result is inconsistent with Bowers and Wolf's (1993) conjecture that deficits in rapid naming are uniquely associated with deficits in orthographic coding.

Two previous studies have shown that subjects' rapid naming scores account for independent variance in word recognition beyond that accounted for by measures of phonological awareness (Cornwall, 1992; Bowers & Swanson, 1991). This finding was confirmed in the present sample. A hierarchical regression analysis was performed with our composite measure of word recognition as the dependent variable. Subjects' Verbal IQ and the three measures of phonological awareness were entered in the first step, accounting for 41% of the variance. (Verbal IQ accounted for only 1% additional variance beyond that accounted for by phonological awareness.) Subsequent entry in the second step of subjects' rapid naming scores for numbers and letters accounted for an additional 6% of the variance in word recognition ($p < .001$). Entry of rapid naming in the first step accounted for 18% of the variance in word recognition. Thus, two thirds of the rapid naming variance in word recognition overlapped with phonological awareness and one third was independent. This result is quite remarkable in view of the very brief test time in the letter and number tasks (15 sec for numbers, 15 sec for letters). Regression analyses were also performed with naming speed for pictures and colors. Their combined independent contribution to variance in word recognition was significant ($p < .01$) but much smaller (1%).

2.3.5. Correlation Between Orthographic and Phonological Factors. The oblique rotation allows for a correlation to emerge between the orthographic and phonological factors ($r = .43$). The strongest link between the factors is based on the nearly equal and high loadings of word recognition. But moderate cross-loadings of the orthographic and phonological coding variables are also apparent. Oral and silent nonword reading load on the orthographic factor at .57 and .52 respectively. Of the orthographic tasks, PIAT spelling shows the strongest loading on the phonological factor of .54, perhaps due to phonological differences in some of its foil items. But for the word-pseudohomophone task with homophonic foils, there is still a modest loading of .42 on the phonological factor.

It is interesting to note that the phonological awareness measures, particularly phoneme deletion, show very modest correlations with the orthographic factor. It has often been suggested that subjects perform phonological awareness tasks by consulting an orthographic image. This may be true in some cases, but the relatively low phonological-awareness-task loadings on the orthographic factor suggest a small role for orthographic processes in the present sample.

2.4. Independent Contributions to Word Recognition

We have seen that the phonological and orthographic factors are moderately correlated and that subjects' word recognition loads strongly on both. Much of the correlation between the factors appears to be due to the phonological decoding and orthographic coding measures. We now turn to the results of regression analyses to assess the *independent* contributions of these hypothesized component skills in word recognition to subjects' levels of word recognition.

Two hierarchical regression analyses revealed the independent contributions of orthographic and phonological coding. In both analyses, the composite measure of word recognition was the dependent variable. In the first analysis, the silent and oral nonword reading measures of phonological coding were entered in the first step and the three orthographic coding measures were entered in the second step. The second analysis reversed this order of entry. The results are shown in the top half of Table 2.

Three main results are apparent. First, both phonological and orthographic coding account for significant independent variance in subjects' word recognition. Second, the independent variance is about twice as large for phonological coding. Third, the majority of variance accounted for in word recognition is shared by phonological and orthographic coding.

Table 2

Hierarchical Regressions Predicting Word Recognition

Step	Predictor	R^2	R^2 Change	p
1	Phonological Coding	.698	.698	<.001
2	Orthographic Coding	.799	.101	<.001
1	Orthographic Coding	.582	.582	<.001
2	Phonological Coding	.799	.217	<.001
1	Phonological Coding	.698	.698	<.001
2	Print Exposure	.725	.027	<.001
3	Orthographic Coding	.805	.080	<.001
1	Phonological Coding	.698	.698	<.001
2	Orthographic Coding	.799	.101	<.001
3	Print Exposure	.805	.006	<.01

A second set of regression analyses focused on the contribution of print exposure (Title Recognition Test) to variance in word recognition after controlling for phonological coding in the first step. Print exposure was then entered as the second step and as the third step after orthographic coding (see the bottom half of Table 2). It is clear that print exposure does account for a modest (2.7%) amount of independent variance after phonological decoding. However, it makes only a very small (0.6%) but significant contribution when entered as the third step after orthographic coding. It appears that the contribution of print exposure to word recognition is almost entirely subsumed under the contribution of orthographic coding.

The relatively small contribution of print exposure to variance in word recognition, after phonological coding, should be viewed in the context of the measure's psychometric limitations. The forty yes-no forced-choice trials are likely to result in much error variance associated with guessing. Also, children vary in their exposure to specific books whose titles may or may not appear on this brief test. In view of these limitations, it is remarkable that the title recognition test accounts for as much variance as it does. We hypothesize that the full influence of print exposure is likely to be much larger than that revealed by the title recognition test. Ideally we should have diary information on children's absolute levels of print exposure (Anderson, Wilson, & Fielding, 1988), but we do not have the resources to apply this type of measure in our large sample.

2.5. *Summary of Factor Analyses and Regression Results*

It is clear that the phonological and orthographic factors are distinct yet substantially correlated. Beyond the phonological and orthographic coding tasks, the distinction between the factors appears to be primarily in the uniquely high loading of phonological awareness measures on the phonological factor and the uniquely high loading of print exposure on the orthographic factor. The phonological and orthographic factors were quite similar in their correlations with measures of visual-perceptual processes, rapid naming, and verbal IQ.

The regression analyses with word recognition as a dependent variable showed that the contributions of phonological and orthographic coding were largely overlapping, but there were significant independent contributions as well. The latter result raises the possibility that these two component coding skills in word recognition could show different patterns of deficit and different developmental etiology. The severities of disabled readers' deficits in orthographic and phonological coding are compared in the next section.

3. READING-LEVEL-MATCH (RLM) COMPARISONS

When same-age groups of disabled and normal readers are compared, the disabled group is typically significantly lower in performance on a wide variety of component reading and language skills (Stanovich, 1986). Some skills may appear to be more deficient than others, but the psychometric characteristics of different measures (e.g., different variance and reliability) often make it difficult to compare the different degrees of deficit. An additional problem for researchers attempting to locate potential causal influences on reading disability is that reading skill may have a reciprocal influence on other skills (e.g., vocabulary, phonological awareness). One popular approach for dealing with these problems has been to equate groups of younger normal and older disabled readers, usually on a measure of word recognition, and then compare the group's profiles on other reading, language, and perceptual skills. If the reading-level-matched (RLM) disabled and normal groups' cognitive profiles are significantly different, this at least suggests that "...the developmental paths by which the two groups came to their similar reading levels must be different" (Stanovich & Siegel, 1994). Converging evidence would be required to determine the causal role and etiology of any significant deficits.

3.1. *Phonological Coding and Phonological Awareness*

Previous RLM comparisons in the CLDRC have revealed significant phonological coding deficits for the older disabled group (Conners & Olson, 1990; Olson et al., 1985, 1989). A number of other studies have reported similar deficits in phonological coding but some studies have reported no differences. (No studies have reported superior phonological coding in disabled groups.) Rack, Snowling and Olson (1992) recently conducted a meta analysis of RLM studies on phonological coding and argued that some of the failures to find deficits were due to methodological problems such as inaccurate matches on word recognition or small sample sizes. Manis (personal communication) subsequently suggested that the use of reading disabled groups from special schools with intense phonics remediation might eliminate their phonological coding deficit in RLM comparisons.

Rack et al. speculated that some RLM studies did not find phonological coding deficits because the disabled groups' IQ scores were low. The low IQ groups might have a different basis for their reading deficit (Stanovich, 1988). However, recent studies by Felton and Wood (1992), Siegel (1988, 1992), and Stanovich and Siegel (in press) have shown essentially the same significant phonological deficits in disabled groups with low and normal IQ. In addition, behavioral-genetic analyses have shown similar levels of genetic influence on reading deficits in low and normal IQ groups (Pennington, Gilger, Olson, & DeFries, 1992).

Some of the most convincing evidence for disabled readers' phonological coding deficits and their independence from IQ has been reported by Stanovich and Siegel (in press). In order to avoid potential regression artifacts that may arise in RLM designs (Jackson & Butterfield, 1989), Stanovich and Siegel used a continuous regression-based procedure to control for subjects' level of word recognition. Their large sample included disabled and normal readers whose word-recognition-grade levels ranged from 1 to 5.8. Three subject groups were defined that included normal readers, disabled readers performing significantly below their IQ level, and disabled readers performing at a level that was consistent with their low IQ. When phonological coding was the criterion variable and variance associated with word recognition was regressed out, the regression weights for the group contrasts indicated a similar phonological coding deficit for both of the reading disabled IQ groups, compared to the normal readers.

Disabled readers' deficits in phonological coding have been shown to coexist with deficits in phonological awareness. Several recent RLM studies have followed the lead of Bradely and Bryant (1978) and have included measures of both phonological coding and phonological awareness (Bowey, Cain, & Ryan, 1992; Bruck, 1992; Manis, Custodio, & Szeszulski, 1993; Manis, Szeszulski, Holt, & Graves, 1990; Olson et al., 1989; Pennington, Van Orden, Smith, Green, & Haith, 1990). The disabled groups in these studies were deficient in both skills. Converging evidence for a causal influence of phonological awareness on phonological decoding and word recognition comes from the positive influence of pre-schoolers' training in phonological awareness on later reading ability (c.f., Byrne & Fielding-Barnsley, 1993; Lie, 1991; Lundberg, Frost, & Peterson, 1988). Also, Wagner et al. (1994) reported the results of causal models of longitudinal data from the beginning of kindergarten to the end of the second and first grades that were consistent with the causal influence of phonological awareness on later reading.

3.2. *Orthographic Coding*

A few RLM studies have compared disabled and normal subjects' orthographic coding skills. Olson et al. (1985, 1989) found no significant difference between disabled and normal groups' accuracy in the word-pseudohomophone choice task, but the older disabled groups were significantly faster. This greater speed yielded a modest but significant advantage for the disabled group when the accuracy and latency scores were combined. Manis (1993) recently reported a study that included measures similar to our word-pseudohomophone and homophone choice tasks. No significant differences between the reading-level-matched groups were found for these orthographic measures. However, as in the studies by Olson et al., the disabled group did show significant deficits in phonological coding and phonological awareness.

Disabled readers in an RLM comparison have shown *superior* performance on accuracy in a non-lexical forced-choice orthographic task. Siegel, Geva, and Share (1993) presented pairs of nonwords, one of which contained letter sequence/positions that were common in words, the other not. Subjects were asked to select the nonword that was most like English words (e.g., filv-filk; moke-moje; vism-visn; powl-lowp). In contrast to earlier studies of word-likeness judgments, both choices in the Siegel et al. study were pronounceable nonwords. This task is quite interesting because it does not require a response to words and it may get at a more general level of orthographic knowledge than the previous tasks that used words. Disabled readers were significantly more accurate in this task than a younger normal group matched on word recognition. Stanovich and Siegel (in press) recently confirmed this result using their continuous regression procedure that we discussed earlier. Stanovich and Siegel also found that disabled readers performed above their level of word recognition on the forced-choice PIAT spelling recognition test. Inexplicably, their disabled readers showed a small but significant deficit on accuracy in an adaptation of the Olson et al. (1985) word-pseudohomophone choice task.

Analyses of spelling errors in spelling-level-matched groups have also suggested that disabled readers have a higher level of sensitivity to certain orthographic features. Pennington, McCabe, Smith, Lefly, Bookman, Kimberling, and Lubs (1986) reported that disabled readers' spelling errors on the WRAT were significantly more accurate in some complex aspects of English orthography. Lennox and Siegel (1993) found that while the misspellings of poor spellers tended to be less phonologically accurate, their errors were more visually similar than those of good spellers at the same spelling age.

The evidence reviewed so far supports superior or at least equal performance for disabled readers' orthographic reading and spelling processes when compared to younger normal subjects at the same reading or spelling levels. However, a seemingly minor change in orthographic-task procedure yields strikingly different results. Manis et al. (1990) had subjects listen to a word (e.g., "street") and subsequently press a yes or no button to indicate if a letter string presented on the computer screen was the correctly spelled word. Foils presented on 50% of the 42 trials were pseudohomophones of the target word (e.g., "streat"). Unlike the Olson et al. (1985, 1989) and Manis (1993) results with a forced-choice between a target and foil, disabled readers in the Manis et al. (1990) task were significantly less accurate than their younger normal comparison group, primarily due to a higher number of false-positive responses. Manis et al. (1990) included a second orthographic task wherein subjects listened to a sentence ("It is the last day of the week"), and then a word was presented on the screen that was either the correct word for the sentence (week) or an incorrect homonym (weak). Subjects pushed a yes or no button to indicate if the trial contained the correct word. As in the above word-pseudohomophone task, the dyslexic subjects showed a significant accuracy deficit in a RLM comparison with younger normal readers, again because of too many false-positive responses.

Manis, Custodio, and Szeszulski (1993) reported a replication of their earlier results for the above tasks in a new sample, so their finding of an orthographic coding deficit appears to be robust for the "yes-no" tasks. Again, the disabled readers' deficit was primarily due to a higher number of false-positive responses. It appears from these results that the orthographic representations disabled readers typically use for word recognition may be less precise than those of younger normal readers at the same reading level. Perfetti (1992) has argued that there is a developmental continuum from low to high precision in lexical representations and the development of this precision is linked to development in the precision of phonological representations. From this point of view, it is not surprising to find similar deficits in phonological and orthographic coding. Such a result is consistent with a highly integrative view of development in phonological and orthographic processes (Ehri, 1992).

On the other hand, the absence of an orthographic deficit when targets and foils are presented simultaneously seems to support a more separatist view of orthographic and phonological coding processes. Perhaps disabled readers typically approach the reading task with a lower criterion for orthographic precision, but they can demonstrate reading-level-appropriate recognition memory for target words' orthography when the words can be simultaneously compared with foils. Future reading-level-match comparisons should include both types of orthographic measures with the same subjects to be sure that sample differences or regression artifacts are not leading to different results. It would also be helpful to include other converging measures of orthographic precision in reading and spelling. For the present, the reading-level-match studies yield conflicting evidence regarding disabled readers' cognitive profiles for orthographic coding.

4. BEHAVIORAL-GENETIC EVIDENCE

A fundamental question about the development of individual differences in reading and related skills is their genetic and environmental etiology. In this section we present evidence from identical and fraternal twins concerning the balance of genetic and environmental influences on disabled readers' deficits in word recognition, orthographic coding, phonological coding, and phonological awareness. In addition, a series of bivariate analyses will assess the degree to which the correlated deficits in different skills are due to the same genes.

4.1. *Methods and Assumptions for Behavioral-Genetic Analyses of Twin Data*

Identical and same-sex fraternal twins are being tested in the CLDRC to obtain estimates of the proportion of genetic, shared-environment, and non-shared environment influence on twin similarities in reading and related cognitive skills. Identical twins develop from the same sperm and egg (they are monozygotic or MZ), and thus share all their genes. Fraternal twins are derived from two different sperm-egg combinations (they are dizygotic or DZ), just as ordinary siblings, and they share half their segregating genes on average.

The behavioral-genetic interpretation of data from MZ and DZ twins is based on several assumptions, including additive influence from any relevant genes, no assortative mating, and an equal degree of shared environment for MZ and DZ pairs (Plomin, DeFries, & McClearn, 1990). If these assumptions are not violated to a significant degree, comparing MZ and DZ within-pair differences provides valid estimates for the proportions of genetic, shared-environment, and non-shared environment influences on average twin resemblance.

Traditional twin studies of the full range of individual differences across the population may compare the correlations for MZ and DZ pairs. A significantly higher correlation for MZ pairs provides evidence for a genetic etiology. Different methods are used to assess the heritability of extreme deviations from the normal population, such as reading disability. Earlier twin studies of reading disability (c.f., Hallgren, 1950; Stevenson, Graham, Fredman, & McLoughlin, 1987) compared the "concordance rates" (the proportion of twin pairs that share the categorical deficit) between MZ and DZ twins. However, a more appropriate and powerful statistical approach can be used to assess the group heritability for varying degrees of deviance in characteristics such as reading disability that fall on a continuous dimension (DeFries & Fulker, 1985). In DeFries and Fulker's approach, an affected twin (the "proband") is identified based on a severity criterion for deviation from the mean of the normal population. (In the analyses described here, probands included those individuals who were at least 1.5 sd below the mean of the control group). Genetic and shared-environment influence is then assessed by comparing the MZ and DZ cotwins' regression toward the control group mean. For example, suppose that the average proband deficit for both MZ and DZ twins is 2 sd below the population mean for a particular measure. If there is no test error and individual differences in performance on that measure are completely heritable, the MZ cotwins should show no regression to the population mean because they share identical genes. DZ cotwins should regress half way (1 sd) to the population mean because they share half their segregating genes, on average. On the other extreme, if there is no heritability for a particular measure, MZ and DZ cotwins would show equal regression to the population mean. Differential cotwin regression between these two extreme examples would indicate an intermediate level of heritability.

Twin data are also informative about the degree to which shared environment is important for individual differences. If *both* MZ and DZ cotwins showed no regression to the population mean, this would indicate that shared family environment accounted entirely for individual differences across the twin pairs. In the more likely case in which MZ cotwins regress somewhat to the mean due to test error and non-shared environment, and DZ cotwins regress more, but somewhat less than half way to the mean, the combined influence of shared environment and genetic factors is indicated for the probands' group deficit.

The multiple-regression procedure developed by DeFries and Fulker (1985) yields estimates and standard errors for the proportion of genetic influence on the probands' group deficit (h^2_g). Related procedures reveal the proportion of shared-environment influence (c^2_g). The difference between the sum of these estimates and 1.0 indicates the proportion of twin differences due to non-shared environment and/or test error.

4.2. *Results of Behavioral-Genetic Analyses*

DeFries, Fulker, and LaBuda (1987) reported the first evidence from the CLDRC for the heritability of reading disability. They selected probands based on their low performance on a composite variable that included the word recognition, spelling recognition, and reading comprehension scores on the PIAT. The resulting heritability estimate for the composite variable was $h^2_g = .29 \pm .10$ SE; $p < .05$ (SE is the standard error of the estimate and the p value indicates the probability that the population h^2_g is greater than zero). Subsequent estimates of heritability for the group deficit on the composite reading variable have increased as the twin sample has become larger. The most recent heritability estimate from a sample of 133 MZ and 98 DZ pairs was $h^2_g = .51 \pm .10$ SE (Gillis, 1993). The estimate of shared-environment influence on the group deficit was also highly significant ($c^2_g = .41 \pm .10$ SE).

We have been particularly interested in possible differences in the patterns of genetic and environmental influence on different reading and related language skills. Table 3 includes results from separate heritability analyses for the individual PIAT measures incorporated in the composite score discussed above. For each variable independently, MZ and DZ pairs were selected wherein at least one member of the pair was below -1.5 sd from the comparison group mean.

The number of MZ and DZ twin pairs entered in each analysis is presented under each variable name on the left side of Table 3. The sample sizes differ across the different variables depending on the variance in the normal comparison sample and the degree to which the variables correlate with the initial group assignment from school records. PIAT Word Recognition has the highest correlation with group assignment and is the most reliable of the three measures. Thus, it has a larger sample than the other two variables.

It can be seen in Table 3 that for PIAT Word Recognition and PIAT Spelling, the MZ cotwin's regression toward the population mean is substantially less than that observed for the DZ cotwins. These patterns of differential regression yield substantial estimates for both genetic and shared-environment influence. However, the regression pattern is somewhat different for the PIAT Reading Comprehension variable. The difference between MZ and DZ cotwin regression is smaller, yielding a lower estimate for genetic influence and a higher estimate for shared-environment influence on the group deficit in PIAT Reading Comprehension. With the present sample size, the differences between the heritabilities for PIAT Reading Comprehension and PIAT Word Recognition or Spelling Recognition are not statistically significant ($p > .05$). If the present trend is statistically confirmed in a larger sample, it would indicate that the pattern of genetic and environmental etiology for group deficits is different across the PIAT subtests.

Separate heritabilities for deficits in orthographic coding (word-pseudohomophone choice) and phonological coding (oral nonword reading) were first reported by Olson et al. (1989; also in Olson, Wise, Conners, & Rack, 1990). The results were word recognition $h^2_g = .40 \pm .12$, orthographic coding $h^2_g = .28 \pm .16$, and phonological coding $h^2_g = .47 \pm .14$. From these preliminary analyses it appeared that the heritability of phonological coding was higher than that for orthographic coding, although the contrast was not statistically significant.

There were several problems with this initial study (Olson et al., 1989). One was the small sample size. Another was the way in which probands were selected for the regression analyses. The lowest scoring twin was always selected as the proband and the higher scoring twin was the cotwin. This procedure introduces too much regression associated with error variance and it is not appropriate for "truncate" selection wherein our twin subjects were ascertained based on a deficit in either member of the pair (see Thompson & Thompson, 1986; DeFries & Gillis, 1991). With "truncate" selection, it is appropriate to "double enter" a twin pair if both members fall below the deficit criterion level. In this case, each twin is entered twice, once as the proband and once as the co-twin. The standard errors are subsequently adjusted to reflect the single-entry sample size. This was the procedure followed for the analyses presented in Tables 3, 4, and 5.

Table 3

Genetic (h^2_g) and Shared Environment (c^2_g) Influence on Group Deficits in Disabled Readers' PIAT Word Recognition, PIAT Spelling Recognition, and PIAT Reading Comprehension

Task	MZ Proband	MZ Cotwin	DZ Proband	DZ Cotwin	h^2_g (SE)	c^2_g (SE)
PIAT Word (MZ=174,DZ=126)	-2.59	-2.37	-2.55	-1.75	.46 (.10)*	.45 (.11)*
PIAT Spell (MZ=155,DZ=107)	-2.31	-1.94	-2.33	-1.39	.48 (.11)*	.36 (.11)*
PIAT Comp. (MZ=151, DZ=96)	-2.35	-1.84	-2.27	-1.48	.27 (.12)*	.52 (.11)*

NOTE: The numbers of MZ and DZ pairs for each measure are presented in parentheses.
* = $p < .01$ for estimates significantly greater than 0. $h^2_g = 2 * CMZ/PMZ - CDZ/PDZ$; $c^2_g = 2CDZ/PDZ - CMZ/PMZ$.

Our most recent behavioral-genetic analyses included a much larger twin sample and employed the "double entry" procedure described above. The new results for word recognition (combined PIAT and TWRT), phonological coding (combined accuracy and latency in the oral nonword reading task), orthographic coding (combined accuracy and latency in the word-pseudohomophone choice task), and Phonological Awareness (Phoneme Segmentation and Transposition) are presented in Table 4.

It can be seen in Table 4 that for the group deficit in word recognition, genetic and shared-environment influences are both substantial and approximately equal, while non-shared environment influence is very low (1 - (.47 + .48) = .05). For phonological coding, orthographic coding, and phonological awareness, the genetic influence appears to be somewhat stronger than the influence of shared environment. However, with the present sample size and standard errors, there are no statistically significant contrasts with the genetic and shared-environment effects for word recognition.

Table 4

Genetic (h^2_g) and Shared Environment (c^2_g) Influence on Group Deficits in Word Recognition, Phonological Coding, Orthographic Coding, and Phonological Awareness

Task	MZ Proband	MZ Cotwin	DZ Proband	DZ Cotwin	h^2_g (SE)	c^2_g (SE)
Word Recog. (MZ=183,DZ=129)	-2.65	-2.52	-2.62	-1.87	.47 (.09)*	.48 (.11)*
Phonological (MZ=151,DZ=105)	-2.63	-2.28	-2.62	-1.50	.59 (.12)*	.27 (.12)*
Orthographic (MZ=132,DZ=92)	-2.77	-2.37	-2.71	-1.56	.56 (.13)*	.29 (.13)*
Pho. Awareness (MZ=93,DZ=68)	-3.37	-2.67	-2.79	-1.39	.60 (.17)*	.20 (.16)

In relation to our previous reports (Olson et al., 1989, 1990), the most surprising result in Table 4 is the nearly identical patterns of genetic and shared-environment effects for phonological and orthographic coding. Although contrasts were not significant in previous reports, there was a trend toward higher heritability for phonological coding. Now with a substantially larger sample and more appropriate analyses of the twin data, the patterns are very similar. Our other measures of orthographic coding (PIAT Spelling Recognition, see Table 3, and Homophone Choice) and phonological coding (Silent Nonword Reading) yielded very similar results.

There was a strong genetic influence on deficits in phoneme awareness (Phoneme Segmentation and Transposition) and no significant effect of shared environment. A similar result was found for the Phoneme Deletion measure ($h^2_g = .70 \pm .19$; $c^2_g = .16 + .18$). Because this measure was recently introduced in the test battery, the sample was much smaller (68MZ, 49DZ), resulting in larger standard errors.

Even though deficits in the different reading and language skills in Table 4 are similarly heritable, it cannot be assumed that the same genes are operating to produce these deficits. For example, we might find that individual differences in height and word recognition have similar heritability levels, but they are most certainly influenced by different genes. Of course height and word recognition are not likely to be correlated at the phenotypic level. But even though the variables in Table 3 are significantly correlated, it does not follow that these correlations arise primarily through genetic influence. They could just as likely arise primarily through the influence of shared environment.

The degree of common genetic influence across different variables can be assessed by a bivariate extension of the DeFries and Fulker (1985) univariate multiple-regression procedure. In the bivariate extension, the proband is selected for a deficit on one variable and cotwin regression to the population mean is assessed for the second variable (Stevenson, Pennington, Gilger, DeFries, & Gillis, in press). The resulting bivariate estimate of h^2_g is a function of the group heritabilities for the two variables and the degree to which these group heritabilities are influenced by the same genes. Furthermore, the ratio of the bivariate heritability to the observed standardized covariance between the variables yields an estimate of the proportion of the correlation between the variables that is due to the same genes. For example, the bivariate heritability could be low between two variables because their covariance is low, but most of the variables' shared variance could be due to the same genes. Examples of this situation are in Table 5.

Table 5 presents the results of a series of bivariate heritability estimates. For each estimate, the proband is selected on the variable that is most highly correlated with the initial group designation of school history. This selection is least likely to violate significantly the assumptions of the DeFries and Fulker (1985) multiple-regression procedure. The first column in Table 5 presents the estimate of bivariate heritability with its standard error. The second column presents the regression coefficient between the two variables within the proband sample, which provides an unbiased estimate of their linear relationship in selected samples. The third column includes the estimates and their standard errors for the proportion of the correlation between the two variables that is due to common genetic factors.

The first three analyses in Table 5 all involve proband selection on deficits in word recognition and cotwin regression on a second variable. The bivariate heritability estimates were significantly greater than zero ($p < .05$) for phonological coding, orthographic coding, and phonological awareness. After dividing these estimates by the regression coefficient, the estimates in the right column represent the proportion of the correlation due to common genetic influences. These estimates are all quite high, indicating that the observed covariances are due primarily to heritable influences.

The lower block of bivariate heritability estimates in Table 5 includes a proband selection on phonological coding and cotwin regression on orthographic coding. It is clear that there is also significant bivariate heritability for these two variables, as there is between each of the variables and phonological awareness.

Table 5

Genetic Influence on Bivariate Relations

Proband Variable		Cotwin Variable	Bivariate Heritability	Regression Coefficient	Genetic Proportion
Word Rec.	-	Phonological	.43 ± .10	.742	.58 ± .14
Word Rec.	-	Orthographic	.29 ±.12	.420	.69 + .29
Word Rec.	-	Ph. Awareness	.46 ±.16	.613	.75 + .26
Phonological	-	Orthographic	.43 ± .14	.649	.66 + .22
Phonological	-	Ph. Awareness	.51 + .18	.656	.78 + .27
Orthographic	-	Ph. Awareness	.44 + .20	.515	.85 + .39

5. GENERAL DISCUSSION AND CONCLUSIONS

5.1. *Important Qualifications of Heritability Estimates*

Regarding the genetic effects reported in this chapter, it is important to remember that the estimates of h^2_g do not pertain to any individual in the sample. Individual deficits could be mostly due to genetic factors or mostly due to environment. What we are observing here are the average genetic and shared-environment effects on deficits in the disabled group.

The specific *type* of genetic as well as shared environment influence could also vary widely across individuals. For example, different individual reading disabilities could be variously caused by different single genes or by different combinations of multiple genes. Genetic linkage analyses within several extended families containing reading disabled probands have suggested heterogeneity in the apparent mode of genetic transmission (Smith, Kimberling, & Pennington, 1991). (The genetic linkage procedure relates reading deficits to specific loci on the chromosomes.) Thus, there may be different genetic mechanisms in different individuals leading to the same or similar reading deficits.

A third important qualification of the behavioral-genetic results is that estimates of the relative balance of genetic and environmental influence depends jointly on the amount of relevant genetic variation and the amount of relevant environmental variance in the sample. Compared to a sample that might be drawn from some large cities with an extremely broad range of educational and socioeconomic environment, the environmental variation in the Colorado sample may be relatively homogeneous. Nevertheless, there was a significant influence of shared family environment for all the group deficits except phonological awareness. Part of the environmental variance may be associated with the varying quality of reading instruction in the Colorado schools that we have observed in our studies of computer-based remediation (Olson & Wise, 1992). Some environmental variance may also be linked to differences in print exposure in the home (Anderson, Wilson, & Fielding, 1988; Cunningham & Stanovich, 1993).

5.2. A Shared Genetic Etiology for Correlated Orthographic and Phonological Deficits

The patterns of genetic and shared-environment influence on the group deficits were very similar across all measures of orthographic and phonological coding. Moreover, the estimate of bivariate heritability was highly significant, indicating a substantial common genetic etiology for correlated deficits in phonological and orthographic coding. Thus, within twin pairs, the specific genetic mechanisms tend to be the same for correlated deficits in phonological and orthographic coding.

The new results are inconsistent with earlier reports of apparently strong trends toward higher heritability for phonological coding deficits (Olson et al., 1989, 1990). However, the sample size for those estimates was much smaller and the contrast between orthographic and phonological coding heritabilities was never statistically significant.

Our new results are also inconsistent with those of the only other twin study to assess the differential heritability of group deficits in orthographic and phonological coding. Stevenson, Graham, Fredman, and McLoughlin (1987) studied the reading and spelling skills of 275 pairs of 13 year-old London twins. In this initial report, they found significant differences in the MZ and DZ concordance rates for deficits in spelling production but not for deficits in word recognition. However, because the twin sample in this study was a representative sample of London twins and was not initially selected for deficits in reading or spelling, the number of twin probands expressing deficits was quite small. The contrast in MZ-DZ concordance patterns between word recognition and spelling deficits would not have been statistically significant.

A more recent set of analyses from the London twin study used the same continuous twin regression method that we have used here (DeFries & Fulker, 1985). Because his sample size was too small to use our more severe 1.5 sd cut-off for disabled probands, Stevenson (1991) selected twin probands who were -1 standard deviation below the sample mean on the respective measures. As in the earlier concordance analyses, the heritability for deficits in word recognition was not significant ($h^2_g = .03 \pm .37$). The heritability for spelling production was significant but only after regressing IQ variance from the subjects' spelling scores ($h^2_g = .58 \pm .34$). The standard errors are quite large because there were only about 20 MZ and 40 DZ pairs in these analyses.

Stevenson (1991) also assessed the heritabilities for deficits in orthographic and phonological coding. The phonological coding task involved the untimed oral reading of a list of 30 three-letter nonwords. The orthographic task involved the untimed oral reading of a list of 39 irregular or exception words (e.g., answer, break, yacht, gross). For phonological coding, 27 MZ and 36 DZ twin pairs yielded a moderate but statistically insignificant heritability estimate (h^2_g = .41 ± .39). For orthographic coding, 6 MZ and 30 DZ twin pairs yielded a strongly *negative* heritability estimate (h^2_g = -.91 ± .53). A negative heritability estimate indicates there was more average cotwin regression for the MZ than for the DZ pairs. Such a result is not consistent with the basic theory of twin designs. The result is most likely due to error variance and the very small MZ sample size. In any case, the contrast between the heritabilities for deficits in Stevenson's measures of orthographic and phonological coding is not statistically significant.

Of course, the lack of statistical significance for the difference between Stevenson's (1991) orthographic and phonological heritabilities does not prove the null hypothesis. The trend toward higher heritability for phonological coding observed in Stevenson's sample could be a real difference without necessarily contradicting the results of our analyses. The samples in the London and Colorado studies were different, as were the measures of phonological and particularly orthographic coding. Stevenson's orthographic coding measure involved the oral reading of exception words. If there was a wider range of environment for print exposure in the London sample, previous exposure to some of the uncommon exception words that would be required for their correct reading may have been more strongly linked to this environmental variance.

Stevenson (1991) speculated that the low heritability he observed for deficits in word recognition may have been due to the large number of exception words in the Schonell Graded Word Reading Test (Schonell & Schonell, 1960). On the other hand, our word recognition tests and the three orthographic choice tasks also contained a number of exception words that would require previous print exposure for correct performance.

To resolve the difference in results for the London and the most recent Colorado twin analyses, it would be necessary to employ both the exception-word-reading and orthographic-choice tasks in the same samples. For now, we are left with a strong but statistically insignificant contrast in heritabilities from the small sample in the London study, and nearly identical genetic and shared-environment profiles with small standard errors in the much larger Colorado study. Results from the larger sample suggest that if there is any real difference between the *amount* of genetic and shared environmental influence on the group deficits in orthographic and phonological coding, that difference is not likely to be very large.

It is important to remember that the relative amount of genetic and shared-environment influence on phonological and orthographic deficits may vary widely across *individual* proband twins within the disabled group. Furthermore, although the bivariate analysis suggests a strong common genetic etiology for the *covariance* between phonological and orthographic coding deficits within twin pairs, the specific genetic etiology for any reliable *independent* variance in phonological and orthographic coding could be different. Thus, it is possible that one proband's specific genetic defect could have a stronger impact on phonological coding, while another proband could have a genetic defect that has greater influence on orthographic coding.

The twin sample has become large enough for us to begin exploring the heritability of residual patterns of deficit for phonological and orthographic coding. When orthographic coding is regressed on phonological coding, subjects low on the residual variable are relatively deficient in orthographic coding. When phonological coding is regressed on orthographic coding, a different group of subjects low on the residual variable are relatively deficient in phonological coding. Significant heritability estimates for deficits on both residual variables support the possibility of different genetic and environmental mechanisms for specific deficits in phonological and orthographic coding. However, we are concerned that the residual analyses may violate some population assumptions of the DeFries and Fulker (1985) method for assessing the heritability of group deficits. Different biologically based genetic-linkage markers for specific orthographic and phonological deficits would provide more convincing support.

5.3. *Implications for Dual Route vs. Connectionist Models*

We began with a "dual-route" perspective on individual differences among disabled readers that guided our choice of the orthographic and phonological coding tasks (Olson et al., 1985). Early trends in the behavior-genetic analyses seemed to support differences in the absolute amount of genetic influence on deficits in phonological (indirect route) and orthographic (direct route) processing (Olson et al., 1989, 1990). It appeared that deficits in phonological coding were more heritable, although the contrast was not statistically significant. We had thought this apparent trend supported a "dual-route" perspective by indicating a fundamentally different developmental etiology for deficits in phonological and orthographic coding.

The present univariate results suggest that there is little if any difference in levels of heritability for the group deficits in phonological and orthographic coding. The bivariate results suggest further that the covariance between the deficits is largely due to the same genetic mechanisms. Therefore, the new results seem more supportive of Ehri's (1989, 1992) integrative view of the development of phonological and orthographic coding skills for most disabled readers. However, there is some preliminary evidence that some disabled readers may have unique genetically based deficits in either phonological or orthographic coding.

Even the integrative view does not necessarily contradict the "dual-route" model. It is possible that the developmental-genetic etiology for deficits in phonological and orthographic processes could be similar within most individuals, but the two processes could still involve somewhat different mechanisms and anatomical substrates. For example, brain mechanisms associated with good phonological processing could be linked to the development of anatomically separate, more visually related processing mechanisms for the accurate representation of orthographic images. This view is consistent with some analyses of the apparently selective loss of phonological or orthographic processes due to brain damage (Coltheart et al., 1993, but there are other less modular interpretations of the acquired dyslexia literature). The hypothesis that there are anatomical differences in the location of orthographic and phonological reading processes is currently being tested by functional neural-imaging techniques (Carr & Posner, in press; Rumsey, personal communication, 1993).

Connectionist models have raised the possibility of a developmentally *and* anatomically integrated mechanism for orthographic and phonological coding (Plaut & McClelland, 1993; Seidenberg & McClelland, 1989; Van Orden, Pennington, & Stone, 1990). Computer simulations have demonstrated that codes for nonwords, regular words, and exception words can be learned and represented in the same artificial neural network consisting of orthographic input units, hidden association units, and phonological output units. Moreover, Plaut and McClelland have found that after learning a corpus of words, specific association units participated in the processing of both exception words, regular words, and nonwords.

Coltheart et al. (in press) and Besner, Twilley, McCann, and Seergobin (1990) have criticized Seidenberg and McClelland's (1989) model for its "dyslexic" performance in reading nonwords, but Plaut and McClelland's (1993) modifications in the structure of the orthographic input and phonological output units seems to have solved this problem. A number of researchers are now attempting to simulate reading and spelling disabilities within connectionist models (c.f., Brown, Loosemore, & Watson, 1993; Hulme, Snowling, & Quinland, 1991; Seidenberg, 1992). A clue to the simulation of phonological coding deficits may be taken from the better performance apparently associated with Plaut and McClelland's more precise representation of phonological structure in the output units. In the following section we emphasize the importance of deficits in disabled readers' awareness of phonological structure for the development of deficits in phonological and orthographic coding.

5.4. A Genetic Etiology From Phonological Awareness To Reading

Deficits in two phonological awareness measures were highly heritable and demonstrated significant bivariate heritability with proband deficits in word recognition, phonological coding, and orthographic coding. Although there is certainly a reciprocal influence on phonological awareness from learning to read (Morais, 1991; Wagner et al., in press), phonological awareness training studies and causal models of longitudinal data mentioned earlier have provided strong support for the causal influence of early phonological awareness on later reading. Our data are consistent with the hypothesis that the genetic influence on reading disability arises through genetically influenced deficits in phonological awareness. Of course, a more reductionist approach might reveal more fundamental genetically based deficits in brain processes, such as poor temporal resolution (Tallal, 1984), that ultimately lead to deficits in phonological awareness. (We are currently introducing temporal measures in the ongoing twin study.) The importance of phonological awareness is that it may be the main proximal cause of most genetically-based deficits in word recognition, and thus it may be the most appropriate focus for diagnosis and remediation.

Although heritabilities were high and shared-environment influences were not significant for the group deficit in phonological awareness, training studies have shown significant improvement in both phonological awareness and reading. This demonstrates that high heritability does not imply that a skill can not be significantly improved by training. It might suggest that some extraordinary environmental intervention may be required to significantly improve a deficit that is highly heritable. Our current approaches to the remediation of phonological awareness in disabled readers are exploring the training of articulatory awareness as an intermediate step to phonological awareness (Alexander, Anderson, Heilman, Voeller, & Torgesen, 1991; Lie, 1991; Wise, Olson, & Lindamood, 1993), in addition to computer-based reading practice (Olson & Wise, 1992).

5.5. *Independent Variance Between Phonological and Orthographic Coding*

In spite of the significant correlation between the phonological and orthographic factors, and the substantial genetic covariation between orthographic and phonological coding deficits, the fact remains that phonological and orthographic coding accounted for significant independent variance in word recognition. The factor loadings for other variables suggested the basis for these separate contributions to word recognition. There were no differences in factor loadings for visual processing, naming speed, or verbal IQ. Thus, there was no support for theories that have proposed a unique relation between orthographic coding and visual perception or naming speed.

Aside from the different loadings for the orthographic and phonological coding variables, the key variables that loaded differentially on the orthographic and phonological factors were phonological awareness (high on the phonological factor) and print exposure (high on the orthographic factor). We noted that previous exposure to the printed target words in the orthographic tasks is a logical necessity for accurate performance. Our results for print exposure confirm the results of earlier studies by Stanovich and his colleagues. We noted that the true contribution of variation in print exposure was probably much larger than indicated by the Title Recognition Test.

Print exposure may explain why many disabled readers' word recognition and some types of orthographic coding are able to rise above their more severe deficits in phonological coding and phonological awareness. Disabled groups in reading-level match designs are often as much as five years older than their younger normal comparison groups. Thus, the older disabled readers may have an advantage in print exposure that fosters greater orthographic knowledge in spite of their phonological deficit. The extreme phonological dyslexic described by Campbell and Butterworth (1985) is a case in point. This individual was extremely poor in reading nonwords, but through an extraordinary amount of reading practice, she was able develop her orthographic knowledge and had a word-recognition vocabulary that was above normal. Variation in print exposure may also be related to individual differences in the balance of orthographic and phonological skills *within* groups of disabled (c.f., Castles & Coltheart, 1993) and normal readers (c.f., Baron, 1979).

We conclude with a puzzle. Preliminary behavior-genetic analyses for deficits in print exposure (Title Recognition Test) have revealed no significant heritability ($h^2_g = .17 \pm .17$), but the estimate of shared-environment effects was highly significant ($c^2_g = .54 = \pm .15$). Of course, the nonsignificant heritability estimate could be wrong, with only 61 MZ and 39 DZ pairs in the analysis. (We have learned to be cautious about estimates from small samples.) The review by Plomin and Bergeman (1991) revealed strong genetic effects on some measures of environment (e.g., a genotype-environment correlation). But assuming that the present low heritability and high shared-environment estimates for print exposure are correct, the relatively high loading of print exposure on the orthographic factor would be consistent with a higher shared-environment influence on orthographic coding. This we did not find, but the unique influence of print exposure on orthographic coding deficits may be relatively weak in this sample, compared to the substantial genetic influence.

FOOTNOTE

1. This work was supported in part by program project and center grants from the NICHD (HD-11681 and HD-27802), and RO1 HD-22223. The contributions of staff members of the many Colorado school districts that participate in our research, and of the twins and their families, are gratefully acknowledged. Co-investigators on the Colorado Reading Project are John DeFries, David Fulker, Richard Olson, Bruce Pennington, and Shelly Smith.

REFERENCES

Adams, M.J. (1990). *Beginning to read: Thinking and learning about print*. Cambridge, MA: MIT Press.

Alexander, A.W., Anderson, H.G., Heilman, P.C., Voeller, K.S., & Torgesen,J.K. (1991). Phonological awareness training and remediation of analytic decoding deficits in a group of severe dyslexics. *Annals of Dyslexia, 41*, 193-206.

Anderson, R.C., Wilson, P.T., & Fielding, L.G. (1988). Growth in reading and how children spend their time outside of school. *Reading Research Quarterly, 23*, 285-303.

Barker, T.A., Torgesen, J.K., & Wagner, R.K. (1992). The role of orthographic processing skills on five different reading tasks. *Reading Research Quarterly*, 334-345.

Baron, J. (1979). Orthographic and word-specific mechanisms in childrens' reading of words. *Child Development, 50*, 60-72.

Baron, J., & Strawson, C. (1976). Orthographic and word-specific mechanisms reading words aloud. *Journal of Experimental Psychology: Human Perception and Performance, 2*, 386-393.

Barron, R.W. (1986). Word recognition in early reading: A review of the direct and indirect access hypothesis. *Cognition, 24*, 93-119.

Besner, D., Twilley, L., McCann, R.S., & Seergobin, K. (1990). On the connection between connectionism and data: Are a few words necessary? *Psychological Review, 97*, 432-446.

Boder, E. (1973). Developmental dyslexia: A diagnostic approach based on three atypical reading and spelling patterns. *Developmental Medicine and Child Neurology, 15,* 663-687.

Bowers, P.G., & Swanson, L.B. (1991). Naming speed deficits in reading disability: Multiple measures of a singular process. *Journal of Experimental Child Psychology, 51,* 195-219.

Bowers, P.G., & Wolf, M. (1993). Theoretical links among naming speed, precise timing mechanisms and orthographic skill in dyslexia. *Reading and Writing, 5,* 69-85.

Bowey, J.A., Cain, M.T., & Ryan, S.M. (1992). A reading-level design study of phonological skills underlying fourth-grade children's word reading difficulties. *Child Development, 63,* 999-1011.

Bradely, L., & Bryant, P.E. (1978). Difficulties in auditory organization as a possible cause of reading backwardness. *Nature, 271,* 746-747.

Brown, G., Loosemore, R., & Watson, F. (1993). Normal and dyslexic spelling: A connectionist approach. Manuscript under review.

Bruce, D.J. (1964). The analysis of word sounds by young children. *British Journal of Psychology, 34,* 158-170.

Bruck, M. (1992). Persistence of dyslexics' phonological awareness deficits. *Developmental Psychology, 28,* 874-886.

Byrne, B., & Fielding-Barnsley, R. (1993). Evaluation of a program to teach phonemic awareness to young children: A 1-year follow-up. *Journal of Educational Psychology, 85,* 104-111.

Carr, T.H., & Posner, M.I. (in press). The impact of learning to read on the functional anatomy of language processing. In B. de Gelder & J. Morais (Eds.), *Language and Literacy: Comparative approaches.* Cambridge, MA: MIT Press.

Castles, A.E., & Coltheart, M. (1993). Varieties of developmental dyslexia. *Cognition, 47,* 149-180.

Catts, H. (1989). Defining dyslexia as a developmental language disorder. *Annals of Dyslexia, 39,* 50-64.

Cipielewski, J. & Stanovich, K.E. (1992). Predicting growth in reading ability from children's exposure to print. *Journal of Experimental Child Psychology, 54,* 74-89.

Coltheart, M. (1978). Lexical access in simple reading tasks. In G. Underwood (Ed.), *Strategies of information processing* (pp. 151-216). London: Academic Press.

Coltheart, M., Curtis, B., Atkins, P., & Haller, M. (1993). Models of reading aloud: Dual-route and parallel-distributed-processing approaches. *Psychological Review, 100*, 589-608.

Conners, F., & Olson, R.K. (1990). Reading comprehension in dyslexic and normal readers: A component skills analysis. In D.A. Balota, G.B. Flores d'Arcais, & K. Rayner (Eds.), *Comprehension processes in reading* (pp. 557-579). Hillsdale, NJ: Erlbaum.

Corcos, E., & Willows, D.M. (1993). The processing of orthographic information. In D.M. Willows, R.S. Kruk, & E. Corcos(Eds.). *Visual Processes in Reading and Reading Disabilities* (pp. 163-190). Hillsdale, NJ: Lawrence Erlbaum Associates.

Cornwall, A. (1992). The relationship of phonological awareness, rapid naming, and verbal memory to severe reading and spelling disability. *Journal of Learning Disabilities, 25*, 532-538.

Cunningham, A.E., & Stanovich, K.E. (1991). Tracking the unique effects of print exposure in children: Associations with vocabulary, general knowledge, and spelling. *Journal of Educational Psychology, 83*, 264-274

Cunningham, A.E., & Stanovich, K.E. (1993). Children's literacy environments and early word recognition subskills. *Reading and Writing: An Interdisciplinary Journal, 5*, 193-204.

DeFries, J.C., & Fulker, D.W. (1985). Multiple regression analysis of twin data. *Behavior Genetics, 15*, 467-473.

DeFries, J.C., Fulker, D.W., & LaBuda, M.C. (1987). Evidence for a genetic aetiology in reading disability of twins. *Nature, 239*, 537-539.

DeFries, J.C., & Gillis, J.J. (1991). Etiology of reading deficits in learning disabilities: Quantitative genetic analysis. In J.E. Obrzut & G.W. Hynd (Eds.), *Neuropsychological foundations of learning disabilities: A handbook of issues, methods, and practice* (pp. 29-47). Orlando, FL: Academic Press.

DeFries, J.C., Olson, R.K., Pennington, B.F., & Smith, S.D. (1991). Colorado reading project: An update. In D. Duane and D. Gray (Eds.), *The reading brain: The biological basis of dyslexia* (pp. 53-87). Parkton, MD: York Press.

Denkla, M.B., & Rudel, R.G. (1974). Rapid "automatized" naming of pictured objects, colors, letters, and numbers by normal children. *Cortex, 10*, 186-202.

Dunn, L.M., & Markwardt, F.C. (1970). *Examiner's manual: Peabody Individual Achievement Test.* Circle Pines, MN: American Guidance Service.

Ehri, L.C. (1989). The development of spelling knowledge and its role in reading acquisition and reading disability. *Journal of Learning Disabilities, 22,* 356-365.

Ehri, L.C. (1992). Reconceptualizing the development of sight word reading and its relationship to recoding. In P. Gough, L. Ehri, & R. Treiman (Eds.), *Reading Acquisition* (pp. 107-144). Hillsdale, NJ: Erlbaum.

Felton, R.H., & Wood, F.B. (1992). A reading level match study of nonword reading skills in poor readers with varying IQ. *Journal of Learning Disabilities, 25,* 318-326.

Freebody, P., & Byrne, B. (1988). Word-reading strategies in elementary school children: Relations to comprehension, reading time, and phonemic awareness. *Reading Research Quarterly, 23,* 441-453.

French, J.W., Ekstrom, R.G., & Price, L.A. (1963). *Manual for a kit of reference tests for cognitive factors.* Princeton, NJ: Educational testing service.

Gillis, J.J. (1993). Comorbidity of reading and mathematics disabilities: Genetic and environmental etiologies. Doctoral Dissertation, Department of Psychology, University of Colorado.

Goswami, U., & Bryant, P. (1990). *Phonological Skills and Learning to Read.* Hove, England: Lawrence Erlbaum.

Gough, P.B., Juel, C., & Griffith, P.L. (1992). Reading, spelling, and the orthographic cipher. In P. Gough, L. Ehri, & R. Treiman (Eds.), *Reading Acquisition.* Hillsdale, NJ: Erlbaum. Pp. 35-48.

Goulandris, N., & Snowling, M. (1991). Visual memory deficits: A plausible cause of developmental dyslexia? Evidence from a single case study. *Cognitive Neuropsychology, 8,* 127-154.

Hallgren, B. (1950). Specific dyslexia: A clinical and genetic study. *Acta Psychiatrica et Neurologica Scandinavica, 65,* (Suppl.), 1-287.

Hulme, C., Snowling, M., & Quinland, P. (1991). Connectionism and learning to read: steps towards a psychologically plausible model. *Reading and Writing, 4,* 19-31.

Jackson, N.E., & Butterfield, E.C. (1989). Reading-level-match designs: Myths and realities. *Journal of Reading Behavior, 21,* 387-412.

Jastak, J., & Jastak, S. (1978). *The wide range achievement test-revised*. Wilmington, DE: Jastak Associates.

Kaufman, A.S. (1975). Factor-analysis of the WISC-R at eleven age levels between 6 1/2 and 16 1/2 years. *Journal of Consulting and Clinical Psychology, 43*, 135-147.

Lennox, C., & Siegel, L.S. (Submitted). The development of phonological rules and visual strategies in good and poor spellers.

Liberman, I., Shankweiler, D., & Liberman A. (1989). The alphabetic principle and learning to read. In D. Shankweiler & I. Liberman (Eds.), *Phonology and reading disability: Solving the reading puzzle* (pp. 1-33). Ann Arbor, MI: University of Michigan Press.

Lie, A. (1991). Effects of a training program for stimulating skills in word analysis in first-grade children. *Reading Research Quarterly, 26*, 234-250.

Lindamood, C.H., & Lindamood, P.C. (1979). *Lindamood auditory conceptualization test*. Hingham, MA: Teaching Resources Corporation.

Lundberg, I. Frost, J., & Peterson, O. (1988). Effects of an extensive program for stimulating phonological awareness in preschool children. *Reading Research Quarterly, 23*, 263-284.

Manis, F.R. (1993). Personal communication.

Manis, F.R. (1993). *A longitudinal study of print exposure, phonological skill and orthographic skill in normal and disabled readers*. Paper presented at the SRCD Convention, New Orleans, March, 1993.

Manis, F.R., Custodio, R., & Szeszulski, P.A. (1993). Development of Phonological and Orthographic Skills: A two-year longitudinal study of dyslexic children. *Journal of Experimental Child Psychology, 56*, 64-86.

Manis, F.R., Szeszulski, P.A., Holt, L.K., & Graves, K. (1990). Variation in component word recognition and spelling skills among dyslexic children and normal readers. In T. Carr & B.A. Levy (Eds.), *Reading and its development: Component skills approaches* (pp. 207-259. New York: Academic Press.

Mitterer, J.O. (1982). There are at least two kinds of poor readers: Whole word poor readers and recoding poor readers. *Canadian Journal of Psychology, 36*, 445-461.

Morais, J. (1991). Phonological awareness: A bridge between language and literacy. In D Sawyer & B. Fox (Eds.), *Phonological awareness in reading: The evolution of current perspectives* (pp. 31-71). New York: Springer-Verlag.

Morton, J. (1969). The interaction of information in word recognition. *Psychological Review, 76*, 165-178.

Olson, R., Forsberg, H., Wise, B., & Rack, J. (1994). Measurement of word recognition, orthographic, and phonological skills. In G.R. Lyon (Ed.) *Frames of reference for the assessment of learning disabilities: New views on measurement issues* (pp. 243-277). Baltimore: Paul H. Brookes Publishing Co.

Olson, R. K., Kliegl, R., Davidson, B.J., & Foltz, G. (1985). Individual and developmental differences in reading disability. In G.E. MacKinnon and T.G. Waller (Eds.), *Reading research: Advances in theory and practice, Vol. 4* (pp. 1-64). New York: Academic Press.

Olson, R.K. & Wise, B.W. (1992). Reading on the computer with orthographic and speech feedback: An overview of the Colorado Remedial Reading Project. *Reading and Writing: An Interdisciplinary Journal, 4*, 107-144.

Olson, R.K., Wise, B., Conners, F., & Rack, J. (1990). Organization, heritability, and remediation of component word recognition and language skills in disabled readers. In T.H. Carr and B.A. Levy (Eds.), *Reading and its development: Component skills approaches* (pp. 261-322). New York: Academic Press.

Olson, R.K., Wise, B., Conners, F., Rack, J., & Fulker, D. (1989). Specific deficits in component reading and language skills: Genetic and environmental influences. *Journal of Learning Disabilities, 22*, 339-348.

Patterson, K.E., Marshal, J.C., & Coltheart, V. (1985). *Surface dyslexia: Neuropsychological and cognitive studies of phonological reading*. Hillsdale, NJ: Lawrence Erlbaum Associates.

Pennington, B.F., Gilger, J., Olson, R.K., & DeFries, J.C. (1992). The external validity of age- versus IQ-discrepancy definitions of reading disability: Lessons from a twin study. *Journal of Learning Disabilities*, *25*, 562-573.

Pennington, B.F., McCabe, L.L., Smith, S., Lefly, D., Bookman, M., Kimberling, W., & Lubs, H. (1986). *Child Development, 57*, 1001-1013.

Pennington, B.F., Van Orden, G.C., Smith, S.D., Green, P.A., & Haith, M.M. (1990). Phonological processing skills and deficits in adult dyslexics. *Child Development, 61*, 1753-1778.

Perfetti, C.A. (1985). *Reading Ability*. New York: Oxford University Press.

Perfetti, C.A. (1992). The representation problem in reading acquisition. In P. Gough, L. Ehri, & R. Treiman (Eds.), *Reading Acquisition* (pp. 145-174). Hillsdale, NJ: Erlbaum.

Perfetti, C.A., & Bell, L. (1991). Phonemic activation during the first 40 ms. of word identification: Evidence from backward masking and masked priming. *Journal of Memory and Language, 30*, 473-485.

Plaut, D.C., & McClelland, J.L. (1993). Generalization with componential attractors: Word and nonword reading in an attractor network. In *Proceedings of the 15th annual conference of the Cognitive Science Society*. Hillsdale, NJ: Erlbaum.

Plomin, R., & Bergeman, C.S. (1991). The nature of nurture: Genetic influences on environmental measures. *Behavioral and Brain Sciences, 14*, 373-427.

Plomin, R., DeFries, J.C., & McClearn, G.E. (1990). *Behavior Genetics: A Primer.* San Francisco: W.H. Freeman and Company.

Rack, J.P., Snowling, M.J., & Olson, R.K. (1992). The nonword reading deficit in developmental dyslexia: a review. *Reading Research Quarterly*, 27(1), 28-53.

Rosner, J., & Simon, D. (1971). The Auditory Analysis Test: An initial report. *Journal of Learning Disabilities, 4*, 384-392.

Rumsey, J.M. (1993). Personal Communication.

Schonell, F.J., & Schonell, P.E. (1960). *Diagnostic and attainment testing*. Edinburgh: Oliver and Boyd.

Seidenberg, M.S. (1992). Dyslexia in a computational model of word recognition. In P. Gough, L. Ehri, & R. Treiman (Eds.), *Reading Acquisition*. Hillsdale, NJ: Erlbaum. Pp. 35-48.

Seidenberg, M.S., & McClelland, J.L. (1989). A distributed, developmental model of word recognition and naming. *Psychological Review, 96*, 523-568.

Seymour, P.H.K. (1986). *Cognitive analysis of dyslexia*, London: Routledge & Kegan Paul.

Seymour, P.H.K., & Evans, H.M. (1993). The visual (orthographic) processor and developmental dyslexia. In D.M. Willows, R.S. Kruk, & E. Corcos (Eds.). *Visual Processes in Reading and Reading Disabilities*. Hillsdale, NJ: Lawrence Erlbaum Associates. pp. 347-376.

Siegel, L.S. (1988). Evidence that IQ scores are irrelevant to the definition and analysis of reading disability. *Canadian Journal of Psychology, 42*, 201-215.

Siegel, L.S. (1992). An evaluation of the discrepancy definition of dyslexia. *Journal of Learning Disabilities, 25*, 618-629.

Siegel, L.S., Geva, E., & Share, D. (1993). The development of orthographic skills in normal and disabled readers. Unpublished manuscript.

Smith, S.D., Kimberling, W.J., & Pennington, B.F. (1991). Screening for multiple genes influencing dyslexia. *Reading and Writing: An Interdisciplinary Journal, 3,* 285-298.

Stanovich, K.E. (1986). Cognitive processes and the reading problems of learning disabled children: Evaluating the assumption of specificity. In J.K. Torgesen & B.Y.L. Wong (Eds.), *Psychological and educational perspectives on learning disabilities.* Orlando, FL: Academic Press.

Stanovich, K.E. (1988). Explaining the differences between the dyslexic and garden variety poor reader: The phonological-core variable difference model. *Journal of Learning Disabilities, 21,* 590-612.

Stanovich, K.E. & Siegel, L.S. (1994). The phenotypic performance profile of reading-disabled children: A regression-based test of the phonological-core variable-difference model. *Journal of Educational Psychology, 86,* 24-53.

Stanovich, K.E., & West, R.F. (1989). Exposure to print and orthographic processing. *Reading Research Quarterly, 24,* 402-433.

Stevenson, J. (1991). Which aspects of processing text mediate genetic effects? *Reading and Writing: An Interdisciplinary Journal, 3,* 249-269.

Stevenson, J., Graham, P., Fredman, G., & McLoughlin, V. (1987). A twin study of genetic influences on reading and spelling ability and disability. *Journal of Child Psychology and Psychiatry, 28,* 229-247.

Stevenson, J., Pennington, B.F., Gilger, J.W., DeFries, J.C., & Gillis, J.J. (in press). ADHD and spelling disability: Testing for shared genetic aetiology. *Journal of Child Psychology and Psychiatry.*

Stuart, M., & Coltheart, M. (1988). Does reading develop in a sequence of stages? *Cognition, 30,* 139-181.

Tallal, P., (1984). Temporal or phonetic processing deficit in dyslexia? That is the question. *Applied Psycholinguistics, 5,* 167-169.

Thompson, J.S., & Thompson, M.W. (1986). *Genetics in medicine.* Philadelphia, PA: Saunders.

Treiman, R. (1984). Individual differences among normal children in reading and spelling styles. *Journal of Experimental Child Psychology, 37,* 463-477.

Van Orden, G.C. (1987). A ROWS is a ROSE: Spelling, sound, and reading. *Memory and Cognition, 15,* 181-198.

Van Orden, G.C., Pennington, B.F., & Stone, G.O. (1990). Word identification in reading and the promise of subsymbolic psycholinguistics. *Psychological Review, 97,* 488-522.

Vellutino, F., & Scanlon, D. (1987). Phonological coding, phonological awareness and reading ability: Evidence from a longitudinal and experimental study. *Merril-Palmer Quarterly, 33,* 321-363.

Wagner, R.K., Torgesen, J.K., & Rashotte, C.A. (1994). The development of reading related phonological processing abilities: New evidence of bi-directional causality from a latent variable longitudinal study. *Developmental Psychology, 30,* 73-87.

Wise, B.W., Olson, R.K., & Lindamood, P. (1993). *Training Phonemic Awareness: Evidence Relating to Why and How It Could Be Done.* Paper presented to the American Educational Research Association. Atlanta, April 12, 1993.

Address correspondence to:

Richard K. Olson
Department of Psychology, Box 345
University of Colorado at Boulder
Boulder, CO 80309
U.S.A.

NANCY EWALD JACKSON, WEN-HUI LU, & DAUSHEN JU[a]

READING CHINESE AND READING ENGLISH: SIMILARITIES, DIFFERENCES, AND SECOND-LANGUAGE READING

1. INTRODUCTION

Any theory of the relation of reading processes to orthography must be able to account for the reading of Chinese, an orthography used by more people than any other in the world (Hoosain, 1991). Because Chinese orthography differs radically from the alphabetic systems on which most of our conclusions about the cognitive psychology of literacy have been based, the study of Chinese provides opportunities to test the extent to which universal characteristics of the human mind constrain the way any written language is processed and to identify ways in which readers may have adapted their processing to variations in the language they read. Answers to these fundamental questions are beginning to emerge as more scholars who are fluent in Chinese become involved in literacy research.[1]

Our goal in the present chapter is to summarize and integrate the recent literature on reading Chinese, including a few of our own studies. We have tried to provide a balanced perspective on a literature in which controversy abounds. We begin with a brief description of characteristics of Chinese orthography that seem especially relevant for understanding its processing. We then contrast that processing with the processing of English words and text, describe some aspects of the development of Chinese literacy,[2] and consider how learning to read Chinese as a first orthography might influence a bilingual person's reading of an alphabetic language.

[a]*The second and third authors are Taiwanese and native readers of Chinese. Two of the original studies reported here were supported by grants to the first author from the Iowa Measurement Research Foundation.*

V.W. Berninger (ed.), The varieties of orthographic knowledge I: Theoretical and developmental issues, 73-109.

2. THE CHINESE WRITING SYSTEM

2.1 *Character Construction*

The Chinese writing system usually is described as logographic, that is, as a system in which each graphic symbol represents a word (e.g., Carr, 1986). This description fits classical Chinese better than it does the modern writing system, which might better be described as morphosyllabic (Haynes & Carr, 1990; Hoosain, 1991), because a character generally represents a morpheme and a syllable. Chinese contains a great many homophones, so a character often conveys more precise information than a spoken syllable. A few characters retain pictographic elements, but these have diminished as the writing system has evolved over the centuries, and describing Chinese as a pictographic orthography would be inappropriate.

More than one system of characters exists. Classical Chinese remains in use in literature, and most educated readers of Chinese are familiar with this form of the language. Also, as in other orthographies, characters can be printed or written in several styles. However, the same character system is used to represent the various dialects of Chinese. The traditional character system still in use in Taiwan has been simplified into a variant now used in the People's Republic of China.

Each character occupies a square space. All characters are written with a combination of eight types of stroke, each of which is a straight or curved line, completed without stop, that has a habitual orientation (Wang, 1973). Each stroke has its own name. A character can contain from 1 up to 29 or more strokes, and the information packed within a small space can be very dense (Chen, 1992). The strokes are written in a fixed order and have a two-dimensional structure in which major component parts can be organized in any of several ways (Huang & Wang, 1992). Although the character as a whole almost always corresponds to a single syllable and morpheme, it may have component parts that, when they stand alone, have a different meaning or sound. These principles are illustrated in Figure 1.

In modern Chinese, most words comprise two characters, and, by some estimates, words can range up to six characters in length. However, the most frequently occurring words are single syllables represented by one character (Hoosain, 1991; Huang & Wang, 1992). Most cognitive psychological research on Chinese word identification processes has focused on single characters.

Approximately 80-90% of characters are semantic-phonetic compounds (Hoosain, 1991). One part of a compound character, called the semantic radical,[3] suggests something about its literal or metaphoric meaning. For example, characters containing the semantic radical that means *tree* when it stands alone have meanings that are somehow related to the concept *tree* or *wood*, such as names for parts of a tree or for things that grow on trees or are made from wood. Most semantic radicals have a customary position within the square character space, frequently on the left (Flores d'Arcais, 1992), which may facilitate their identification. Huang and Wang (1992) report that there are 214 possible semantic radicals, and Perfetti, Zhang, and Berent (1992) give an estimate of 188. The difference between these two estimates may reflect differences between traditional and simplified characters.

The phonetic part of a semantic-phonetic compound character provides at least a hint linking pronunciation of the character to the approximately 400 syllables in the Chinese dialects (Taylor & Taylor, 1990). In about 25 percent of semantic-phonetic compounds, the phonetic radical gives the full pronunciation of the character (Hoosain, 1991), and it gives some guidance in about 39% of the compounds (Perfetti et al., 1992). As shown in Figure 1, a phonetic radical may occur alone with one meaning or in compound with various semantic radicals with diverse meanings. Whatever the context in which it occurs, a phonetic radical is likely to be pronounced similarly. When they do not indicate the full pronunciation of a character, phonetic radicals often signal the rime part of a character's sound. However, the pronunciation of some phonetic radicals is quite inconsistent from one character to another (Hue, 1992).

Because semantic and phonetic radicals have customary positions, pseudocharacters can be formed by creating novel combinations that preserve these habitual relations. Similarly, noncharacters can be formed by combining character elements in illegitimate ways. Researchers studying character identification (e.g., Cheng, 1992; Lu, 1992) have used pseudocharacters and noncharacters as stimuli, much as researchers studying alphabetic languages have used pronounceable pseudowords and illegitimate, unpronounceable, letter strings.

Characters Sharing a Phonetic Radical

Character	Pronunciation	Meaning
情	/ts.ɪ.əŋ/	feeling
請	/ts.ɪ.əŋ/	invitation
精	/dʒ.ɪ.əŋ/	essence, good at
倩	/ts.en/	beautiful

Homophone Characters with Different Phonetic Radicals

Character	Pronunciation	Meaning
鮭	/g.u.e/	salmon
規	/g.u.e/	rule
鬼	/g.u.e/	ghost
貴	/g.u.e/	expensive

Characters Sharing a Semantic Radical

Character	Pronunciation	Meaning
洗	/s.ɪ/	wash
海	/h.aɪ/	sea
河	/h.ɚ/	river
池	/č/	pond, pool

Figure 1 Examples of similarities and differences in meanings and pronunciations of semantic-phonetic compound characters with shared and distinct elements. All pronunciations are given in Mandarin.

2.2 *Multi-Character Words*

About 65% of the words in modern Chinese are composed of two characters and two syllables (Huang & Wang, 1992). In some two-character words, each character is of equal importance in determining the word's meaning; in others, one character is the main morpheme and the other provides modifying or supplementary meaning (Zhang & Peng, 1992). The relation between the meaning of a two-character word and the meanings of its components may be obscure.

Word boundaries are not marked in Chinese text. Also, like single characters, multi-character words generally are not marked with lexical category or inflection (Chen, 1992). There is no analog in Chinese to the English system whereby a word ending in *-tion* can be recognized as a noun or a word ending in *-ed* as a past-tense verb. However, there are some characters that change the form class of preceding characters. For example, one character turns a preceding noun, such as *beauty*, into an adjective, such as *beautiful*.

2.3 *Text Structure*

Characters in text can be ordered either from left to right or from top to bottom, and different arrangements may be used within a single document. Right-to-left order also is used on occasion for headlines and logos. The ends of clauses and sentences in modern Chinese are marked by punctuation marks borrowed from Roman script. Word order provides important information for interpreting a sentence (Chang, 1992), but the relation of word order within sentences to syntax is complex (Chen, 1992).

3. HOW CHINESE CHARACTERS ARE READ

3.1 *Efficiency*

Skilled readers can identify the meaning of Chinese characters very rapidly (Hoosain, 1991), possibly because characters elicit meaning more automatically or unavoidably than English words do (Carr, 1986). Factors determining the speed with which an individual character can be identified include frequency of usage (e.g., Hue, 1992; Seidenberg, 1985; Zhang & Peng, 1992), which is inversely associated with number of strokes (Hoosain, 1991), and the extent to which a character's pronunciation is predictable from its phonetic radical (Hue, 1992). These factors interact, so that effects of predictable pronunciation are not observed among high-frequency characters (Hue, 1992).

3.2 Left Or Right Hemisphere Processing?

The processing of alphabetic orthographies, like the processing of oral languages, typically is concentrated in the left hemisphere, which is consistent with interpretation of the reading of alphabetic text as a task that draws heavily on rapid sequential phonological processing. In contrast, many studies of character recognition have been motivated by the interpretation of characters as pictographs or logographs that should be processed in the right hemisphere (Carr, 1986). The literature includes experimental comparisons of responses to characters and two-character words presented to the right visual field (RVF), which is served by the left hemisphere (LH), and to the left visual field (LVF) served by the right hemisphere (RH). It also includes studies of aphasia and acquired dyslexia in patients who have suffered localized brain damage.

A substantial clinical case literature indicates that, for readers of Chinese, just as for readers of alphabetic languages, lesions in the LH (of right-handed patients) are far more likely than RH lesions to be associated with acquired dyslexia (Hoosain, 1991; Yin & Butterworth, 1992). For example, Yin and Butterworth (1992) describe 11 right-handed acquired dyslexia cases whose brain damage was documented by CT scans and other imaging techniques. One patient was a 12-year-old boy, but the remainder were adults, most over 50 years of age. Only the child had RH damage. Hoosain's (1991) summary of earlier case studies of aphasic patients also supports the broad conclusion that language functions, including reading and writing, are lateralized in speakers and readers of Chinese much as they are in readers of alphabetic languages. The clinical literature does raise the possibility that the localization of processing within the left hemisphere may be somewhat different for Chinese and alphabetic orthographies, with lesions in the parietal-occipital cortex more likely to occur in Chinese dyslexics (Hoosain, 1991; Yin & Butterworth, 1992).

The experimental literature is less clear-cut, and the conclusions one draws from it about the lateralization of character processing seem to be associated with stimulus and task characteristics. Hoosain (1991) has reviewed a number of studies in which the processing of two-character Chinese words, like the processing of English words and letters, was more efficient if the stimuli were presented to the RVF. The processing of single characters sometimes shows a similar RVF/LH advantage, but a number of investigators have found a LVF/RH advantage, or no advantage, for these stimuli.

Hoosain (1991) suggests that perceptual factors may be more important than orthographic/linguistic ones in producing the single-character results. Studies showing a LVF/RH advantage for single character identification often have a combination of task features, such as very short exposure times and low luminance, that create a degraded visual signal better suited to RH processing. These results remain ambiguous, but the bulk of the experimental and clinical evidence does suggest that reading Chinese, like reading an alphabetic language, is an activity dominated by LH functioning.

3.3 *Character Recognition*

3.3.1 Strokes and Sequences in Character Processing. To individuals accustomed to alphabetic scripts and unfamiliar with Chinese, each character appears to be a much more integrated whole than, say, an English word. The square shape is constant; the pattern of strokes within that shape may be very dense; and there is no dominant unidimensional order such as the left-to-right string pattern of words written in English. However, there is structure, and the potential for sequential processing, within a character. Recent research suggests that for Chinese, within-character scanning patterns are likely to be multi-dimensional and related to the various possible two-dimensional within-character configurations (Huang & Wang, 1992).

In reading a Chinese character, as in reading an English word (Healy, Conboy, & Drewnowski, 1987), skilled readers may process information at various levels simultaneously and identify the whole unit before completing processing of its components (Huang & Wang, 1992). However, readers of Chinese are aware of, and can use if necessary, sequential information that is apparent to them in a character's stroke pattern. Recall that the strokes in a character are produced in a standard order when written by hand. Writing characters is emphasized in teaching Chinese, so this order has been well learned by all skilled readers. Huang and Wang (1992) occasionally observed subjects mimicking the stroke-writing order with hand movements as they struggled to recognize some briefly presented characters.

Individual strokes are not the only subcharacter units that may receive attention during character identification. In the very common semantic-phonetic compound characters, the independent meanings and sounds of the two components, which may be different from their composite meaning and sound, are recognized (Flores d'Arcais, 1992; Cheng, 1992). Unfamiliar characters are identified more rapidly if they contain a phonetic radical that indicates their pronunciation (Seidenberg, 1985).

3.3.2 Orthographic, Phonological, and Semantic Activation. Cognitive psychological studies of the roles of orthographic, phonological, and semantic information in character identification have drawn on several classical experimental techniques. In most of these studies, the independent variable has been the relation between two characters (or pseudocharacters) paired so as to have meaning, sound, or orthographic characteristics either the same or different. The dependent variable typically is accuracy or latency to pronounce or make a lexical decision about one of the characters, but also has been latency to make a judgment about whether a pair of characters have the same meaning or pronunciation (Perfetti & Zhang, 1992).

In priming studies (e.g., Cheng, 1992; Perfetti & Zhang, 1991), the question is whether information activated during presentation of a priming character reinforces or interferes with information in a target character. If, for example, phonological information from the prime has been activated, that information should facilitate identification of a briefly presented target character that has the same sound. Similarly, in backward masking studies, a mask presented immediately after a briefly presented target character should interfere less with the target's identification if information common across the two characters has been activated during the very brief exposure of the mask. Perfetti et al. (1992) discuss some of the strengths and limits of these techniques.

One view of character recognition (e.g. Smith, 1985) is that characters are identified by direct linkage of orthographic with semantic information. This view is most compatible with a traditional dual-route model of the identification of words in alphabetic orthographies, in which irregularly spelled words are identified by direct access to a lexicon (Coltheart, 1978).

Early studies of the roles of orthographic and phonological information in character identification did not directly challenge this view, but they did confirm that phonological activation has occurred by some time soon after a character has been recognized (Seidenberg, 1985). This activation is important, because it provides phonological codes that can be used, in any orthography, for recall and integration of information in working memory during text comprehension (Tzeng, Hung, & Wang, 1977; Tzeng & Hung, 1980), and for the integration of multi-part words (Hue, 1992). However, recent research suggests that phonological information plays a role in character identification as well as in recall.

Much of the recent research has been guided by the principles that (1) "across writing systems, encounters with most printed words ... automatically lead to phonological activation, beginning with phoneme constituents of the word and including the word's pronunciation"; (2) "writing systems constrain the extent to which this activation includes sublexical phonology, but not whether activation occurs"; and (3) "activated phonology serves memory and comprehension, with phonological rehearsal but not the activation itself under reader control" (Perfetti et al., 1992, p. 231).

Backward masking studies have indicated that both graphemic and phonological information are available very early in the process of identifying a written English word, before the word's meaning is available (Perfetti, Bell, & Delany, 1988). Although the graphic information available in a character cannot be described as consisting of a set of graphemes, early activation of graphic information also would be expected in character identification, and such activation has been found in both backward masking and priming studies (Ju, 1992; Perfetti & Zhang, 1991). For example, when a target character and a subsequently presented mask share strokes, the extent to which the mask interferes with identification of the target is reduced. Although this graphic overlap is in visually presented information, it is not overlap at the level of the physical signals. Just as upper and lower-case letters are typically used to differentiate the members of target-mask or target-prime pairs in English word identification studies, different styles of print have been used in studies of character identification. Therefore, the graphic effects must be due to the perception of the shared strokes as orthographic patterns.

Because characters cannot be sounded out letter by letter, sublexical phonological information would not be expected to be available as early in the identification of characters as it is in identification of English words (Perfetti et al., 1988). Indeed, in backward masking studies of character identification processes, activation of graphic information has been detected well before activation of phonological information (Ju, 1992; Perfetti & Zhang, 1991). When a briefly presented target character and a subsequent briefly presented mask share the same pronunciation, the overlap in phonological information does not reduce interference with identification of the target. This finding holds both when the target and mask are identical only in pronunciation (Perfetti & Zhang, 1991; Ju, 1992) and when phonological information shared between target and mask could, if available, be used to increase the effect of shared graphic information (Ju, 1992).

In a priming study, Perfetti and Zhang (1991) found that phonological information has become available immediately at identification of a character. In subsequent research, these and other investigators demonstrated that phonological activation occurs automatically, even when the dependent variable is not naming and when phonological information actually interferes with the required response. Cheng (1992) found that phonological similarity between a prime and target character influenced the latency of a lexical decision about the target, even when the interval between onset of the prime and onset of the real or pseudocharacter target was only 50 ms. Similarly, Perfetti and Zhang (1992) found that phonological similarity between two characters made it more difficult for readers to judge that two words were not synonyms. Interference in the latter study occurred when the interval between onset of the first and second characters was only 90 ms. Phonological interference appeared at shorter presentation intervals than semantic interference.

Results have been consistent across the studies reviewed above in indicating that graphic information is available relatively early in the identification of characters and that semantic information is not available until relatively late, either at about the same time as, or after, phonological information is available. Because findings have varied across experimental tasks, the exact time at which phonological information becomes available during the process of character identification remains unspecified. Indeed, the variation in findings across studies may suggest that the availability of phonological information increases gradually. Some phonological information may be available to skilled readers as soon as 50 ms after the onset of character presentation, and this information may even be described as mediating, rather than accompanying, a connection between the character and its meaning (Cheng, 1992; Flores d'Arcais, 1992).

3.4 *Multi-Character Word Identification*

To adult readers of an alphabetic language, the concept *word* is familiar and clear-cut. Although a single English word may contain more than one morpheme (e.g., *walk/ed, child/ren*), its boundaries are clearly marked in the orthography and an understanding of the concept develops as young children are exposed to print (Roberts, 1992). The word is the fundamental unit in a literate English speaker's mental lexicon as well as in English dictionaries. The meaning and role of *word* is less clear-cut in Chinese, which is consistent with the lack of marking of boundaries between multi-character words in Chinese text.

Hoosain (1992) asked 14 native speakers of Cantonese, all undergraduates at the University of Hong Kong and bilingual in English, to segment nine sentences by drawing slashes between words. The subjects differed from one another and from the author of the sentences on many word boundaries. Hoosain suggests that this uncertainty reflects the history and structure of the Chinese language: individual morphemes (characters) that functioned independently in classical Chinese have become bound in bisyllabic words, and whether a character can stand alone varies across dialects and contexts.

As one might expect in a language in which words are not the clearly dominant unit, the constituent characters in a multi-character Chinese word "have a life of their own" (Hoosain, 1992, p. 120). The word as a unit does have some psychological reality in Chinese, as it does in English. In both languages, component parts (letters or characters) are generally perceived more easily if they are presented as parts of real words rather than in a nonsense string. This is the classic word superiority effect. However, for readers of Chinese, the effect can disappear under some circumstances (Hoosain, 1992).

Other evidence also suggests that component characters

within multi-character words can be accessed from a mental lexicon (Hoosain, 1991). In a lexical decision task in which university students were asked to decide whether a two-character stimulus was a word, reaction times and accuracy sometimes varied with characteristics of the component characters as well as of the composite words. This effect was dependent upon the position of the component character and the nature of the relation between the components (Zhang & Peng, 1992).

Because multi-character Chinese words arouse associations both as wholes and from the meanings of their components, associative responses may be more varied than for English words, and the associations given to a word presented orally may be different from those to a written word (Hoosain, 1991). Hoosain (1991) suggests that Chinese words might be more likely than English words to remembered in terms of a visual code rather than, or in addition to, a phonological code.

3.5 Text Comprehension

Most Western researchers, intrigued by the obvious differences between Chinese characters and alphabetic text, have formulated hypotheses about cross-linguistic differences in reading processes at the level of character or word recognition. However, a few recent studies of Chinese text reading suggest important cross-linguistic similarities and differences at this level as well.

In discussing the role of phonological information in character recognition (section 3.3.2), we cited studies of readers of English which have demonstrated that phonological representations of words are automatically activated and used in text reading. A key finding in this literature is McCutchen and Perfetti's (1982) demonstration of a tongue-twister effect in the silent reading of English. Silent reading is slowed when stories contain sentences with repeated word-initial phonemes. Recently, Zhang and Perfetti (in press) have shown that this same tongue-twister effect occurs when native speakers of Mandarin read stories written in Chinese. They found that this effect occurred in both oral and silent reading and that it was evident in reading times, articulation errors, and written recall errors. Furthermore, the materials permitted measurement of phonological interference completely independent of graphic interference, which enabled Zhang and Perfetti to evaluate their subjects' relative use of graphic and phonological codes in their recall. The errors made in written free recall of the texts were much more likely to be homophonic than graphic. Thus, this study does not support Hoosain's (1991) suggestion that Chinese words are likely to be remembered in a graphic code.

The reading of Chinese text does differ in at least some ways from the reading of English. Some key differences are more directly related to the syntax and semantics of Chinese than to its orthography. Because inflection is almost nonexistent, word order has been regarded as an important device for interpreting Chinese sentences (Chang, 1992). However, Chen (1992) and Li, Bates, Liu, and MacWhinney (1992) suggest that word order often does not give the reader information sufficient for sentence comprehension, which is a context-dependent process.

The interpretation of the comprehension of Chinese text as a highly integrative process is consistent with the results of a study reported by Chen (1992) in which native Chinese-speaking Hong Kong undergraduates read passages presented on a computer screen with a moving window that revealed a single character at a time. Subjects controlled the pace at which they moved the window along the text, and the question of interest was the extent to which various attributes of a character contributed to the time spent viewing it. Some of these attributes were intrinsic to the character itself, such as its visual complexity or frequency; others were attributes of the word or text of which the character was a part, including the character's position in a sentence or clause, whether the present character was part of a noun introducing an argument new to the reader and whether it was one of a number of such new argument nouns in the sentence, the character's position in the text as a whole, and its position in the visual layout of the text on the screen.

When the students in Chen's study read a passage in order to prepare to answer comprehension questions, mean reading speed was very fast (397 ms per character) and relatively little of the variance in exposure time across characters could be accounted for. The only variables that contributed to how long a character was viewed were those related to its status as a new argument noun and whether the character appeared at the end of a line on the screen. When the students read in anticipation of being asked to recall the passage verbatim, average reading speed (859 ms per character) and allocation of attention across characters changed. In that condition, more attention was paid to words at the end of clauses and sentences, and word and character features were more important.

In general, these results suggest that the word-level predictors that are major contributors to reading times for English text are less important sources of variance in the time allocated to processing Chinese text. Instead, readers of Chinese tend to pause at physical or syntactic boundaries, perhaps to integrate what they have read so far. Indeed, Chen (1992) also found that, when reading an English text that contained a lexical, syntactic, or semantic violation, readers of English were likely to pause at the point of the violation. In contrast, readers of Chinese did not pause at any particular position before or after encountering a syntactic or semantic violation. They did show a modest disruption two words after the introduction of a lexical violation.

4. LEARNING TO READ CHINESE

4.1 *Correlates Of Children's Success In Learning To Read Chinese*

Hoosain (1991) reviews a number of studies in which Chinese children and adults have been found to be generally strong on tests of visual-spatial perception and reasoning, a pattern that could be attributed to practice in reading Chinese. He also reports some findings suggesting a relation between individual differences in reading success and performance on several different visual-spatial measures. However, not all investigators have found a special pattern of association between visual-spatial task performance and children's success in learning to read Chinese.

The most extensive studies of children's acquisition of Chinese have been conducted in Taipei, Taiwan by Stevenson and his colleagues (Stevenson, Stigler, Lucker, Lee, Hsu, & Kitamura,1982; Stevenson, Stigler, Lee, & Lucker, 1985). In two studies, children's reading achievement was measured with an individually administered test that yields scores for sight reading of vocabulary, oral reading of meaningful text, and comprehension of text.

In their 1982 study, Stevenson et al. compared the reading achievement of fifth graders in Taipei; Minneapolis; and Sendai, Japan. They concluded that there was no relation between orthography and incidence of specific reading disability. However, the Taiwanese children were more likely than the

Americans to have difficulty with the comprehension of text and less likely to have difficulty pronouncing individual words. Stevenson et al.'s results also suggest that reading disability among Chinese children is more likely than English reading disability to be part of a pervasive learning problem that includes mathematics achievement. Furthermore, within the subgroups of poor readers in Taiwan and Japan, those whose scores were lowest also performed less well on a test in which they were asked to draw a spatial array by following verbal instructions.

In their 1985 study of Taipei first and fifth graders, Stevenson et al. found that the cognitive abilities associated with reading achievement were similar in Taiwan, Japan, and the United States. In all three countries, a general information test score was among the strongest correlates of reading achievement at both grade levels. Among first graders in all of the countries, scores on a visual-spatial representation test also contributed to variance in achievement. However, the regression equations for the Taiwan and United States' samples were different in several ways.

Among the fifth graders in Stevenson et al.'s (1985) study, the set of ten cognitive test scores accounted for substantially less variance in the Taiwanese children's achievement than in the achievement of the American or Japanese children. Also, among the Taiwanese first graders, scores on a test of serial memory for digits and a test of recall of an orally presented story also contributed to the regression equation. The story recall test retained its predictive power in the fifth-grade Taiwanese sample. In contrast, an auditory memory test in which children were asked to reproduce sequences of pencil taps separated by short or long intervals predicted reading achievement only among the American children at both grade levels.

The Taiwanese children generally performed well above the other groups on the digit recall test but less well than the Japanese and American children on the tapping series recall. On the story recall task, the Taiwanese first graders earned scores at about the same level as the Japanese children, but lower than the American children. At fifth grade, the Taiwanese group performed at the same level as the Americans and above the level of the Japanese on story recall. These results are difficult to interpret because of the possibility that the scores were not valid indicators of the constructs they were assumed to measure, particularly when considered across cultures. However, Stevenson et al.'s (1985) findings do raise the possibility that different kinds of memory for sequential auditory information may be involved in the reading of Chinese and alphabetic languages.

As a whole, the results of studies of individual differences in children's reading achievement are tantalizing but do not permit firm conclusions about the kinds of cognitive skills or processes involved in learning to read Chinese. One possible, tentative synthesis is that visual-spatial processing is more likely to be associated with severe developmental disability in reading Chinese than in reading English. Difficulty in some aspect of auditory-sequential memory may be a more common source of difficulty in learning both orthographies. However, when children learning to read Chinese have difficulty with auditory-sequential memory, that difficulty may be more manifest in text comprehension than in word identification.

4.2 Taiwanese Children's Understanding Of Character Construction

Much less is known about how literacy in Chinese is acquired than about the process of character identification by skilled readers. Although children learning to read Chinese do not have to abstract and apply the grapheme-phoneme correspondence principles that underly the reading and writing of an alphabetic language, they do have to master principles of character construction that permit identification of a visual pattern as a potentially legitimate character. They also must be able to apply their understanding of character structure to learning new characters.

Lu (1992; Lu & Jackson, 1993) described the development of children's recognition and application of character construction principles in a cross-sectional study of 297 children selected from kindergarten to sixth grade classes in Taiwan. She administered four tests, all of which were highly reliable and showed performance increases with age. Performance on the tests was most consistently correlated with individual differences in reading achievement among the second graders.

Taiwanese children's ability to identify the correct orientation of a character developed in a sequence reminiscent of how children learn to recognize the correct orientation of letters in the English alphabet. The kindergartners, who, unlike the older children in this study, attended a private school, had not yet received formal instruction in reading characters. However, they would have had extensive exposure to environmental print, and may have been taught some characters by their parents. Therefore, like children learning to read English, they were expected to show some knowledge of how print in their language should look.

Even in kindergarten, children performed well above chance level on the character orientation test. By third grade, about half earned perfect scores on the 20-item, 5-alternative, multiple-choice test. Most of the errors children made were in accepting mirror-image reversals as correct characters, rather than in misidentifying upside-down characters (within which strokes would look wrong) or characters rotated 45 degrees.

Lu's second test required children to accept pseudocharacters, in which the semantic and phonetic radicals were in their accustomed positions, as unfamiliar but legitimate characters and to reject noncharacters whose radicals were reversed. Children were expected to begin showing success on this 40-item test in second grade, when semantic-phonetic compound characters and the concept of the semantic radical are introduced. Most of the children's errors were incorrect acceptances of noncharacters. Kindergartners scored below chance on the noncharacter items, but, by third grade, children correctly identified more than 90 percent of the noncharacters as invalid. Age differences were not attributable to age changes in response bias.

Lu's third and fourth tests also focused on the structure of semantic-phonetic compound characters. The key to success on both of these tests was to use the principles for constructing semantic-phonetic compound characters to create an analogy (Goswami & Bryant, 1990) between a target pseudocharacter and another novel character. In the pronunciation transfer test, children were asked to identify which of a set of novel characters would be pronounced the same as a pseudocharacter whose pronunciation they were given. The correct choice was a novel character containing the same phonetic radical as the target. Among children above kindergarten level, the most common errors on these 4-alternative multiple choice items involved choosing the character sharing a semantic radical with the target. Accurate responses rose sharply from kindergarten until grade three and then leveled off at about 85–90 percent correct.

The final test in Lu's battery was a meaning transfer test in which children had to choose the response alternative that shared meaning with a pseudocharacter target. On this test, the most common error was to choose the response alternative that shared a phonetic, rather than a semantic, radical with the target. In general, performance was less accurate than it was on the pronunciation transfer test. The fourth grade results for the meaning transfer test were higher than those for any other grade. However, this group's data are suspect because one child in the class shouted out the correct principle for identifying the answer. Scores for kindergartners and first graders were very low; those for second and third graders at about 50 percent correct, and those for fifth and sixth graders about 70 percent correct.

Although the format of the meaning transfer test was the same as that of the pronunciation transfer test, it had been expected to be more difficult. Teachers in Taiwan emphasize pronunciation before meaning. Also, in most cases, the phonetic part of a character contains more strokes and is therefore a more salient base from which to draw an analogy. Yet another factor that might have made this task especially difficult is that analogic meaning relations across characters are less constrained than sound relations.

4.3 How Readers Of English Begin To Learn To Read Characters

Phonological information plays a role in the identification and recall of characters, but readers of Chinese do not have to match a string of graphemes with a string of phonemes. Therefore, reading-disabled English-speaking children, who often have difficulty with identification and manipulation of phoneme sequences (Olson, Wise, Conners, Rack, & Fulker, 1989) might be expected to have less trouble learning to read Chinese than English. This hypothesis led Rozin, Poritsky, and Sotsky (1971) to teach a small number of characters to reading-disabled American children. This study has been cited widely, but their successful demonstration provides little information about how characters are learned. The characters were associated with English words, apparently at random, and the report does not suggest that the children learned anything about the orthographic structure of characters.

In an attempt to determine whether specific aspects of English reading skill might be related to success in learning to read Chinese (Jackson, Ju, Lu, & Forte, 1992), we recently studied 24 American ninth graders whose English reading skills had been assessed with Form F of the Nelson-Denny Reading Test (Brown, Bennett, & Hanna, 1981) and four orthographic and phonological processing tasks that had been used in a number of previous studies (Olson et al., 1989). None of these students were disabled readers, and their mean Nelson-Denny score was above average for their grade level. They were taught a 24-word vocabulary of single-syllable Chinese words and then taught the characters for half of the words. The students learned to read the remaining 12 words represented in *zhuyin fuhao*, an alphabet-like, phonological symbol system used in beginning reading instruction in Taiwan. Unlike the *pinyin* system used in the People's Republic of China, *zhuyin fuhao* consists of symbols that bear no resemblance to the Roman alphabet. Therefore, we could contrast individual differences in the students' ability to learn to read characters with individual differences in their ability to read a novel alphabetic orthography.

The vocabulary words and their written forms are shown in Figure 2. All oral vocabulary and reading instruction was done as drill with no mention of meaning or sound relations among words.

We gave the students study time sufficient to bring their learning of the characters and *zhuyin fuhao* words to near ceiling. Our interest was in the extent to which they were able to identify the structure we had built into each set of words--semantic structure within the character set and phonological structure within the *zhuyin* set. For example, the character set in Figure 2 includes three *mouth* characters that mean *shout*, *cry*, and *eat*, and the set of *zhuyin fuhao* words contains three words that share an /u/ sound.

Abstraction of the meaning of the semantic radicals repeated within the character set was tested with a sorting and naming test. The students were given cards on which the characters they had learned were written and told, "There are some characters that go together. Put them in piles and tell me why you put them that way." If the student did not sort the cards perfectly according to their semantic radicals, additional prompts and opportunities to sort again were given. The students then were asked to "show...the parts in each character that you think are shared by other characters." Finally, they were asked to suggest meanings for the common parts. Performance was well below ceiling on both parts of the test.

English Meaning	Chinese Character	Pronunciation
Die	死	/s/
Hungry	餓	/ə/
Sun	日	/ž/
(The characters above are unrelated.)		
Tree	樹	/š,u/
Orange	桔	/z,yu/
Branch	枝	/j/
(The characters above share the *tree* radical 木.)		
Strawberry	莓	/m,e/
Vegetable	菜	/ts,ay/
Bean	荳	/d,o/
(The characters above share the *grass* radical 艹.)		
Shout	喊	/h,an/
Eat	吃	/č/
Cry	哭	/k,u/
(The characters above share the *mouth* radical 口.)		

English Meaning	Zhuyin Fuhao	Pronunciation
Ear	ㄦ	/r/
Father	ㄅㄚ	/b,a/
Fat	ㄆㄤ	/p,aŋ/
(The one- and two-symbol words above are unrelated.)		
Jump	ㄊㄧㄠ	/t,ɪ,æw/
Rock	ㄧㄠ	/ɪ,æw/
Bird	ㄋㄧㄠ	/n,ɪ,æw/
Cat	ㄇㄠ	/m,æw/
(The words above share the symbol ㄠ, pronounced /æw/.)		
Tail	ㄨㄟ	/u,e/
Turtle	ㄍㄨㄟ	/g,u,e/
Mosquito	ㄨㄣ	/u,n/
(The words above share the symbol x, pronounced /u/.)		
Bee	ㄈㄥ	/f,əŋ/
Fly	ㄧㄥ	/ɪ,əŋ/
(The words above share the symbol ㄥ, pronounced /əŋ/.)		

Figure 2.

English Chinese vocabulary taught orally and written either in characters or in *zhuyin fuhao*. Pronunciations were anglicized to make them easier for American students to learn. Because each *zhuyin* symbol may correspond to more than one English phoneme, pronunciations are written with the phonemes corresponding to each symbol separated by commas.

The sorting and naming scores, which correlated $r = .24$, were summed to yield a total score.

Ability to use the grapheme-phoneme correspondence rules that could be induced from the *zhuyin fuhao* word set was tested with a single-symbol and new-combination pronunciation test, hereafter called the new symbol test. In the first part of this test, the students were asked to pronounce in isolation the single *zhuyin fuhau's* that they had learned in two- or three-symbol words. In the second part of the test, students were asked to pronounce the symbols in novel two-symbol combinations. The two subtests correlated $r = .61$, and the 26-item test as a whole had an acceptable level of internal consistency (alpha = .81).

As one might expect from the difference in sound emphasis between the tests we used to assess mastery of the two orthographies, performance on a Chinese oral vocabulary pronunciation test administered just prior to reading instruction was correlated with performance on the new symbol test ($r = .41$)[4], but not with performance on the meaning oriented character sorting test ($r = .15$). Several measures of English reading were associated with the Chinese reading measures, but not always in the ways that we had predicted.

Reasonably enough, the best English word-reading predictor of performance on both Chinese reading tests was Nelson-Denny Vocabulary score ($r = .57$ for character sorting and $r = .48$ for the new symbol test). Accuracy in performance on one of the two English phonological processing tasks predicted performance on both the Chinese reading tests ($r = .40$ for character sorting and $r = .41$ for new symbols). We had not predicted this finding, but it is consistent with the research summarized in section 3.3.2 showing that phonological encoding does play a role in character identification and memory.

Interestingly, the phonological processing measure that correlated with Chinese reading was not our pseudoword pronunciation test. Instead, it was the test that assessed the students' ability to read three simple pseudowords and then decide which one, *as a whole*, sounded like a real English word. We had hypothesized that English orthographic processing might be associated with ability to learn characters. However, accuracy on the two English orthographic tasks was negatively associated with performance on the character sorting task.

As a whole, these results suggest that students who are better readers of an alphabetic language are also more likely to succeed at the short-term initial learning of a small foreign language vocabulary presented in either an alphabet-like or morphosyllabic orthography. Accuracy in making phonological judgments about English words also predicts the learning of both kinds of new orthography, which is consistent with Perfetti's conclusion that phonological coding is universally important in reading. However, these results also raise a possibility that is consistent with Rozin et al.'s conclusion and with more recent emphasis on the importance of phonemic awareness for learning alphabetic languages (e.g., Rack, Snowling, & Olson, 1992): learning the sound pattern of a new language may be less critical for understanding the structure of a morphosyllabic orthography than for mastering a new grapheme-phoneme correspondence system. The extent to which the results of this study would generalize to other populations and to more sustained instruction of larger reading vocabularies, in which students could learn to identify both semantic and phonetic radicals, merits investigation.

5. CHINESE READERS OF ENGLISH

The many dramatic differences between Chinese and English as orthographies and as oral languages have led a number of researchers, including ourselves, to ask whether any of the skills or strategies developed in becoming a fluent reader of Chinese might transfer to the reading of an alphabetic second language, such as English. This issue has been investigated in several studies of bilingual university students or scholars whose first language was Chinese.

5.1 English Text-Reading Speed

Native readers of Chinese who are students at American universities, including the second and third authors of this chapter, often report that they take an enormous amount of time to complete their English reading assignments, relative to the time used by their American counterparts. The results of several studies suggest that these anecdotal reports represent a consistent pattern.

Haynes and Carr (1990) compared the text-reading rates of 28 freshman and 32 senior science majors at a selective university in Taiwan with that of 15 American undergraduate volunteers from an introductory psychology class. The mean reading comprehension score of the Taiwanese seniors was about 0.7 *SD* below that of the Americans, and the freshmen's mean score was about 1.25 *SDs* below. However, the American-Taiwanese differences in reading rate for the same passages were much more extreme. The Taiwanese freshman read about 83 words per minute (wpm) and the seniors about 88 wpm. The seniors' mean rate was more than 4 *SDs* below the American students' mean of 254 wpm.

These results are consistent with the findings of a study of 25 Taiwanese graduate students, 17 women and 8 men, at The University of Iowa (Jackson, Ju, Lu, & Reitz, 1993). Fifteen of these students had arrived in the United States within two months of the test session, 9 had been in the United States for 1 to 4 years, and 1 had been in the United States for 12 years. The students were enrolled in graduate programs in 14 different departments. The mean age at which the students had begun instruction in reading English was 12 years, 10 months (range 104 to 248 months). As part of a larger study whose other results are described in section 5.2, these Taiwanese students were administered Form F of the Nelson-Denny Reading Test (Brown et al., 1981) in a group session under standard conditions. This test includes a Vocabulary subtest in which 100 multiple-choice items are presented within a time limit of 15 minutes, a highly speeded Comprehension test consisting of text passages followed by comprehension questions, and a self-reported reading rate score computed at the beginning of the Comprehension test.

The Taiwanese students' mean reading rate was 152 wpm (*SD* = 45 wpm), well below the 256 wpm (*SD* = 85 wpm) mean reading rate of 24 American ninth graders who served as a comparison group in this study.[5] The Taiwanese graduate students' slow reading rates appeared to have affected their performance on the Vocabulary and Comprehension subtests, on which most students left a great many items unanswered. The Taiwanese students' mean grade-equivalent scores of 9.6 (*SD* = 2.5) for the Vocabulary subtest and 10.2 (*SD* = 2.6) for the Comprehension subtest also were well below what one would expect for graduate students who were native readers of English, but they show less disadvantage than the measure of reading rate.

Are native readers of Chinese slower than other students who also are reading English as a second language and whose untimed comprehension levels are similar? The possibility that many differences between cultural/linguistic groups could create differential speed-accuracy tradeoff or other confounds make this question extremely difficult to answer. However, Haynes and Carr (1990) compared the English text-reading speed and comprehension of their Taiwanese undergraduates with the performance of Spanish ESL students in an earlier study (Henderson, 1983 in Haynes & Carr, 1990) who had read the same passages. The Taiwanese undergraduate group's comprehension scores approached those of Henderson's Spanish group, but their reading rates were much slower than the Spanish students' 110 wpm.

Haynes and Carr interpret the inefficient text reading of Chinese readers of English as a manifestation of difficulty in rapid processing of an unfamiliar orthography, dismissing other possibilities such as difficulty with English phonology or sentence structure. The evidence they use to support this interpretation is included in the following discussion of Chinese readers' word-processing strategies.

5.2 English Word-Reading Processes

Difficulty in reading words in a second language could be attributed to difficulty with the orthography, the phonology, or even the semantics or morphology of the new language. Research to date has focused on Chinese readers' mastery of English orthography and phonology.

Whatever model of English word identification one prefers, the evidence is clear that native readers of English (1) process both orthographic and phonological information automatically as they identify words (e.g., Perfetti et al., 1988) and (2) differ from one another in the extent to which they are skilled at processing one or the other kind of information (e.g., Rack et al., 1992; Coltheart, Curtis, Atkins, & Haller, 1993). These individual differences can be observed among successful beginners and fluent readers as well as among disabled readers (Jackson, Donaldson, & Mills, 1993). Therefore, the task of English word identification is sufficiently flexible to permit the expression of differences in orthographic and phonological processing that might arise from differences in English reading history and transfer of word-identification strategies from a first language.

Haynes and Carr (1990) have argued that experienced

readers of a new alphabetic orthography remain inefficient in processing the visual patterns of that orthography, even though learning to identify its letters accurately is a relatively trivial task. In the study introduced above, they compared Taiwanese and American undergraduates' efficiency in making visual same-different judgments about orthographically irregular (i.e., illegitimate) four-letter strings, orthographically legitimate four-letter pseudowords, and real four-letter words. As one would expect, both groups judged the real words most efficiently and the illegitimate letter strings least efficiently. However, the investigators' primary interest was in the extent to which the groups differed in efficiency gains as the stimuli became more familiar. They computed difference scores which they labeled as a lexicality effect (word - pseudoword efficiency) and an orthography effect (pseudoword - letter string efficiency).

Relative to the American comparison group, the native readers of Chinese gained relatively little advantage from what Haynes and Carr called orthography and relatively more advantage from lexicality. They interpret this finding as evidence that native readers of Chinese are inefficient at detecting legitimate but novel orthographic sequences within English words, a conclusion that is consistent with their belief that reading unfamiliar orthographies is difficult even when phonology is not an issue. However, making a judgment about the visual similarity of letter strings may not be a purely orthographic task for Chinese readers of English.

Although orthographically legitimate letter strings (i.e., pseudowords) can be matched without phonological encoding (Carr, 1986), there is no evidence in Haynes and Carr's study about the processes that actually were used by these readers. Therefore, what Haynes and Carr interpret as an orthography effect might also be a phonology effect, and their Chinese readers' deficit in matching English pseudowords also could be attributed to difficulty in phonologically coding unfamiliar letter strings. Fortunately, Haynes and Carr's finding that these Chinese readers gain a considerable processing advantage from lexicality is more clear-cut and more directly relevant to other research in which orthographic processing has been operationalized as identification of lexicality.

Among native readers of English, individual differences in reading history have been found to be related to individuals' skill in using orthographic information to make lexical judgments about English words (e.g., Stanovich & West, 1989). Extensive exposure to English print may help a reader to build a large lexicon of both regular and irregular words associated with letter strings. Even among Chinese readers of English, there is evidence that exposure to English print is associated with individual differences in this kind of orthographic processing. The 25 Taiwanese graduate students described in section 5.1 (Jackson et al., 1993) completed a questionnaire in which they were asked to identify titles of American magazines. This estimate of their exposure to English print correlated moderately (*r*'s = .36 and .45) with the students' accuracy on two orthographic processing tasks that are described below.

As a group, Chinese readers of English would be expected to have had limited exposure to English print, relative to native readers. However, even among native readers, a substantial amount of variation in orthographic processing skill remains unexplained after exposure to print and other variables have been entered as predictors. This unexplained variance may reflect individual differences in strategic preference (Barker, Torgesen, & Wagner, 1992) such as a Chinese adult might build up in many years of reading an orthography in which words cannot be sounded out one phoneme at a time. Chinese readers of English could be especially well able to take advantage of orthographic patterns when reading English words with sound patterns they find difficult (Newport, 1990).

In our study (Jackson et al., 1993) of orthographic and phonological processing among Chinese readers of English, we hypothesized that, relative to a comparison group of native readers of English, Taiwanese graduate students at an American university would show greater skill in orthographic than in phonological processing of English words and pseudowords. However, we also considered the alternative hypothesis that the emphasis on grapheme-phoneme correspondence rules in the English curriculum of Taiwan schools, together with lack of exposure to English print, might make Taiwanese graduate students relatively better at phonological than at orthographic processing of English words.

The four computer-administered word identification tasks we used were all developed by Olson and his colleagues (Olson et al., 1989). Orthographic processing was measured in two tasks: one requiring lexical decision for pseudohomophone pairs such as *rain/rane*, and the other, choice of which of two homophones answered an oral question such as "Which is used to smell? *(knows/nose).*" Note that both of these tasks tap knowledge similar to that responsible for the lexicality effect in Haynes and Carr's (1990) study. Phonological processing was measured in one task by pronunciation of one- and two-syllable pseudowords (e.g., *derl, bremick)* and in another by choice of the pseudohomophone (related to a real word) from sets of three pseudowords (e.g., *beal/bair/rabe).* Accuracy and latency for correct responses were measured for all tasks.

Again, our research participants were the 25 Taiwanese graduate students and 24 American ninth graders described in section 5.1. Ninth graders had been chosen as the comparison group in the expectation that their timed Nelson-Denny word-reading ability would be comparable to the 9.6 mean grade-equivalent level of the Taiwanese graduate students. However, relatively few of the available ninth graders volunteered, and their mean Nelson-Denny Vocabulary grade-equivalent score was 11.9 (*SD* = 2.1). This large group difference in overall performance levels complicated interpretation of our orthographic and phonological processing results. Because the two groups were 1 *SD* apart in their Nelson-Denny Vocabulary raw scores, we used that difference as a benchmark against which to evaluate group differences in performance on the orthographic and phonological processing measures.

Speed and accuracy scores were not consistently correlated with one another. Therefore, composite speed/accuracy scores would have had no consistent meaning, and we looked separately at the accuracy and speed results pictured in Figure 3. The accuracy results are clear-cut: The Taiwanese graduate students performed as well or better on measures of orthographic processing accuracy as on the Nelson-Denny subtests, while their phonological processing accuracy scores were considerably lower. These results are consistent with the hypothesis that native readers of Chinese can use relatively strong knowledge of English orthographic patterns to compensate for difficulty with phonological processing of English words.

The pattern in the speed scores in Figure 3 at first appears to be the inverse of the accuracy pattern, with phonological processing stronger than orthographic processing. However, the two kinds of scores cannot be interpreted in the same way. Because the American students got many more items correct on the phonological processing tasks, the group difference in

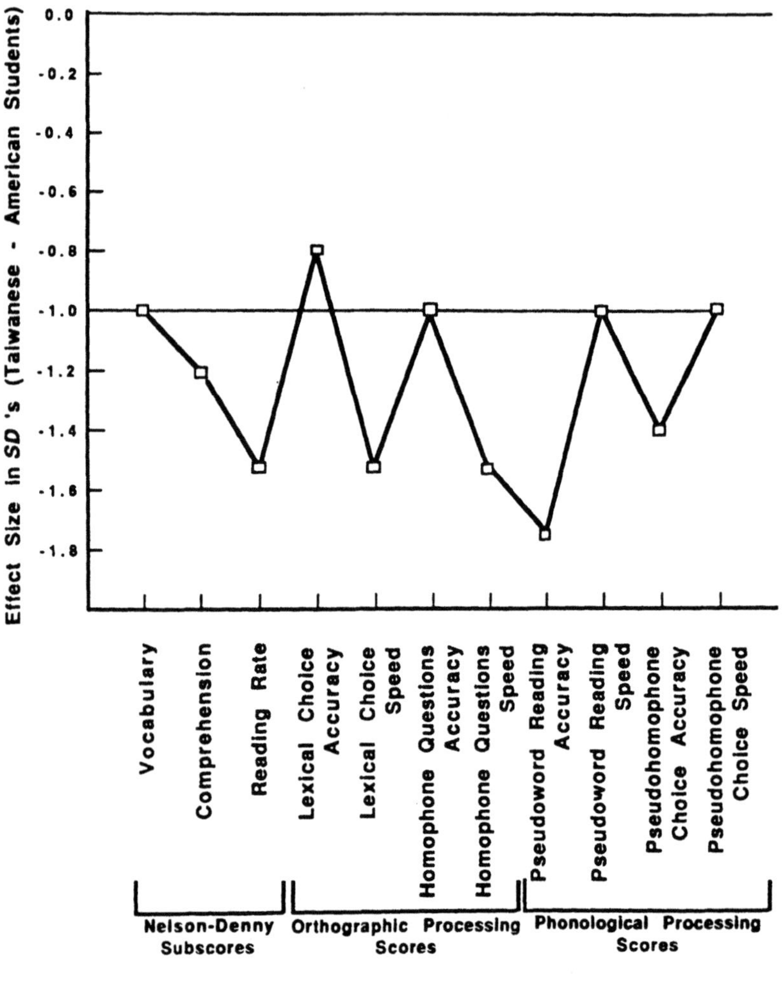

Figure 3 Mean performance levels for Chinese-English bilingual Taiwanese (n = 25) graduate students on three scores from the Nelson-Denny Reading Test and eight measures of orthographic and phonological processing. Each score is plotted in pooled within-group *SD* units, relative to the performance of the comparison group of American readers (n = 24). The horizontal line approximately at effect size -1.0 indicates the Chinese readers' performance deficit on the Nelson-Denny Vocabulary subtest, which was used as the primary benchmark for interpreting other scores. The Nelson-Denny Reading Rate score also was used as a benchmark for interpretation of the orthographic and phonological processing speed scores.

phonological processing speed scores is uninterpretable. Looking only at orthographic processing speeds, one can see that, relative to the American comparison group, the Taiwanese students were no slower at orthographic processing than at reading text (Nelson-Denny Reading Rate). This last finding is consistent with the argument that native readers of Chinese are not at any special disadvantage in ability to use orthographic information to identify English words.

A preliminary conclusion that Chinese readers of English are relatively stronger in orthographic processing, or more specifically, in making orthographic-semantic connections, than they are in phonological processing is consistent with both our own results and the large lexicality effect for the Chinese readers of English in Haynes and Carr's (1990) study. However, this conclusion needs to be evaluated further in studies involving other word identification tasks, preferably tasks in which the balance of Chinese readers' orthographic and phonological processing strategies could be assessed as they read English text. The possibility that Chinese readers of English actually do use what Baron and Strawson (1976) called a "Chinese" strategy to identify words merits further investigation.

5.3 *English Text-Reading Processes*

The slow English text reading of native readers of Chinese might reflect word-level processing, but it might also be attributed to negative transfer of text-level processing strategies across the two orthographies. Characteristics of a reader's first language or orthography might influence the way second-language text is processed.

In the study introduced in section 5.1, Haynes and Carr (1990) found that individual differences in 60 Taiwanese undergraduates' English text-reading speeds were associated with only three other scores: efficiency in visual matching of three-digit numbers, efficiency in English synonym/antonym matching, and accuracy on a written test of English grammar proficiency. Together, these variables accounted for less than 40% of the variance in text-reading speed, but no significant additional variance was accounted for by the students' Chinese reading proficiency or efficiency in visual matching of English words or letter strings. These results suggest that knowledge of English word meanings and sentence structure, together with individual differences in what may be a measure of elementary processing efficiency (number matching), contribute to the speed with which a native reader of Chinese reads English text. None of the significant predictor variables in this analysis directly assessed orthographic or phonological processing. However, the possibility remains that mastery of English orthography or phonology contributes to mastery of English vocabulary and sentence structure.

Another approach to understanding cross-linguistic transfer in text-reading strategies is to monitor readers' eye movements. We already have reviewed literature suggesting that eye movements and processing strategies may differ for Chinese and English text. Experience reading Chinese text arrayed both horizontally and vertically gives Chinese-English bilinguals some advantage in acuity for scanning vertical arrays of English letters (Freeman, 1980). However, there is no strong evidence that more subtle cross-language differences in scanning strategies transfer across orthography. Some results that appear to suggest shorter saccades for Chinese readers of English are confounded by other processing disadvantages of the Chinese group (Chen, 1992; Hoosain, 1991).

Fluent Chinese readers of English may adapt their text-scanning patterns to the language they are reading. In the study of Hong Kong undergraduates' Chinese and English text-reading processes using the moving-window technique introduced in section 3.5, Chen (1992) found that the Chinese students' viewing strategies differed depending on which language they were reading. Furthermore, the overall distribution of their viewing times across words occurring before and after a violation introduced into the text was consistent with results for native readers of English who had performed an oral-reading production task in another investigation. Chen interpreted his results as evidence that "readers are sensitive to the differences in the cognitive demands imposed by different linguistic structures in reading comprehension and that they adapt their processing strategies to meet the cognitive demands of the situation" (1992, p. 199). However, the English-reading strategies of Chen's Hong Kong sample, members of a bilingual community, might differ from the strategies of adult Chinese readers whose exposure to oral and written English has been less intense or started later.

The possibility that the profound differences between Chinese and English syntax affect the overall speed and possibly the processes used by Chinese readers of English merits further investigation, despite Chen's null finding. Li et al. have suggested that "Chinese speakers, in the absence of inflectional morphology, make use of almost all possible cues and integrate them interactively in identifying the functional roles of different linguistic constituents. In a language like Chinese, speakers cannot rely on one type of information, either because single pieces of information would not give unique answers to the processing task, or because some of them...although highly reliable, are not always available." (1992, p. 229).

Among readers who are not yet fluent enough to think in English as they read, the burden of mental translation across languages with radically different syntactic structures could conceivably be a major factor influencing text-reading speed and ease of comprehension. The automatic formation and retention of phonological codes may be critical to text comprehension and recall in any language (Perfetti et al., 1992). Native speakers of Chinese who have not been immersed in English in childhood or early adolescence have enduring difficulty with English phonology and morphology (Newport, 1990). If a reader cannot easily access and retain English phonological codes, an obvious strategy would be to read English with a word-by-word translation to Chinese. However, the syntactic differences between the two languages could make such a strategy highly inefficient.

As we learn more about the cognitive psychology of reading English as a second language, we also may become better able to identify correlates of individual differences in readers' effectiveness and strategies. Individual differences in elementary cognitive abilities, instructional histories, and reading experience may influence the word identification and text comprehension strategies of Chinese readers of English, just as they do the strategies of native readers.

6. CONCLUSIONS

On the whole, the results of recent studies of Chinese reading are consistent with a conclusion that universal properties of the human mind are more important than specific properties of different orthographies in determining how written language is processed. As researchers have learned more about the cognitive psychology, neuropsychology, and development of

Chinese reading, claims for cross-linguistic differences related to differences in orthography have become progressively more modest.

There are some differences in how alphabetic and morphosyllabic words are processed, but these differences may be gone by the time a word has been exposed for less than 100 milliseconds. The cognitive characteristics associated with success in learning to read Chinese may differ to some extent from those associated with success in learning to read an alphabetic orthography but, again, the differences are not as sweeping as one might expect. As we learn more about the reading of Chinese text, important cross-linguistic differences in text processing may be identified as products of differences in oral language structure rather than orthography.

The accumulating research may soon be sufficient to support the formulation of comprehensive models of Chinese word identification and text reading. Ideally, these models will be based on converging evidence from different measures and different paradigms. We see a particularly strong need for more studies of the development of Chinese literacy. Process models that emerge from experimental studies of skilled readers should be evaluated in terms of their ability to account for developmental and individual differences in first and second language reading.

NOTES

1. The literature on reading Chinese contains many research papers published only in Chinese as well as many available in English. However, comprehensive English summaries of the literature have only recently become available. In preparing this chapter, we found two books especially helpful: Rumjahn Hoosain's (1991) *Psycholinguistic implications for linguistic relativity: A case study of Chinese* and Hsuan-Chih Chen and Ovid J.L. Tzeng's (1992) edited collection, *Language processing in Chinese*.
2. Studies of other writing systems, such as Japanese, that incorporate Chinese characters in a complex orthography are not considered here. The combination of kanji (characters) and kana (a syllabary) in Japanese orthography presents interesting opportunities to contrast the processing of two different orthographies in within-language, within-subject designs. However, characters do not function the same way in Chinese and Japanese.
3. Different authors use different terms to denote the parts of compound characters. What we call the semantic radical is also called the radical (Huang & Wang, 1992) or the signific (Flores d'Arcais, 1992), and what we call the phonetic radical is also called the phonetic (Hoosain, 1991), or the stem (Huang & Wang, 1992).
4. All correlations with absolute values of at least .41 were significant at or beyond the .05 level, two-tailed.
5. American students in the comparison group for this study subsequently

participated in the Chinese learning study described in section 4.3.

REFERENCES

Barker, T.A., Torgesen, J.K., & Wagner, R.K. (1992). The role of orthographic processing skills on five different reading tasks. *Reading Research Quarterly*, 27, 334-345.

Baron, J. & Strawson, C. (1976). Use of orthographic and word-specific knowledge in reading words aloud. *Journal of Experimental Psychology: Human Perception and Performance*, 2, 386-393.

Brown, J.I., Bennett, J.M., & Hanna, G. (1981). *The Nelson-Denny Reading Test*. Chicago: Riverside Publishing.

Carr, T.H. (1986). Perceiving visual language. In K.R. Boff, L. Kaufman, & J.P. Thomas (Eds.), *Handbook of human perception and performance*. Vol. 2. *Cognitive processes and performance* (pp. 29-1 to 29-91). New York: Wiley.

Chang, H.W. (1992). The acquisition of Chinese syntax. In H.-C. Chen & O.J.L. Tzeng (Eds.), *Language processing in Chinese* (pp. 277-312). Amsterdam: North Holland.

Chen, H.-C. (1992). Reading comprehension in Chinese: Implications from character reading times. In H.-C. Chen & O.J.L. Tzeng (Eds.), *Language processing in Chinese* (pp. 175-206). Amsterdam: North Holland.

Chen, H.-C. & Tzeng, O.J.L. (Eds.) (1992). *Language processing in Chinese*. Amsterdam: North Holland.

Cheng, C.-M. (1992). Lexical access in Chinese: Evidence from automatic activation of phonological information. In H.-C. Chen & O.J.L. Tzeng (Eds.), *Language processing in Chinese* (pp. 175-206). Amsterdam: North Holland.

Coltheart, M. (1978). Lexical access in simple reading tasks. In G. Underwood (Ed.), *Strategies of information processing* (pp. 151-126). London: Academic Press.

Coltheart, M., Curtis, B., Atkins, P., & Haller, M. (1993). Models of reading aloud: dual-route and parallel-distributed-processing approaches. *Psychological Review*, *100*, 589-608.

Flores d'Arcais, G.B. (1992). Graphemic, phonological, and semantic activation processes during the recognition of Chinese characters. In H.-C. Chen & O.J.L. Tzeng (Eds.), *Language processing in Chinese* (pp. 37-66). Amsterdam: North Holland.

Freeman, R.D. (1980). Visual acuity is better for letters in rows than in columns. *Nature*, *286*, 62-64.

Goswami, U. & Bryant, P. (1990). *Phonological skills and learning to read*. East Sussex, UK: Erlbaum.

Haynes, M. & Carr, T. (1990). Writing system background and second language reading: A component skills analysis of English reading by native speaker-readers of Chinese. In T.H. Carr & B.A. Levy (Eds.), *Reading and its development: Component skills approaches*. San Diego: Academic Press.

Healy, A.F., Conboy, G.L. & Drewnowski, A. (1987). Characterizing the processing units of reading: Effects of intra- and inter-word spaces in a letter detection task. In B. Britton & S. Glynn (Eds.), *Executive control processes in reading* (pp. 279-296). Hillsdale, NJ: Erlbaum.

Hoosain, R. (1991). *Psycholinguistic implications for linguistic relativity: A case study of Chinese*. Hillsdale, NJ: Erlbaum.

Hoosain, R. (1992). Psychological reality of the word in Chinese. In H.-C. Chen & O.J.L. Tzeng (Eds.), *Language processing in Chinese* (pp. 111-131). Amsterdam: North Holland.

Huang, J.-T. & Wang, M.-Y. (1992). From unit to gestalt: Perceptual dynamics in recognizing Chinese characters. In H.-C. Chen & O.J.L. Tzeng (Eds.), *Language processing in Chinese* (pp. 3-36). Amsterdam: North Holland.

Hue, C.-W. (1992). Recognition processes in character naming. In H.-C. Chen & O.J.L. Tzeng (Eds.), *Language processing in Chinese* (pp. 93-110). Amsterdam: North Holland.

Jackson, N.E., Donaldson, G., & Mills, J. (1993). Components of reading skill in post-kindergarten precocious readers and level-matched second graders. *Journal of Reading Behavior, 25*, 181-208.

Jackson, N.E., Ju, D., Lu, W.-H., & Forte, E. (1992). *First test of a measure of ability to learn new orthographic and phonologically based orthographies*. Paper presented at the annual convention of the American Educational Research Association, San Francisco.

Jackson, N.E., Ju, D., Lu, W.-H., & Reitz, E. (1993). Chinese readers of English: *Orthographic and phonological processing, word identification, and exposure to print*. Paper presented at the biennial meeting of the Society for Research in Child Development, New Orleans.

Ju, D. (1992). *The process of Chinese character identification*. Paper presented at the annual convention of the American Educational Research Association, San Francisco.

Li, P. Bates, E., Liu, H., & MacWhinney, B. (1992). Cues as functional constraints on sentence processing in Chinese. In H.-C. Chen & O.J.L. Tzeng (Eds.), *Language processing in Chinese* (pp. 207-236). Amsterdam: North Holland.

Lu, W.-H. (1992). *Children's developing metalinguistic awareness of properties of Chinese characters*. Unpublished master's thesis. College of Education, University of Iowa, Iowa City, IA.

Lu, W.-H. & Jackson, N.E. (1993). *Children's developing metalinguistic awareness of properties of Chinese characters*. Paper presented at the biennial meeting of the Society for Research in Child Development, New Orleans.

McCutchen, D. & Perfetti, C.A. (1982). The visual tongue-twister effect: Phonological activation in silent reading. *Journal of Verbal Learning and Verbal Behavior, 21*, 672-687.

Newport, E. (1990). Maturational constraints on language learning. *Cognitive Science, 14*, 11-28.

Olson, R.K., Wise, B., Conners, F., Rack, J. & Fulker, D. (1989). Specific deficits in component reading skills: Genetic and environmental influences. *Journal of Learning Disabilities, 22*, 339-348.

Perfetti, C.A., Bell, L.C. & Delaney, S.M. (1988). Automatic prelexical phonetic activation in silent word reading: Evidence from backward masking. *Journal of Memory and Language, 27*, 59-70.

Perfetti, C.A. & Zhang, S. (1991). Phonological processes in reading Chinese words. *Journal of Experimental Psychology: Learning, Memory, and Cognition, 17*, 633-643.

Perfetti, C.A. & Zhang, S. (1992, November). *In reading Chinese there is no semantics without phonology*. Paper presented at the 33rd annual meeting of the Psychonomic Society, St. Louis.

Perfetti, C.A., Zhang, S., & Berent, I. (1992). Reading in English and Chinese: Evidence for a "universal" phonological principle. In R. Frost & L. Katz (Eds.), *Orthography, phonology, morphology, and meaning* (pp. 227-248). Amsterdam: North-Holland.

Rack, J.P., Snowling, M.J., & Olson, R.K. (1992). The nonword reading deficit in developmental dyslexia: A review. *Reading Research Quarterly, 27*, 28-53.

Roberts, B. (1992). The evolution of the young child's concept of *word* as a unit of spoken and written language. *Reading Research Quarterly, 27*, 125-138.

Rozin, P., Poritzky, S. & Sotsky, R. (1971). American children with reading problems can easily learn to read English represented in Chinese characters. *Science, 171*, 1264-1267.

Seidenberg, M.S. (1985). The time course of phonological code activation in two writing systems. *Cognition, 19*, 1-30.

Smith, F. (1985). *Reading without nonsense* (2nd ed.). New York: Teachers College Press.

Stanovich, K.E. & West, R.F. (1989). Exposure to print and orthographic processing. *Reading Research Quarterly, 24*, 402-433.

Stevenson, H.W., Stigler, J.W., Lee, S.Y., & Lucker, G.W. (1985). Cognitive performance and academic achievement of Japanese, Chinese, and American children. *Child Development, 56*, 718-734.

Stevenson, H.W., Stigler, G.W., Lucker, G.W., Lee, S.Y., Hsu, C.C. & Kitamura, S. (1982). Reading disabilities: The case of Chinese, Japanese, and English. *Child Development, 53*, 1164-1181.

Taylor, I. & Taylor, M.M. (1990). *Psycholinguistics: Learning and using language*. Englewood Cliffs, NJ: Prentice-Hall.

Tzeng, O.J.L., & Hung, D.L. (1980). Reading in a nonalphabetic writing system: Some experimental studies. In J.F. Kavanagh & R.L. Venezky (Eds.), *Orthography, reading, and dyslexia*. Baltimore: University Park Press.

Tzeng, O.J.L., Hung, D.L., & Wang. S.-Y. (1977). Speech recoding in reading Chinese characters. *Journal of Experimental Psychology: Human Learning and Memory, 3*, 621-630.

Wang, W.S.-Y. (1973). The Chinese language. *Scientific American, 228* (2), 51-63.

Yin, W. & Butterworth, B. (1992). Deep and surface dyslexia in Chinese. In H.-C. Chen & O.J.L. Tzeng (Eds.), *Language processing in Chinese* (pp. 349-366). Amsterdam: North Holland.

Zhang, B. & Peng, D. (1992). Decomposed storage in the Chinese lexicon. In H.-C. Chen & O.J.L. Tzeng (Eds.), *Language processing in Chinese* (pp. 131-150). Amsterdam: North Holland.

Zhang, S. & Perfetti, C. A. (in press). The tongue-twister effect in reading Chinese. *Journal of Experimental Psychology: Learning, Memory, and Cognition*.

Address Correspondence to:

Nancy Ewald Jackson
Division of Psychological and Quantitative Foundations
University of Iowa
Iowa City, IA 52242
USA

EGBERT M. H. ASSINK & GÖRAN KATTENBERG

HIGHER-ORDER LINGUISTIC INFLUENCES ON DEVELOPMENT OF ORTHOGRAPHIC KNOWLEDGE: ILLUSTRATIONS FROM SPELLING PROBLEMS IN DUTCH AND ASSESSMENT TOOLS

1. INTRODUCTION

Alphabetic writing systems vary considerably as to their use of higher-order linguistic principles at the morphological and syntactic levels in spelling. This use of higher-order principles adds to the complexity of the orthography, which is not just related to phonology. As discussed in this chapter, Dutch orthography is characterized most distinctly by its specific use of analogy rules in polymorphemic words. The analysis that we will present here further elaborates and extends the work reported in empirical studies published by Verhoeven (1979), Assink (1987a), and Assink, Van der Linden, and Kattenberg (1990). The first study is central for sections 2-3, while the other studies form the basis of sections 4-9.

2. INVENTORY OF DUTCH ORTHOGRAPHY PROBLEMS

An interesting point in studies on spelling problems is the observation that some spelling problems seems to disappear more or less spontaneously in the course of development, while other problem types appear to remain. The implication is that spelling problems differ in their persistence. Psychologically, persistence of spelling problems may give us an important clue concerning the cognitive processes involved in learning to spell. The following categories of spelling problems in Dutch provide such clues: (a) Analogy problems; (b) Congruence problems; (c) Etymology problems; (d) Spelling of vowels and consonants in polysyllables; (e) Interference of pronunciation options; (f) Dialect interference; and (g) Spelling of loan words.

The *principle of analogy* demands uniformity in the orthography of flexion morphemes in polymorphemic words.

V.W. Berninger (ed.), The varieties of orthographic knowledge I: Theoretical and developmental issues, 111-136.

Analogy is applicable in words like "meisjesschool" (girls' school), where the first *s* is spelled on the analogy of words like "meisjesboek" (girls' book). A second instance in which the analogy principle must be used is the orthography of verb forms. Analogy requires here that equivalently constructed verb forms must be dealt with analogously in spelling, for example, the suffix *-t* in "hij speelt" (he plays) has to be written analogously in "hij vindt" (he finds), although in the latter case its function is purely orthographic. In verb orthography this principle is very dominating. In that case it expresses a number of specific syntactic functions in writing. Verb orthography will be discussed in more detail further on in this chapter.

The *congruence principle* demands uniformity in the orthography of stem morphemes. To illustrate, *paard* [pa:rt] "horse" is written with final *-d*, in congruence with its plural *paarden* [pa:rdən]. Likewise *staart* [sta:rt] "tail" is written with final -t because of its plural staarten [sta:rtən]. In the case of *paard* the final "morphological *-d*" overrules the phonological principle.

The *etymological principle* demands that different letter codings with identical sound values must be employed to capture acoustic distinctions that existed in older stages in the development of the language. To illustrate, the diphthong [əu] is represented in spelling by *au* or *ou* (e.g., *blauw* "blue" and zout "salt"). Another example is [ɛi], which is represented by *ei* or *ij* (e.g., klein "small" and *lijn* "line").

Another source of spelling problems is the spelling of *consonants and vowels in polysyllabic words.* In Dutch polysyllables there is a complicated letter-phoneme conversion rule, pertaining to the spelling of vowels and single letter consonants (to be referred to as *CV-problems* in the remaining part of this article, cf. Van Heuven, 1980). In Dutch monosyllables, a long vowel is normally spelled with reduplication *(aa, ee, oo, uu),* unless it is in final position, or, as it is traditionally called, in an "open syllable." In monosyllables with the long vowel in final position reduplication is simplified (reduced to one letter, e.g., compare *naar* "towards" [na:r] and na "after" [na:]). A basic principle of Dutch syllabification is that, unless a word boundary intervenes, a single intervocalic consonant is the first element of the next syllable. This principle implies that when, for example, *beek* "brook" is pluralized (by adding -en

[- n]), the syllable division is *bee-ken,* leaving ee in the final position of the syllable. Consequently, the stem vowel is now spelled with a single *e* : *beken.* To complicate matters further, vowel simplification does not take place when the next syllable begins with a digraph consonant: *goochelen* [χo:χələn] "juggle." Conversely, a single letter consonant grapheme is reduplicated in the intervocalic position after a short vowel. Thus, the plural of *gek* "fool" is spelled *gekken* and *stok* "stick" as *stokken.* Understandably, this rule is a direct consequence of the vowel simplification rule. If the intervocalic consonant grapheme were not reduplicated, the stem vowel would be assigned the value of a long vowel. CV-problems are a notoriously difficult topic in Dutch spelling instruction.

Pronunciation options and dialect interference both refer to the phenomenon that peculiarities observed at the level of speech may penetrate into the level of writing. The term *pronunciation options* refers to the phenomenon that in Received Standard Spoken Dutch there exist some equally acceptable pronunciation options, such as the final *-n* in the plural suffix of verbs and nouns. This -n is not pronounced in the central and western parts of the country. Other examples are vowel reduction (e.g., *banaan* [bəna:n] for [bana:n] "banana"), and schwa insertion (e.g., melk [mɛlək] for [mɛlk] "milk"). For *dialect interference* analogous examples may be given, such as *t*-deletion in Southern Limburgian *vrien* for *vriend* "friend."

In the case of *loan words,* the spelling difficulties originate primarily from the unfamiliar orthographic conventions present in the words that have been incorporated in Dutch from other languages. The majority of Dutch loan words comes from French, English, Latin and Greek. Examples are *horloge* "watch," *couvert* "envelope," and *taxateur* "valuer."

3. DEVELOPMENTAL TRENDS IN LEARNING TO SPELL

Verhoeven (1979) collected a vast corpus of written materials, such as compositions, papers and essays, in various types of schools. The texts were produced predominately in the course of regular teaching activities. The investigator's main interest was the construction of an inventory of spelling errors based on "spontaneous" texts. The study was designed primarily to demonstrate that standard dictation tests give a biased and inaccurate picture as to the frequency and occurrence of spelling problems in "real life" texts. The materials were collected in six types of school, selected as prototypes or representatives for the principal schooling levels in the Dutch educational system:

(1) Elementary school, initial grades (1-3);
(2) Elementary school, advanced grades (4-6);
(3) Secondary school, introductory class;
(4) High school, final grades;
(5) High school (introductory to university[1]), final grades;
(6) University students, freshmen.

The spelling errors detected in the corpus were categorized into the spelling problem types described in the previous paragraph. The results obtained are summarized in the histogram presented in Figure 1. This histogram presents an overview of the contribution of the problem categories (expressed as relative proportions) to the total amount of spelling errors detected in the corpus.[2] Inspection of the histogram shows that a rising education level[3] coincides with a striking shift in the relative contributions of the various problem types to the total amount of spelling errors present in the corpus.

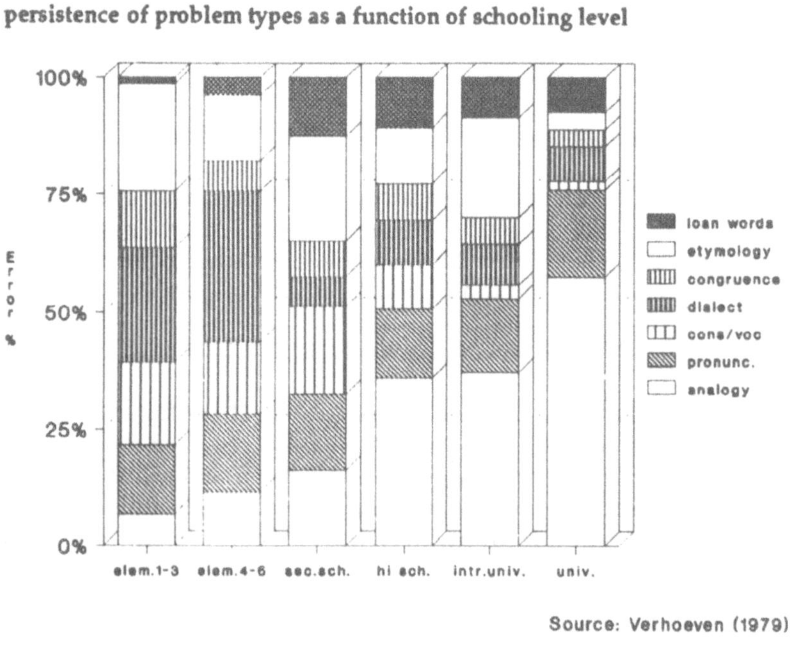

Figure 1 Persistence of Problem Types in Dutch Orthography

There must, of course, be no misunderstanding about the fact that in the higher education levels there is a dramatic drop in the absolute number of spelling errors present in the data. With this fact in mind the picture is very clear: there is a strong decline in problems relating to the vowel/consonant rule in polysyllables and to problems associated with dialect interference. A similarly declining category is congruence, which on the whole turns out to be rather unproblematic. In sharp contrast to this declining trend are problems concerning the analogy principle and loan words which increase over development. Finally, there are some categories that appear to remain relatively constant across the various education levels. These are problems associated with pronunciation options in Dutch and, to some degree, etymology problems. Next we offer some interpretative comments on the trends observed in the presented data.

First, the decreasing influence of dialect interference is one of the most prominent trends in the data. The most plausible explanation of this trend is that with an increasing education level it becomes easier to discriminate between formal standard language and spoken dialect options. Especially in the elementary education levels the effect of dialect interference (relative proportions of 18 to 25%) turns out to be remarkably strong in Verhoeven's data. In this respect it is inconsistent with other specially designed dialect studies, such as the investigation published by Hagen (1981). This study was concerned with the Southern Limburgian dialect.[4] The written materials analyzed were collected in elementary schools, and comparable to Verhoeven's data. Hagen found in the lower grades a relative proportion of 12.1% dialect interference errors, and a corresponding value of 6.6% in the higher grades.[5] The most convincing explanation for this discrepancy with Verhoeven's data has been presented by Hagen (1985), who suggests that differences between the dialects involved in both studies produced the discrepancies. The implication of Hagen's suggestion is that the dialects involved (provincial idioms of Limburg and Utrecht) differed as to their potential capabilities to produce interference on the level of orthography. This explanation is convincing, since the Utrecht dialect, associated with Verhoeven's study, corresponds to the standard language to a much larger degree than does the Limburgian dialect. Another possibility is that the discrepancy between the two studies is due to differences in the categorization criteria employed in both studies.

Second, there is a comparable sharp decrease in the contribution of CV-problems. A similar trend, but less articulated, is present in the case of congruence problems. In our view, these trends offer a major clue to uncover system-inherent difficulties present in Dutch orthography. Both categories are prototypical "rule problems," taught in the initial phase of the learning process. Congruence problems, as well as CV-problems, are taught by practicing these rules explicitly. However, this teaching practice does not mean that pupils continue to use these rules consciously and explicitly when they grow into more proficient spellers. The use of phoneme-grapheme rules is specially important in the initial stage of the learning process, when unfamiliar words are often encountered. In subsequent developmental stages of the reading/spelling process fluency and speed are enhanced by making use of larger orthographic units, such as memorized spellings of individual words (often referred to as word images), or memorized word segments and their pronunciations, or the use of analogies, etc. These new possibilities, incorporated into the pupils' inventory of strategies, have similar effects on both congruence problems and CV-problems. The pupil who is beyond the introductory stage of learning to spell has got optional strategies at his disposal to handle both types of problems. If accessible, he or she will apply explicit rules, but shift to more economic memory strategies if this shift is feasible. The declining influence of both problem categories is probably produced by this developmental shift in strategy use. Thus, the pupil may shift to more efficient direct search routines in his developing orthographic memory, possibly in combination with automatically performed rule strategies.

With the exception of analogy problems, only loan words show an increasing relative contribution to the total amount of errors in the corpus. There is a gradual increase of this category, followed by a slight decrease at the higher education levels, a tendency which in my view must be attributed to the point that this category of words plays a rather specific role in the language learning process. Initially, pupils only occasionally encounter these words. In the course of development, however, the number of loan words incorporated into the pupil's vocabulary strongly increases. These new words are not only used passively in reading, but also actively in writing. The observed trend in the contribution of loan words thus reflects the proportional growth of this class, combined with predictable initial spelling problems. The following decline most probably indicates a gradual familiarization to exotic orthographic conventions. Verhoeven (1979) presents a similar interpretation of this trend in the data.

Overall, analogy problems produce the most dramatic increase over development. As is shown by Figure 1, analogy is the only category with a rising trend up to the highest education level. This category demands special discussion so the next section will be dedicated to this subject.

4. GRAMMATICAL OPERATIONS IN SPELLING VERB HOMOPHONES

One of the most prominent features in Dutch orthography is the analogy principle (Assink, 1987a). Of all principles, analogy is undoubtedly the most difficult one to learn. The problems connected with analogy in Dutch verb orthography must be associated with the type of linguistic information involved and the intricacies of Dutch orthography.

Verb orthography demands the expression, or encoding, of certain syntactic relations, which is realized by applying the analogy principle. In a large number of verbs, however, application of this principle creates *homophones*. Homophones are words with equivalent acoustic forms regardless of spelling (e.g., *scale*=pair of scales / *scale*=fish-scale). However, the great majority of homophones are distinguished in print by different spellings, e.g., *sun/son*, *bear/bare* in English and Dutch *leiden/lijden* ("to lead"/"to suffer"), *nood/noot* ("need"/"note"). As the homophones occurring in Dutch verb orthography express grammatical distinctions, they are often referred to as *grammatically defined homophones*. This type of homophones should clearly be distinguished from cases like son/sun, where the difference in spellings is associated with a *lexical* distinction. In the following instances Dutch orthography expresses grammatical functional distinctions where, acoustically, there is no difference.

1. Distinctions in *grammatical person*, for example, ik *vind*/hij *vindt* (I find/he finds). This homophonic distinction occurs in the present tense singular. Orthography expresses here a distinctions between finite forms in the first person singular and forms in the second and third person singular, which take an extra suffix *-t*. This type of problem occurs in the present

tense singular of verbs with a stem ending in *-d*.

2. Distinctions in *grammatical tense*, for example, wij *wachten* nu/wij *wachtten* toen (we wait now/we waited then). In the past tense, Dutch weak verbs generally take a suffix *-te(n)* or *-de(n)* after the verbal stem. This pattern also holds for the set of weak verbs with a stem ending in *-d* or *-t*. For this set of verbs, application of the general past tense suffix rule leads to purely orthographic homophone distinctions like *wachten/wachtten* and *branden/brandden* (burn/burned).

3. Distinctions in *grammatical aspect* (imperfect/perfect). In Dutch, there is a large class of verbs, characterized by the presence of an unstressed prefix in the verbal stem, known as prefix verbs. The weak members of this verb class that have a voiced stem ending induce aspect-type homophones that have a present tense singular (second/ third person) with a suffix *-t* and a corresponding acoustically identical past participle with a suffix *-d*, for example, hij *verandert*/hij is *veranderd* (he changes/he has changed).

4. *Voice-type homophones*. The same class of verbs described just now also produces voice-type homophones, expressing active/passive distinctions in syntax, for example, hij *verdedigt* /hij wordt *verdedigd* (he defends /he is defended).

5. Homophones, expressing *attributive/predicative* distinctions in syntactic structure. A subset of the weak prefix verbs induces an additional homophone problem. Weak prefix verbs with a stem ending in *-t* or *-d* have a past tense singular that is acoustically equivalent to its corresponding, attributively used past participle, for example, hij *verwachtte*/de *verwachte* brief (he expected/ the expected letter).

6. *Grammatical number*-type homophones, expressing singular-plural distinctions, as in: hij *maakte*/wij *maakten*. It should be kept in mind here that most Dutch native speakers do not pronounce the final *-n* of the plural suffix *-en*, a circumstance which may produce confusion in writing.

5. ASSESSING LEARNING POTENTIAL FOR LITERACY SKILLS

Dutch orthography is characterized by its close relationship with syntax. Unlike related languages, such as English and German, Dutch orthography contains syntactic information which is not represented in oral language (Assink, 1987b). Linguistically, it is a highly expressive orthography (Klima, 1972). An orthography is more expressive of the language if it distinguishes between lexical items which, while identical at the sound-level, are distinct at the lexical level. For example, compare *meat* "flesh" and *meet* "encounter" in English.

Dutch orthography is particularly expressive in its verb spelling. The existing orthographic rule system expresses grammatical functions which are absent in the spoken language, such as in: wij *wachten/wachtten* "we wait/waited." A negative aspect of this informative written code, however, is its complexity for the novice learner. Educators disagree on the question of what age is most suitable to begin formal instruction of the complex grammatical rules involved. To gain more insight regarding this issue and in order to track the developmental relationship between syntactic and orthographic skills (Bowey 1986a; 1986b; Tunmer, Nesdale, & Wright, 1987) we designed a computerized test. This test will be described next. Subsequently, the results of two standardization and validation studies of the test are presented.

6. AN OUTLINE OF THE DIAGNOSTIC TEST

The test sentences used are skeletons, in which two of the basic types of orthographic problems in Dutch can be inserted. The most difficult spelling problems are *homophones*. Homophones represent orthographic distinctions, expressing syntactic information which is not present in the oral language. Correct choice must be based on grammatical knowledge. The second type are *non-homophones*, expressing a simple sound-spelling correspondence. In that instance word-specific memory may be used to make the correct choice.

In addition to both types of orthographic skill, indices of syntactic and word imaging skills are assigned. *Syntactic skill* is the ability to select syntactically legal options regardless of correct spelling. *Word-image* refers to implicit knowledge of orthographic structure. It is the ability to detect and reject "system-illegal" orthographic options, regardless of context. Word-image skill should be clearly distinguished from spelling ability. Incorrect spellings are not necessarily violations of existing spelling options in a language. Word image mistakes only refer to "system-illegal" letter combinations, options that could never occur in writing. Thus, word image refers to a specific type of spelling error, violating graphotactic constraints. To illustrate, in English orthography the option "bcat" for *boat* is system-illegal, whereas *"boap"* is not. Skilled readers are able to discriminate any input letter string from thousands of other letter patterns by making use of the characteristics of redundancy in the written language (Seidenberg & McClelland, 1989). This skill of utilizing constraints on the forms of written words enables the subjects in our test to detect system-illegal alternatives.

Subjects who perform very poorly on orthography tests are not necessarily dyslexics. There are several possible causes for poor performance in spelling. Only one of them is dyslexia, and psychologists should be cautious to come too easily to that conclusion (Treiman & Hirsh-Pasek, 1985; Vellutino, & Scanlon, 1982). Basically there are two possibilities. One possibility is that the subject is the victim of poor or inadequate instruction. Another possibility is that there may be some malfunctioning mechanism in the pupils's cognitive system causing poor reading and spelling performance. Dyslexics have problems with the use of orthographic redundancy, and consequently will perform poorly on tasks demanding the detection of system-illegal forms.

In order to comprehend the conceptual basis of our test it is important to note here that a clear distinction should be made between poor spellers who perform at a normal level on the word-image scale on the one hand, and poor spellers who combine poor spelling with poor word-image skills on the other. The first type of student has much better prospects for improvement provided by remedial instruction.

The test was computerized to enable individual teachers to test and diagnose verbal skills in classroom settings. One advantage of computerized testing is that the test can be optimally tuned for ease of use with regard to the specific test situation. Another advantage of computerized testing is the immediate availability of the results and comparisons with reference groups.

The program was designed as an interface facilitating the choice process. Inserting an alternative in the skeleton sentence is enabled by pressing the UP and DOWN keys of the numeric keypad (figure 2). This process may be repeated until a satisfactory option has been found. It enables the subject to evaluate the alternative within the frame of the sentence context. In a paper and pencil version this is simply impossible.

After finishing the test a scoring program is invoked. This program recodes the subject's raw scores into numerical scores. In the next step the mean scores on the four different measures are calculated. The program also presents test scores of the correct reference group and makes corrections for guessing. Finally, the subject's difference scores with his reference group are calculated and presented.

make
maakt
maken

De monteurs . . . de raceauto weer snel in orde.

73/192 ____________________

1a Sample Test Item. Initial position.

make
maakt

De monteurs maken de raceauto weer snel in orde.

73/192 ____________________

1b Inserting an alternative

Figure 2. The Test Program

7. TEST STANDARDIZATION RESULTS

The diagnostic test was standardized on a group of elementary school pupils (n=97). The results on the test were used as a reference to evaluate individual test profiles based on grade norms. Standardization data not only included final grade pupils (see schooling levels in the Dutch educational system earlier in this chapter), but also younger groups of subjects who comprehended the test instructions (i.e., grades 5, 6 and 7). This large sample of subjects enabled us to investigate developmental trends. As is shown in figure 3, three of the indices demonstrate monotonously rising linear curves: syntax, non-homophones, and homophones. The word-image index however, shows a curvilinear, U-shaped trend. This finding is in agreement with more general findings in cognitive development research, as discussed later on. Our interpretation is that initially words are spelled holistically by using word-images. During further development of orthographic knowledge the efficient use of word-images in spelling is negatively affected by the growing knowledge of grammar and syntax, thus producing spelling errors. In this phase when conceptual knowledge is restructured, grammatically based spelling rules are often overgeneralized to instances where they do not apply. In the final stage of development the positive relationship between word-image and spelling ability is reestablished.

The developmental trend described here has also been demonstrated by other investigators for a variety of content domains (Strauss, 1982). Curvilinear trends across age development have been reported in Piaget style conservation studies (Stavy, Strauss, Orpaz & Carmi, 1982), language development (Bowerman, 1982, 1985) and the development of artistry (Gardner & Winner, 1982). To illustrate, Strauss (1982) reported a curvilinear developmental trend in an experiment investigating the development of the concept of temperature. His subjects were children, varying in age from three to nine years. The subjects were shown three cups of water (A, B and C) each containing the same amount of water of identical temperature. Cups A and B were emptied into an empty cup D. Then they were asked to compare the temperatures of cup C and D. Three-to-five year olds solved the problem correctly, whereas six-to-nine year olds made lots of mistakes. Children older than nine experienced no problems any more. The general explanation for this phenomenon may well be found in the development of the underlying representations that are being built up under the influence of different sources of information. While subjects are accommodating their knowledge to new sources of information, such as the grammatical and syntactic knowledge involved in our study, performance drops temporarily because the subject has to

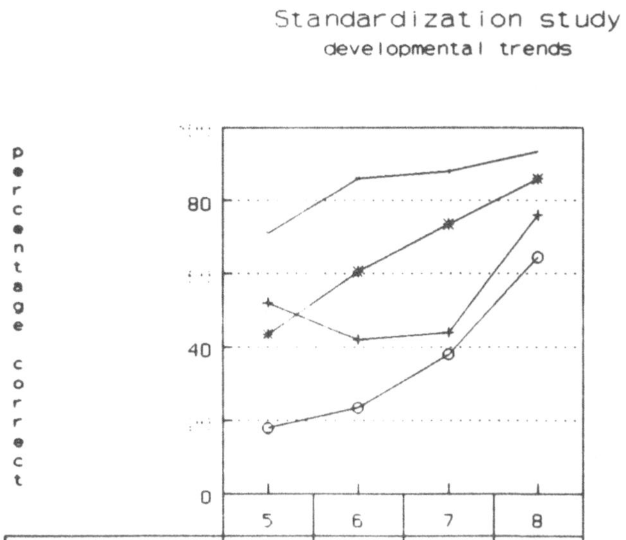

	5	6	7	8
syntax	71	86	88	93.5
word image	52	42	44	76
non homophones	43.5	60.5	73.5	86
homophones	18	23.5	38	64.5

grade

corrected for guessing

- syntax
- word image
- non homophones
- homophones

Figure 3 Developmental Trends: Standardization Study

reorganize his knowledge base. When this information finally has been assimilated performance improves again.

Reliability measures of the four test indices are presented in Table 1. The relatively low reliablity of syntax must probably be attributed to the circumstance that even young children performed relatively well on this index. Little test variance and poor discriminating power across grade levels contributed to the low reliability.

Table 1

Reliability Coefficients[b] of Test Indices

1. Non Homophones	:	.87
2. Homophones	:	.87
3. Syntactic skill	:	.67
4. Word image	:	.76

[b]Cronbach's alpha

8. TWO CASE STUDIES

Earlier we argued that subjects who perform very poorly on orthography are not necessarily dyslexics. The point to be stressed here is that students performing very poorly in spelling, but with an average to normal score on the word-image scale of our diagnostic test, may be expected to profit more from specially provided instruction than poor spellers who combine this below average performance with an extremely low score on the word-image scale. These predictions were tested with two cases diagnosed by us with the test. These case studies will be presented next.

The first subject was a girl. We saw her for the first time in the initial test session. A few days later we saw the second subject, a boy. Compared with their age reference group, both subjects performed below average in spelling, confirming their negative classroom experiences. Especially the girl produced extremely low scores on all scales, with the exception of word-image. The same held for the boy, although his performance was less extreme.

Very notable, however, was that both subjects scored beyond average, as compared with their age reference group, on the word-image scale. This observation allowed us to assume that both subjects were probably not dyslexics. This was confirmed by a standard reading test (Brus & Voeten, 1972). We advised the children's parents to make appointments for additional individual instruction on the subject matter that proved to be most problematic. They followed our advice. Remedial instruction was provided for a period of one year. Remedial instruction was focused on the explicit training of the most complex aspects of Dutch orthography. These are the rules for the orthography of vowels and consonants in closed and open syllables, the training of word-specific letter codings in homophones, and mastering the complex rules of verb orthography (Assink, 1987b). Pupils were taught to correct their own work. An essential aspect of the training was that the subjects were taught to reflect on their own decision process. After a period of one year the results of the training were evaluated by retesting the subjects. The results of this retest are graphically presented in Figure 4. More detailed information on the test scores is presented in table 2. Figure 4 shows that both subjects considerably improved their syntactic and orthographic skills. As a matter of fact, the boy even succeeded to outperform the reference group.

The final grade results of the standardization study were used as a reference to evaluate the individual test score profiles of the girl and boy. The developmental trends found in the standardization study should be kept in mind when interpreting the profiles presented in fig. 4. Both subjects had poor grammatical and syntactic spelling skills. The boy had attained a higher performance than the girl, but both compensated their poor spelling ability by relying on the use of word-images, as if they were intuitive spellers. When, during remedial teaching, the boy learned more about syntax and grammar his new knowledge had a negative impact on his use of word- images as might be predicted from the developmental trend. Conversely, the girl still had so much to learn about grammar and syntax that she did not attain the word-image interference stage. She even improved her word-image based spelling strategy, while learning a lot about grammar and syntax. Unlike the girl, the boy used grammatical and syntactical knowledge actively, leading to rule confusion and domain mistakes, which had a negative effect on his word-image performance.

Table 2

Pretest, Posttest and Reference Group test scores[a]

	Syntax	Word Image	N.-Homoph.	Homophones
Girl				
Pretest	53 (84)	84 (95)	53 (69)	20 (47)
Posttest	69 (90)	91 (97)	80 (86)	44 (62)
Reference	92 (97)	70 (90)	83 (89)	58 (72)
Boy				
Pretest	78 (93)	72 (91)	77 (84)	52 (68)
Posttest	97 (99)	59 (86)	94 (96)	59 (73)
Reference	92 (97)	70 (90)	83 (89)	58 (72)

[a]Percentage scores corrected for guessing. Raw scores are presented in parentheses.

Although the girl's scores increased considerably, she did not catch up with the reference group completely. Her performance level remained slightly below average. This difference between these cases is significant. The word image scores of the two subjects show different test-retest patterns. Whereas the girl's score remains constant over a full one year period, the boy's score drops by 13%. There probably is a quite simple explanation for this phenomenon if it is realized that developmental trends often are non-linear.

After one year of instruction both subjects had made considerable progress in their command of grammatically based spelling rules. Deficits in orthographic skills can be remediated (see treatment studies cited by Berninger & Abbott in chapter 8 of this volume). Our data suggest that spelling deficits related to lack of knowledge of spelling rules are more responsive to remediation than are deficits related to insufficient knowledge of orthographic structure. Their difference with regard to word-image skill is in close agreement with the developmental curvilinear trend in the acquisition of word-images. As has been suggested earlier in this chapter, we think that the general explanation for this phenomenon must be found in the development of the underlying lexical representations that are being built up under the influence of different sources of information, such as semantic knowledge and syntactic rules.

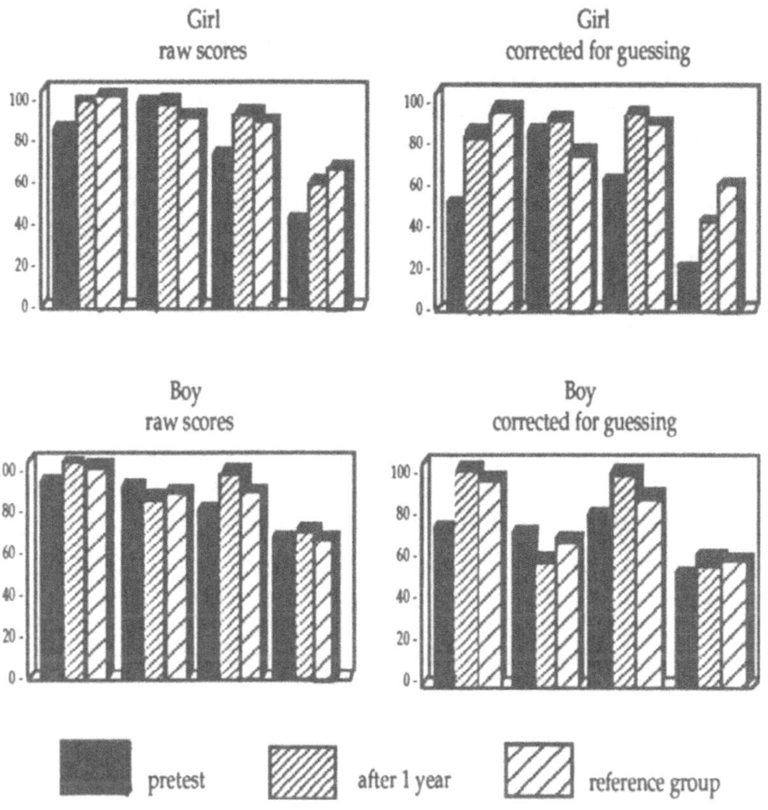

Figure 4 Case Studies:
Test/Retest Score Profiles (% Correct Solutions)

9. TEST VALIDATION RESULTS

The picture emerging from the standardization study was that syntactic knowledge and grammatical skills show a monotonous linear increase, whereas word-image skill has a curvilinear developmental trend. Moreover, syntactic skills seem to be developed quite well at early stages of development. This developmental pattern is sharply in contrast with spelling knowledge, which builds up more slowly. The general picture suggests that spelling ability, syntactic skill and word-image capacity are relatively independent components of learning to read and to spell. The word-image index, measuring the subject's capacity to detect "system-illegal" orthographic structures, might be expected to be a significantly contributing factor to individual differences in reading and spelling ability.

To test this hypothesis we collected data from a reference population of normal (n=52) and poor (n=54) readers and spellers. Grade norms are available for those who might want to use this instrument. Reading level was assessed by a standardized reading test (Brus & Voeten, 1972). Our hypothesis was that in addition to spelling performance, word-image capacity, which is a more general feature of linguistic ability (Young-Loveridge, 1985; Fisher, Shankweiler, & Liberman, 1985), was expected to account for a significant part of the between group variance. A discriminant analysis showed that our test predicted between group differences very well. As is shown in Table 3, 88% of all cases were classified correctly on the basis of their test profiles.

Table 3

Discriminant Analysis: Classification Test Results

Actual group	No. of cases	Correctly Classified
normal readers	52	46 (88 %)
poor readers	54	48 (89 %)

Percentage of grouped cases correctly classified: 88.5 %

The regression analysis demonstrates the status of word-image ability. It indicates that our test can be used as a screening instrument for diagnosing poorly performing readers and spellers. The independent contribution of word- image found in the regression analysis is not only of interest from a theoretical point of view; it also has practical consequences for instruction. It suggests that poorly spelling pupils performing on the word-image index at the age level norm will profit more from remedial instruction than individuals combining poor spelling performance with a word-image score below the age-norm. Since the studies reported here are correlational, no causal relations can be established. The point we want to make here is that word-image independently accounts for individual differences in acquiring the principles of the written code. These are two distinct types of test score profiles, corresponding with two different levels of proficiency. Therefore both types of student should receive different types of instructional programs. Pupils performing poorly on word-image as compared to their age norm should be given instruction focusing on analyzing written words into their component parts (letters, letter clusters, syllables and morphemes). Poor spellers with a normal word-image index need instruction concentrated on the relevant orthographic rules (sound- spelling correspondences and syntactic rules).

A subsequent stepwise regression analysis showed that word-image and the two spelling indices (homophones and non homophones) are related significantly to group membership, whereas syntactic skill turns out not to contribute additionally to the between group variance. The results of this analysis are presented in table 4.

Table 4

Stepwise Regression Analysis of Test Indices

Step	Variable	Beta	t	Sig t
1	Syntactic skill	.13	1.22	.23
2	Word-image	-.52	-3.51	.00
3	Spelling Nhomoph.	-.40	-2.95	.00
4	Spelling Homoph.	-.31	-2.98	.00

10. DISCUSSION

The basic idea of our diagnostic test found empirical support. Explicit knowledge of spelling rules and implicit knowledge of orthographic structure turned out to be two psychologically distinct types of verbal skill. Our test may be used to diagnose pupils on the effect of remedial teaching. The case study results also suggested that pupils may try to compensate for their deficient orthographic skills by relying exclusively on the strategy of using word-images. The strategy they use is simply matching words to entries in their mental lexicon. Grammatical rule based homophonic spelling skill, however, requires a more detailed grammatical analysis of the sentence context.

It appears that there are two discrete categories of poor readers and spellers. The first category has insufficient command of explicit spelling knowledge, but possesses normal syntactic and word-image abilities. The second category combines poor spelling with below average word-image capacity. Consequently, the last group is more backward in the process of acquiring literacy. The computerized testing materials described in this paper may be readily adapted for research on related verbal skills in the English language area. The dimensions of interest in research are primarily the level of automatized processing of orthographic information in addition to the explicit knowledge and use of rules in reading and writing.

It is our intention to add further technical improvements to our computerized test. These improvements include the option to register decision times, and enlarging format options of stimulus presentation. Additional possibilities for the display of test results are also considered in our updating plans. Our aim is to develop a useful multi purpose tool for computerized testing of verbal skills.

The results obtained on the word-image index in our validation study show a curvilinear trend. This phenomenon appears to fit well in established data on cognitive growth functions. An interesting question is why only word-image shows this trend. An answer might well be found in qualitative aspects of the mental operations involved. A possible explanation for this interesting phenomenon is that the word-image is primarily connected with implicit knowledge of orthographic structure, whereas spelling ability involves the explicit command of orthographic rules. The experienced reader has acquired a considerable body of knowledge about graphemic structure enabling him to accelerate his word perception skills. This knowledge is, however, inadequate to allow the determination of particular spellings (Henderson & Chard, 1980).

We have come across two accounts of U-shaped developmental trends in the literature. The first one is a model for the attainment of skilled word recognition, proposed by Ehri and Wilce (1979; 1983), the second one is a model for the development of language skills and cognitive processes

(Karmiloff-Smith, 1985; 1987). We briefly discuss each of these models here.

According to the model of Ehri and Wilce (1983) skilled word identification develops in three phases. In phase 1 unfamiliar words become familiar and are recognized *accurately* by readers directing their attention to component letters as they map sounds. During phase 2, as a result of more practice, familiar words come to be recognized *automatically* as wholes without attention and without deliberate processing of component letter-sound relation. In phase 3 the *speed* of processing familiar word increases to a maximum as the components involved in stimulus recognition and response production become consolidated or "unitized" in memory.

Studies exploring the conditions when word recognition becomes automatized have used a variant of the Stroop task (Stroop, 1935), the picture-word interference task. In this task subjects' speed in naming pictures is compared to their speed in naming pictures printed with distracting words which they are instructed to ignore. The reduced speed in naming the pictures, caused by interference of the printed words, is used as an automaticity index of word recognition. Ehri and Wilce (1979), as well as other researchers (Schadler & Thissen, 1981) found an inverted U-shaped interference effect, reaching its maximum in phase 2.

Ehri and Wilce (1983) explained this result as a growth effect: the expanding repertoire of printed words of the child accelerates automatization, but while "unitization" has not yet been fully accomplished this same repertoire also becomes an increasing source of interference. This effect is reduced in phase 3, when fast unitized processing eventually immunizes the skilled reader for orthographic interference.

The model of Karmiloff-Smith (1987) describes the dynamics of language development from a more general perspective. Many developmental studies on language skills, such as the acquisition of nominal determiners (definite/indefine article), pronouns, verbs, etc. have shown that children's output initially resembles the adult model. This phase is later followed by a period in which children introduce modifications that deviate from it. Later still, they revert to the adult model. According to Karmiloff-Smith (1987) this temporary *regression* should be interpreted as a sign of representational *progression*. She describes this process in a 3 phase model. In phase 1, the production of a particular linguistic form is essentially dependent on external factors. They are stored as isolated entries in memory.

In phase 2 search for a rule or principle for the implicit knowledge accumulated in phase 1 spurs development. A translation of this implicit knowledge into primary explicit knowledge is the result. However, as a result of this progression to explicit knowledge, out-of-range errors are more common during this phase than during the preceding one. During phase 3, the links or rules, established during the previous phase are reconsidered in the light of external evidence. It is at this point when conscious access becomes possible.

Although both models present a plausible account of the state of affairs, we think Karmiloff-Smith model fits better with our data. The reason for this is that the task demands implied in our word-image index exceed the demands involved in word identification. The word-image task used in our studies addressed the subject's ability to assess the orthographic legality of letter strings expressing suffixes of complex verb conjugations. The knowledge required to accomplish this exceeds a simple unitization process in memory, as described in Ehri and Wilce's (1979) model.

As to the theoretical merit of the orthographic processing indices developed in this study, we think that they may be considered as a more sensitive index for potential growth in learning basic elements of literacy. It also presents a way of looking to the role of conscious control in human language learning processes. We agree with Gombert (1992, p. 194) who argued that affirming the existence of degrees of consciousness does have the merit of directly raising the question of how this consciousness is acquired. According to Gombert (1992) and many others, consciousness should be considered as implicit knowledge which has become explicit. One of the goals in our study has been to uncover parts of the mechanism involved in this interesting transformation process for written language.

APPENDIX

Sample Test items[a] of the Computerized Verbal Ability Test

Grammatical person (1st vs. 2e/3rd):

Hij belt om te vragen wat (ik/jij) van het nieuwe boek *(vint/vind/vindt).*
[He calls to ask what (I/you) think of the new book.]

Grammatical number (singular/plural):

Kun je me zeggen, welke (jongen/jongens) vanmiddag op het plein *(speelde/speelden/speeldden)*?
[Can you tell me, which (boy/boys) (plays/played) on the square this afternoon?]

Grammatical aspect (imperfect/perfect):

Dit is de eerste keer dat me dit *(gebeurt/gebeurd/gebeurdt is)*.
[This is the first time this (happens/happened) to me.]

Grammatical tense (present/past):

Bij het vertrek (staat/stond) hij er op dat we voor de deur op hem *(wachte/wachten/wachtten)*.
[At the departure he (insists/insisted) that we should (wait/waited) for him at the door.]

Grammatical voice (active/passive):

Ik heb niet gehoord of (men) de schade *(herstelt/hersteld/hersteldt* wordt).
[I have not been informed whether the damage will be repaired.]

Attributive/predicative distinction:

Niemand ontdekte tijdens het feest de goed *(verklede/verkleedde/verkleden)* acteur.
[At the party nobody noticed the well (dressed/disguised) actor.]

[a]Homophonic choice options are included in the sample skeletons here.

NOTES

1. The Dutch secondary school system differentiates between final examinations that do or do not qualify the student for university studies.
2. Verhoeven (1979) only presents a summary of participating classes. For each education level category there were at least two participating classes.
3. The trends described in this section might equally well be qualified as "educational." Since the relative contribution of development and schooling cannot be assessed separately here, I prefer the broad term "developmental" here.
4. Hagen's data were collected in the village of Kerkrade.
5. Both the lower and the higher grades were represented by four classes.

REFERENCES

Assink, E.M.H. (1987a). De rol van grammaticale operaties bij het nemen van orthografische beslissingen. [The role of grammatical operations in orthographic decisions]. In *Spektator*, pp. 180-193.

Assink. E.M.H. (1987b). Algorithms in spelling instruction. *Journal of Educational Psychology*, 1987, 79, No. 3, 228-235.

Assink, E.M.H., Van der Linden, J., & Kattenberg, G.P.A. (1990). Syntactische intuïties bij kinderen. [Syntactic intuitions in children.] *Tijdschrift voor Ontwikkelingspsychologie, 17*, 1-16.

Berninger, V., & Abbott, R. (1994). Multiple orthographic and phonological codes in literacy acquisition: An evolving research program. In V.W. Berninger (Ed.), *The varieties of orthographic knowledge I: Theoretical and developmental issues* (pp. 277-317). Dordrecht, The Netherlands: Kluwer Academic Press.

Bowerman, M. (1982). Starting to talk worse: Clues to language acquisition from children's late speech errors. In S. Strauss (Ed.), *U-shaped behavioral growth*. New York: Academic Press.

Bowerman, M. (1985). Beyond communicative adequacy: From piecemeal knowledge to in integrated system in the child's acquisition of language. In K.E. Nelson (Ed.), *Children's language. Vol. 5.* Hillsdale, NJ: Erlbaum.

Bowey, J.A. (1986a). Syntactic awareness and verbal performance in relation to reading skill and ongoing reading comprehension monitoring. *Journal of Experimental Child Psychology, 41*, 282-299.

Bowey, J.A. (1986b). Syntactic Awareness and Verbal Performance from Preschool to Fifth Grade. *Journal of Psycholinguistic Research, 15*, 285-308.

Brus, B.Th. & Voeten, M. (1972). *Eén minuut test* [One-minute test]. Nijmegen: Berkhout.

Bryant, P.E. & Bradley, L. (1983). Why children sometimes write words they do not read. In U. Frith (Ed.), *Cognitive Processes in spelling*. London, etc.: Academic Press.

Ehri, L.C. & Wilce, L.S. (1979). Does word training increase or decrease interference on a Stroop task? *Journal of Experimental Child Psychology, 27*, 252-364.

Ehri, L.C. & Wilce, L.S. (1983). Development of word identification speed in skilled and less skilled beginning readers. *Journal of Educational Psychology, 75*, 3-18.

Fisher, F.W., Shankweiler, D. & Liberman, I.Y. (1985). Spelling proficiency and sensitivity to word structure. *Journal of Memory and Language, 24*, 423-441.

Gardner, H. & Winner, E. (1982). First intimations of artistry. In S. Straus (Ed.), *U-shaped behavioral growth*. New York: Academic Press.

Gombert, J.E. (1992). *Metalinguistic Developent*. New York, etc.: Harvester Wheatsheaf.

Hagen, A. (1981). *Standaardtaal en dialectsprekende kinderen* [Standard language and dialect speaking children]. Muiderberg: Coutinho.

Hagen, A. (1985). De relatie tussen spelvaardigheid en dialect [The relation between spelling ability and dialect]. In E.M.H. Assink & G. Verhoeven (Eds.), *Visies op spelling* (pp. 164-172). Groningen, The Netherlands: Wolters-Noordhoff.

Henderson, L. & Chard, J.(1980). The reader's implicit knowledge of orthographic structure. In U. Frith (Ed.), *Cognitive Processes in Spelling*. London: Academic Press.

Henderson, L, & Chard, J. (1983). The reader's implicit knowledge of orthographic structure. In U., Frith, (Ed.), *Cognitive Processes in spelling*. London: Academic Press.

Karmiloff-Smith, A. (1985). Language and cognitive processes from a developmental perspective. *Language and Cognitive Processes, 1,* 61-85.

Karmiloff-Smith, A. (1987). Function and process in comparing language and cognition. In M. Hickmann (Ed.), *Social and Functional Approaches to Language and Thought*. New York: Academic Press.

Klima, E.S. (1972). How alphabets might reflect language. In J.F. Kavanagh & I. Mattingly (Eds.), *Language by Ear and by Eye*. Cambridge, Mass.: MIT Press.

Schadler, M. & Thissen, D.M. (1981). The development of automatic word recognition and reading skill. *Memory & Cognition, 9,* 132-141.

Seidenberg, M.S. &McClelland, J.L. (1989). A distributed, developmental model of word recognition and naming. *Psychological Review, 96,* 523-568.

Stavy, R., Strauss, S., Orpaz, N., & Carmi, G. U-shaped behavioral growth in ratio comparisons. In S. Straus (Ed.), *U-shaped behavioral growth*. New York: Academic Press.

Strauss, S. (1982). Introduction. In S. Straus (Ed.), *U-shaped behavioral growth.* New York: Academic Press.

Stroop, J.R. (1935). Studies of interference in serial verbal reactions. *Journal of Experimental Psychology, 18,* 643-662.

Treiman, R. & Hirsh-Pasek, K.(1985). Are there qualitative differences in reading behavior between dyslexics and normal readers? *Memory & Cognition, 13,* 357-364.

Tunmer, W.E., Nesdale, A.R. & Wright, A.D. (1987). Syntactic awareness and reading acquisition. *British Journal of Developmental Psychology, 5,* 25-34.

Van Heuven, V., (1980). Aspects of Dutch orthography and reading. In J.F. Kavanagh & R.L. Venezky (Eds.), *Orthography, reading and dyslexia* (pp. 57-73). Baltimore: University Park Press.

Vellutino, F.R. & Scanlon, D.M.(1982). Verbal processing in poor and normal readers. In C.J. Brainerd & M. Pressley (Eds.), *Verbal Processes in Children: Progress in Cognitive Development Research*. New York, etc.: Springer.

Verhoeven, G., (1979). Verbeelding en werkelijkheid; Spelfouten in de opstellen uit verschillende typen van onderwijs. [Facts and fancies; spelling errors encountered in essays collected in various types of education]. In *Tijdschrift voor Taalbeheersing, 1*, pp.146-163.

Young-Loveridge, J.M. (1985). Use of orthographic structure and reading ability: What develops? *Journal of Experimental Child Psychology, 40*, 439-449.

Address correspondence to:

Egbert M. H. Assink
University of Utrecht
Heidelberglaan 2
3584 CS Utrecht
The Netherlands

MARYANNE WOLF, CLAUDIA PFEIL, RUTH LOTZ, & KATHLEEN BIDDLE

TOWARDS A MORE UNIVERSAL UNDERSTANDING OF THE DEVELOPMENTAL DYSLEXIAS: THE CONTRIBUTION OF ORTHOGRAPHIC FACTORS

Goethe wrote that only in the process of learning another language can we begin to understand our own (1810). We suggest in the present chapter that Goethe's insight is as applicable to our understanding of written language, as oral language. There exists an "implicit universalist claim" among many American researchers that their view of the reading development process, which is usually based only on the English language, describes general development of reading in all children (Wimmer & Frith, 1991). We will argue here that a similar, implicit-universalist claim dictates our notions about the causes of reading failure.

There is steadily increasing evidence that there are significant differences across languages with differing orthographies, not only in how children acquire reading, but also in the types of reading disabilities. In this paper we have two goals. First, we wish to discuss a group of studies about reading disabilities in children whose first language possesses a more regular orthography than English. Second, we will describe our own recently completed study of reading acquisition and breakdown in children in Berlin, Germany, and several provocative, preliminary results. The findings will be presented within the "Double-Deficit Hypothesis", an approach to the dyslexias that will be described later in this chapter (see Bowers, Golden, Kennedy & Young, chapter 5, this volume; Bowers & Wolf, 1993a, 1993b; Wolf & Bowers, 1994). We will use these studies to suggest that cross-linguistic comparisons of reading disabilities in languages with divergent orthographies offer a unique vehicle for sorting out some of the underlying sources of reading breakdown in the developmental dyslexias.

V.W. Berninger (ed.), The varieties of orthographic knowledge I: Theoretical and developmental issues, 137-171.

THE CRITICAL ROLE OF ORTHOGRAPHIC REGULARITY IN UNDERSTANDING READING FAILURE

For many years the work of Liberman, Liberman, Mattingly, Shankweiler (1980) and their colleagues have directed our attention to the critical role of phonological processes both in learning to read and in being unable to do so. Recently, in a cross-linguistic comparison of Italian and English-speaking children, Cossu, Shankweiler, Liberman, Katz, and Tola (1988) asked the question "whether variations in phonological structure that affect the ease or difficulty of becoming aware of critical sublexical units, in fact, also affect the ease or difficulty of learning to read" (p. 2). They believed that because different languages vary in phonological structure, there will also be differences in phonological demands on the beginning reader.

We would pose the same question with a more explicit emphasis on the degree of *orthographic regularity* represented by the writing system of a given language. There is a continuum of orthographic regularity. Some languages like Italian, Serbo-Croatian, and Finnish are highly regular and have a consistent, almost one-to-one correspondence between the graphemes or printed symbols and the phonemes, or sounds of the language. These languages are said to possess a more regular or shallow orthography. Other languages, like English, are relatively irregular. The relationships between phonemes and graphemes in such languages are described as opaque, with a given letter capable of representing several possible phonemes and the converse, where several letters can potentially represent the same phoneme (Reitsma, 1989). For example, in English as many as 19 sounds are depicted for five vowels, depending on the geographical region (Näslund, 1990). The advantage, however, of irregular languages like English is that they preserve the underlying etymological roots of given words, thus providing tiny word histories in otherwise idiosyncratically appearing spellings. (See Chomsky, 1972; Chomsky & Halle, 1968)

Based on research by Liberman, Shankweiler and their colleagues in English and on work in several other language bases, we begin this paper with two related assumptions. First, variations in orthographic regularity can affect the ease or difficulty of becoming aware of sublexical units, that, in turn, influences learning to read. In other words, differences in orthographic structure affect the degree of phonological demands placed on the developing reader. Second, in highly regular orthographies, where phonological demands are more controlled for, other, non-phonological sources of reading disruption can potentially become more visible to our investigations.

THE PHONOLOGICAL-DEFICIT HYPOTHESIS, ORTHOGRAPHY, AND THE INCIDENCE OF READING DISORDERS

Perhaps the only near consensual assumption in the field of reading disabilities is that the primary source of reading failure lies in phonological processing. Beginning with seminal work in psycholinguistics by Liberman, Liberman, Shankweiler and their colleagues (Shankweiler & Liberman, 1972; Liberman, Shankweiler, Liberman, Fowler, & Fischer, 1977) through the elegant research programs of Stanovich (1986; 1988), Perfetti (1985, 1992), Ehri (Ehri & Robbins,1992; Ehri & Wilce, 1982) and others, to the most recent reviews (e.g., Wagner, Torgeson & Rashotte, 1993), a theoretically driven conceptualization of reading disabled children has emerged. According to this view, early phonemic insensitivity and other phonologically based problems (e.g., inefficient segmentation skills) are believed to be the basis of later impaired word recognition skills, which, in turn, are seen as the critical basis for reading disability. In a review by Rack, Snowling and Olson (1992) the most typical indicator of disabled readers with impaired phonological decoding abilities is evidenced in their general inability to decode nonsense words (i.e., to apply grapheme-phoneme correspondence rules in a context-free situation).

We have long accepted the critical importance of phonological deficits in reading disabled readers, especially in English. However, we consider current, all encompassing notions about phonological deficits to be necessary, but ultimately insufficient when applied to a process as complex and multicomponential as reading; or when used to explain the extraordinary heterogeneity of impaired readers; or when assumed to explain reading breakdown in other language systems. Indeed, as we have written elsewhere, we believe that a "unified phonological theory" obscures the importance of both other potential deficits, and the presence of "non-phonological" subgroups of reading-disabled children (Bowers & Wolf, 1993a, 1993b; Wolf & Bowers, 1994). It is in the latter areas that studies of reading failure in languages that differ in orthographic regularity and type (i.e., alphabet, syllabary, logographic) are critical.

One of the more fascinating, not fully understood aspects in the comparison of reading failure across different orthographies is that the incidence of severe reading impairment remains relatively constant (from 5 to 10%) despite large differences in orthographic regularity and type of writing system (Aaron & Joshi, 1989). Based on a considerable number of studies on dyslexia across multiple languages, Aaron and Joshi (1989) conclude: "even though their incidence may vary, reading and spelling disabilities can be seen in all languages, regardless of the nature of their orthographies."(p. ix). When, for example, one compares the more irregular English alphabetic system with the relatively regular Dutch alphabetic system, the overall incidence of disorders is approximately the same (5 to 7% range) (Reitsma, 1989; Rutter, 1978).

Similarly, the incidence in the German language, whose orthography is relatively regular, is also reported in the 5 to 7 % range (Valtin, 1989). In the Italian language, whose orthography is one of the most regular of European languages, the reported incidence of severe reading failure appears slightly less than for Dutch and German (Lindgren, DeRenzi, & Richman, 1985). Accurate incidence figures for Italian are, however, complicated by few research studies. Lindgren, DeRenzi and Richman (1985) tested one group of fifth graders from Modena, Italy and one comparable group from the United States and found the incidence of dyslexia to be 3.6% and 7.3%, respectively. Other figures for developmental dyslexia in Italy range from 1.34% to 5.04% (Morchio, Ott & Pesenti, 1989). Without equitable test batteries, these figures must remain only approximations.

A more surprising comparison, perhaps, is between alphabetic and non-alphabetic systems. Stevenson, Stigler, Tucker and Lee (1982) in a cross-linguistic survey of reading problems in Taiwan, Japan, and the United States found a very similar incidence of reading failure. This finding is frequently interpreted as indicating that an alphabetic orthography is not a major source of reading problems. For example, in his reporting of these data, Reitsma concludes "that regardless of type or regularity of the orthography, some children have difficulty learning to read (possibly for different reasons!)" (Reitsma, 1989, p. 57, author's parentheses).

We would emphasize Reitsma's notion of "different reasons" further. That is, the fact that the incidence of reading failure remains relatively constant despite profound differences in orthographic regularity and type—both of which significantly affect the phonological demands placed on the beginning reader—places serious doubts on any "implicit universal" claims about phonological core deficits. Equally importantly, it raises central questions about the general explanatory power of this deficit-hypothesis as it is applied currently with English-speaking readers. If there are approximately as many cases of reading failure regardless of whether phonological demands are heavy or light,[1] then explanations based solely on phonological processes bear further scrutiny, at the least. More importantly, if there are non-phonological reasons why children in other languages fail, why shouldn't those same reasons be potential sources of failure for some English-speaking children?

Let us begin to examine these questions with the extensive evidence reviewed by Rack et al. (1992) that the most common indicator of reading disability is impaired performance on nonsense word reading. These tasks clearly tap the child's ability to apply grapheme-phoneme correspondence (GPC) rules in a context-free situation. The application of this criterion to children in other languages, however, reveals that the acquisition of GPC rules differs greatly across orthographies and by no means distinguishes impaired readers from average readers to the same degree in all languages.

Wimmer's recent (1993) data in the German language system is critical to the task of unpacking orthographic differences between languages and, in the process, uncovering potentially more universal deficit patterns across dyslexic populations. German has a relatively regular orthography; there are approximately 40 phonemes represented by 85 graphemes that consist of one to three letters (Valtin, 1989). Vowel sounds have an almost one-to-one correspondence with their graphemic representations. The more regular German orthography makes the acquisition of sound-symbol correspondence rules a simpler task for the young reader.[2] These characteristics of the German writing system provide researchers with an excellent opportunity to examine reading development and breakdown in a language where the phonological coding factors are, in essence, partially controlled.

For example, Wimmer and Frith (1991) found that the degree of regularity in an orthography made a significant difference in the accuracy with which children in the early reading stages decode real and pseudowords. Comparing English and German 7, 8 and 9 year olds, they found that error rates for German readers at 7 years were 5% (real words) and 14% (pseudowords). English children's error rates were more than triple these rates: 20% (real words); 50% (pseudowords). In addition, Wimmer, Hartl, and Moser (1990) and Näslund and Schneider (1990) showed that young German-speaking children can pronounce pseudowords with approximately the same *speed* as real words, a finding in stark contrast with young English-speaking readers. A fascinating advantage found for young English readers was on a lexical decision task where English and German children had to judge whether a pseudoword or real word was real. English-speaking children were faster to make such judgments, perhaps because our orthographic irregularity prepares the reader for some ambiguity (Wimmer & Frith, 1991)!

The most crucial finding, however, was that their severely impaired readers were not differentiated from average readers on pseudoword accuracy in Grade 2 or Grade 4. In other words, the criterion that is widely accepted as the best discriminator of poor reading in English-speaking populations (Rack, Snowling & Olson, 1992) may be inappropriate in the more regular German language. Wimmer (1993) also demonstrated that young German-speaking dyslexic readers (Grade 2 to Grade 4) have less pronounced difficulties in standard phonemic segmentation tasks (which were "high in absolute terms") and in word recognition accuracy for real words than reported for English-speaking dyslexic children. However, German-speaking dyslexic children did show significant problems in lexical access or naming-speed measures and a "pervasive speed deficit for all types of reading tasks" (p. 2, 1993). Further, digit naming-speed was the best predictor of reading differences in German dyslexic children. One potential problem in interpreting these findings concerns the criteria Wimmer (1993) used to determine dyslexic classification: that is, naming-speed differences. We will return to this issue later in the discussion.

EVIDENCE FOR A SECOND CORE DEFICIT; OR THE "DOUBLE-DEFICIT HYPOTHESIS"

Naming-speed deficits may appear more visible in German dyslexic readers, but they have long been noted in American children. An extensive body of cross-sectional and longitudinal evidence on English-speaking children indicates that the single most noted characteristic of poor readers outside their reading impairment is naming-speed problems: that is, deficiencies or disruptions in the processes underlying the precise, *rapid* access and retrieval of visually presented linguistic information (Rudel, 1985). In a recent review Lovett (1993) wrote that she "has found a deficit in visual naming-speed to be the *only* reliable nonreading correlate of a specific disability in reading speed and of the contextual reading and spelling problems associated with it" (p. 617).

The evidence for deficit-specificity for naming-speed problems in dyslexic readers is extensive and rapidly increasing. Studies include data on a) comparisons with carefully matched groups of children with and without reading disabilities; b) independence from such factors as IQ, reading exposure, and articulation; and c) independence from phonological deficits. More specifically, dyslexic children are significantly slower to name the most basic and most familiar visual symbols (i.e., letters, digits, colors, simple objects) than average peers (Bowers, Steffy & Tate, 1988; Denckla & Rudel, 1976a, 1976b; Spring & Capps, 1974; Wolf, 1982), other learning-disabled children (Denckla & Rudel, 1976b; Felton & Wood, 1989), garden-variety learning-impaired children (Ackerman & Dykman, 1993; Wolf & Obregon, 1992), attention-deficit disorder children (Ackerman & Dykman, 1993), and reading-age match children (Wolf, 1991; Wolf & Segal, 1993). Further, this deficit appears unrelated to IQ (Bowers, Steffy & Tate, 1988; Spring & Davis, 1988), rate of articulation (Ackerman & Dykman, 1993; Ellis, 1981; see, however, Nicholson & Fawcett, 1994; Wolff, Michel, & Ovrut, 1990b), memory (Bowers, Steffy & Swanson, 1986), and reading exposure (Wolf, 1991). The deficit appears differentially more powerful in serial versus discrete (or isolated) presentation (Swanson, 1989; Wagner, Torgeson & Rashotte, 1994; Wolff, Michel, Ovrut & Drake, 1990).

There have been two main problems that have prevented the more general acceptance of naming-speed deficits as core deficits in dyslexic readers: first, the issue of whether deficits are found in non-continuous or discrete naming tasks; and second, the tendency to subsume naming-speed under phonological processes. We will address each of these issues briefly and then examine whether these deficits appear in languages other than German and English.

Discrete Presentation. Perfetti, Finger, and Hogaboam (1978) questioned whether naming-speed findings were limited only to a continuous or serial form of naming-speed or whether dyslexic children were also slower to name individually presented stimuli (e.g., in a computerized, discrete-trial format). Results of their work indicated that naming-speed under discrete-trial conditions failed to differentiate good and poor reading groups. Results of newer, more extensive work (Bowers & Swanson, 1991; Levy & Hinchley, 1990; Wolff, 1992; Wolff, Michel, Ovrut, & Drake, 1990), however, indicate two findings: first, deficits in discrete-trial presentation have been found when the poor reader group is severely impaired (Bowers & Swanson, 1991; Wolff, Michel, & Ovrut, 1990a). Second, comparison between the two types of tasks are quite complex because the requirements underlying the two differ significantly (see discussion in Wolf, 1991), as evidenced in various factor analyses when isolated versus serial naming tasks are included (see Wagner, Torgeson, & Rashotte, 1994).

Perhaps the most interesting findings that bear on this distinction are recent results by a member of our lab who constructed a computerized analysis of the speech stream of dyslexic and average controls on various RAN tasks. Obregón (1994) found that dyslexic readers were remarkably similar to average probands on the duration of name articulation time and the latency required to move from one line to the next. The source of significant group difference was found largely in the time taken between stimuli, that is, the interstimulus intervals. Because discrete presentation does not include interstimulus intervals in its format, it is understandable that serial, continuous naming-speed tasks present a more sensitive index of the locus of group differences in dyslexic readers.

Naming-Speed Deficits as another Manifestation of Phonological Deficits. Although few have ever disputed the clear presence of naming-speed deficits in dyslexic children, the position of many researchers has been to explain the phenomenon of naming-speed as another manifestation of phonological problems. Thus, naming-speed has been variously described as phonological encoding (Näslund & Schneider, 1991), phonological retrieval from memory (Wagner & Torgeson, 1987), etc. My colleagues and I have argued strongly (Bowers & Wolf, 1993a, 1993b; Wolf & Bowers, 1994) against such a categorization. Our arguments have been based on: 1) the independent contribution beyond phonology of naming-speed to reading (see for example, Olson, Forsberg, & Wise, chapter 1, this volume); 2) the relative lack of correlations between naming-speed and most conventional measures of phonological processes; and 3) data from other language systems. A brief overview of these arguments is helpful.

The empirical reasons underlying our desire to differentiate naming-speed from phonological processes begin with an understanding of the complex, interrelated perceptual, cognitive, and linguistic processes underlying naming-speed operations. Briefly (for fuller description, see Wolf, 1982, 1991, 1992), visual naming-speed requires: (1) attention to the stimulus; (2) visual perception and identification; (3) conceptual knowledge of the stimulus; (4) integration of conceptual information with stored lexical (semantic and phonological) information; (5) access and retrieval of phonological label; (6) motoric activation leading to articulation; and 7) precise rapid timing both within individual subprocesses and across them (see discussions of automatic processing as a continuum in Logan, 1988; Wolf, 1991). Within this description, phonological processes clearly play a role in visual naming-speed tasks. It is equally the case that semantic fluency tasks, receptive vocabulary, and syntactic tasks have important input from phonological processes. Yet, these tasks are rarely categorized under phonological processes due to the greater emphasis on other operations. Similarly, we would argue that an increased understanding of the complexity of the underlying subprocesses of naming-speed and the differential emphasis on speed or precise, rapid timing processes (Ojemann, 1983, 1991) dictate a separate categorization.

We would go further. Our slowly evolved position is that the emphasis on phonological representation (rather than on speed of processing linguistic information) in naming-speed findings has camouflaged the fact that the *differences* between most conventional phonological measures (i.e., phonological awareness, segmentation, etc.) and most naming-speed measures (i.e., serial, continuous tasks) are more informative for understanding the complex nature of reading disability *than the shared processes*.

In a study designed in part to evaluate the presence of a large, general, phonological factor in a reading-risk population, Felton and Brown (1990) found no significant correlations between naming-speed and *all* measures of phonological processes tested (i.e., four phonological awareness tasks, one phonetic recoding in memory task, and one other task classified as phonological recoding). Of these measures, only the naming-speed measures predicted reading outcome (word identification) when IQ was controlled. Similarly, naming-speed tasks, but not memory span, were correlated with word identification in a study using a broader population reported by Torgeson, Wagner, Simmons, and Laughon (1990). Cornwall (1992) reported a modest relationship ($r=.35$, $p<.05$) between naming-speed and one measure of phonological awareness (auditory analysis task) in a reading-impaired population and differential prediction capacities for both. She concluded that "these abilities may represent unique aspects of the reading process, as opposed to an overall phonological ability" (1992, p. 537).

To summarize, the deficit in naming-speed appears to be experimentally robust, specific to dyslexic children, and not a function of IQ, articulation, or reading exposure, or subsumable under phonological processes. Thus, we believe the cumulative evidence now supports the presence of two core deficits in developmental dyslexia: one in phonological processes; and one in the processes underlying visual naming-speed. Applying our own criticism of universalist claims by others, we raise the question: what are the findings in other language systems?

NAMING-SPEED DEFICITS IN OTHER LANGUAGE SYSTEMS

Significant naming-speed deficits have been demonstrated in Dutch-speaking (Yap & van der Leij, 1991, 1993), Spanish-speaking (Novoa & Wolf, 1984; Novoa, 1988), and German-speaking children (Näslund & Schneider, 1991; Skowronek & Marx, 1989; Wimmer, 1993). The Dutch study showed that under speeded conditions, dyslexic subjects were found to differ significantly on naming and reading tasks from the reading-age control group, especially for the tasks involving pseudowords (Yap & van der Leij, 1993). Novoa (1988) studied young, bilingual-Spanish-English readers, whose first language was Spanish. She demonstrated that impaired readers in her sample had significant naming-speed deficits when compared to both average reading Spanish speakers and monolingual English children (Novoa, 1988). Within the German language, Wimmer (1993) and his colleagues have demonstrated that German-speaking dyslexic readers differ in significant ways from English-speaking dyslexic readers in their strength in some phonological areas, like phonological segmentation and pseudoword recognition, but share similar characteristics regarding pervasive naming-speed deficits. Within many of these studies the naming-speed measures were only weakly related to the phonological measures, but strongly related to both nonsense and exception word recognition.

In the German language, Wimmer (1993) found little interrelationship between naming-speed and his three measures of phonological awareness processes (i.e., respectively r=.19 with vowel substitution; r=.26 with pseudoword spelling; and r=.06 with rhyme detection). Näslund and Schneider (1990) found a modest (r=.37) relationship between naming-speed and phonological awareness tasks in their study of German readers.

Within both these studies the naming-speed measures were weakly related to the phonological measures, but strongly related to both nonsense and exception word recognition (i.e., both lexical and non-lexical routes). In English the relationship between naming-speed and reading comprehension appears to be the consequence of the shared variance with word recognition (Bowers, 1991; Spring & Davis, 1988). These relationships are yet to be studied in other languages. Such findings underscore both the difference in emphases on phonological processes between the two orthographies, and the pressing need for cross-linguistic studies, as a vehicle for clarifying sources of reading problems (Cossu, *et.al.*, 1988).

AN INVESTIGATION OF THE DOUBLE-DEFICIT HYPOTHESIS IN GERMAN READERS

The present study was designed to investigate more systematically and broadly the "pervasive speed deficit" found by Wimmer (1993) and others in German-speaking readers, using different explanatory models and different criteria for dyslexia. Specifically, we wished to examine how different criteria for dyslexic reader categorization might affect the results. For example, in an effort to test the Double-Deficit

Hypothesis, Bowers and Wolf (1993b; Wolf & Bowers, 1994) conducted a complete re-analysis of their two longitudinal data bases in Canada and the United States. They divided their subjects simply according to subjects' performance on naming-speed deficits and nonsense-word decoding deficits. Four distinct groups emerged: 1) average readers with no deficits on either; 2) a dissociated, decoding-deficit group whose naming-speed was intact; 3) a dissociated, naming-speed-deficit subgroup whose decoding was intact, but whose performance on exception words and reading comprehension was impaired; and 4) a double-deficit subgroup who were also the most severely reading-impaired group in both samples across all reading and naming-speed measures. Within these analyses we wish to emphasize that when the most common American criterion (i.e., performance on nonsense word decoding) was used solely to classify dyslexic reader membership, an entire subgroup of poor readers (with naming-speed and comprehension deficits) was not picked up because of their intact decoding skills.

Conversely, Wimmer (1993) used only a naming-speed deficit criteria in his categorization of German-speaking dyslexic readers, because nonsense words are easier to decode in the regular German orthography and because his dyslexic readers were fairly proficient on these tasks. We designed in the present study a more extensive group of nonsense-word decoding tasks in order to ascertain whether some German poor readers could be categorized on the basis of nonsense-word decoding performance alone. Thus, we sought both to apply a Double-Deficit approach to the categorization of dyslexic readers, and to replicate Wimmer's findings with German-speaking Austrian children in a sample in Berlin.

This study is, therefore, an extension of some aspects of the ground-breaking work by Wimmer (1993; Wimmer, Hartl, & Moser, 1990; Wimmer, Landerl, Linortner, & Hummer, 1991) and by Näslund and Schneider (1990, 1991). At its core are questions about the influence of orthographic regularity on phonological demands on a young reader—questions raised earlier by Liberman, Liberman, Mattingly and Shankweiler (1980) and more recently by Cossu, Shankweiler, Liberman, Katz, and Tola (1988).

In addition to the major tasks used in American research to investigate naming-speed, a series of new naming- and reading-speed instruments were designed to probe different areas of impediment to reading fluency. Performance on these tasks will be compared to performance on newly designed orthographic coding measures and on a variety of phonological measures that are modeled after tasks commonly used in German-speaking and English-speaking populations. Although the data analyses are in beginning stages only, several preliminary results will be discussed following the description of the tasks.

Subjects

In this study 84 German-speaking children from two Berlin schools of mixed SES distribution (43 in Grade 2 and 41 in Grade 4) were administered an extensive battery of naming-speed, phonological and reading measures by a German-American research assistant whose first language is German. Male-female distribution was approximately equal: 22 boys and 21 girls in Grade 2; 23 girls and 18 boys in Grade 4. All children identified by their teacher as possessing emotional, intellectual, or sensory handicaps were tested but excluded from data analyses. After attrition, bilingualism and low IQ factors were accounted for, 79 subjects were analyzed. The mean age for Grade 2 subjects was 8 years; the mean age for Grade 4 was 10 years.

Based on Wimmer's criteria of poor performance on naming-speed tasks, 6 in Grade 2 were classified as impaired readers, and 37 as average-to-able readers; 5 in Grade 4 were classified as impaired readers, 36 as average-to-able readers. Based on impaired nonsense word decoding performance as criterion 6 were classified as impaired readers in Grade 2, 37 as average-to-able readers; 5 in Grade 4 were classified as impaired and 36 as average-to-able.

MATERIALS AND METHODS

Name-Retrieval Tasks

Rapid Automatized Naming Tests (R.A.N.) or continuous-naming tests were used to measure name-access speed during serial processing and to compare retrieval of various automatized categories (letters and numbers) with nonautomatized categories (simple objects and colors). The tests measure many lower-level processes involved in both naming and reading: for example, visual recognition, symbol identification, and rapid scanning of serially presented material. Thus, the tests represent one way of "indexing the effort involved in executing lower level skills" (Swanson, 1989). The tasks included three of the original R.A.N. tests for color, letters, and numbers by Denckla and Rudel (1974, 1976a). A fourth continuous-naming set for objects was designed to control for phonological difficulty and word-frequency, as well as different semantic sets.

Each of the four continuous-naming charts consisted of five items repeated ten times in random sequence totaling 50 items: (1) high-frequency, lower-case letters (a, d, o, s, p): (2) digits (2, 4, 6, 7, 9); (3) high-frequency colors (red, yellow, green, blue, black); and (4) objects (hand, chair, dog, star, book). The objects were each monosyllabic, high-frequency, phonologically age-appropriate words and represented membership in five common semantic sets (body part, furniture, animals, objects in nature, school).

Rapid Alternating Stimulus (R.A.S) (see Wolf, 1986) naming tests were included to measure rate of processing when the extra requirements of set-switching and the use of higher-level contextual information are added. The format of the tests is identical to the R.A.N. task, except that stimuli alternate from one set to the next. Tests were administered and measured according to the Rapid Automatized Naming test format (Denckla & Rudel, 1976a). R.A.S. consisted of two versions, one being a random and the other a patterned set. The patterned R.A.S. naming task was made up of four letters, three numbers, and three colors. The pattern of the set was held constant (ABCABC etc.) to determine the potential use of contextual information to increase overall speed. In addition, the fourth graders were presented a *random* R.A.S. naming task. This test differed from the patterned version, in that a pattern for the set did not exist (ACBBA, etc.).

Phonology Tasks

For the *Kispirli Phoneme Deletion* task, which is adapted from Wimmer's "Vowel Substitution" task (Wimmer & Frith, 1992), the children were asked to replace every vowel in the words they heard with the /i/ sound. This task assesses a variety of phonological skills: auditory analysis; phoneme segmentation; phoneme recognition, deletion, and substitution. A popular

German puppet, called "Kasperle," was introduced to the children at the beginning of this testing section. Kasperle then attempted to teach the children a "Zaubersprache" (English: "secret language"). In this secret language, the sounds, /a/, /e/, /o/, and /u/ were replaced by the /i/ sound, so that the puppet's name was changed to "Kispirli" from the original "Kasperle." Three to four practice trials, which introduced the children to the secret language, began with the transformation of their own names. For example, "Hans" became "Hins" and "Anna" became "Inni." The practice trials incorporated increasingly longer and more difficult phrases. Errors were corrected during this period. The actual phoneme-deletion task consisted of seven words or phrases, which totaled a maximum of twenty-seven phonemes which were to be replaced with the /i/ sound. The responses were measured on their total accuracy and the speed of response.

The *Phonological Oddity* task, which was adapted from Wimmer's Rhyme Oddity Detection task (Wimmer & Frith, 1992), measured the children's ability to discriminate a different or odd-sounding word from a sequence of four words. The odd-sounding word deviated from the other three of each sequence, in that it contained a different sounding phoneme that could be a false rhyme formed by an incorrect consonant or vowel sound. For example, in the sequence "Grube-Stube-*Hupe*-Tube" (English: "pit-room-*horn*-tube"), "Hupe" is the phonologically odd sounding word in this sequence. In the sequence, "Nase-Hase-*Bluse*-Vase" (English: "nose-rabbit-*blouse*-vase"), "Bluse" is the oddity. Two practice trials with consecutive corrections of errors introduced the children to this task, which consisted of a total of ten four-word sequences. Before naming the odd-sounding word, the children listened to a tape recording of each group of four words two times.

Pseudo-word spelling tests involved the children's ability to transcribe phonologically regular nonsense words. The following 11 words were dictated to the children by the classroom teacher to allow maximal auditory familiarity: "dalo," "stendo," "rami," "fip," "nosti," "oplis," "panfilteus," "promechto," "fanena," "pflaunkras," and "heimobond." This spelling test was adapted from Wimmer and Frith (1992). The phonemic distance measure of Bishop (1985) was used to score the test. In this procedure, the minimal score of "zero" indicates a correct or appropriate transcription. For each incorrectly pronounced, deleted, or added phoneme, one point was added to the score. Following Wimmer's procedures, in evaluating the spelling test, phonetically similar vowel pairs (e.g., /e/ and /i/, or /u/ and /o/), which were frequently interchanged, were scored as correct. The total score was comprised of the sum of all misrepresented phonemes for the 11 pseudo-words.

The *Memory Task*, modeled after English word-span tasks (Case, Kurland & Goldberg, 1982; Daneman & Blennerhasatt, 1984), measured the children's short-term phonological memory skills. The children initially heard short and then progressively longer phrases. After hearing the phrase, they repeated it from auditory memory. One to two trial runs introduced the children to this task. The entire set was made up of five sub-sets of three sentences, each of which consisted of either two-, three-, four-, five-, or six-word phrases, totaling fifteen sentences.

Reading Tasks

The *Orthographic Coding* task represented a new measure of orthographic coding skills to assess possible differences at the letter-cluster level between impaired German readers and average cohorts. Modeled in part both after Berninger's (Berninger, 1990; Berninger, Yates & Lester, 1991) two-stimuli letter and word recognition procedures and after Peterson and Raichle's word recognition tasks with adults (Peterson, Snyder, Fox & Raichle, 1990), this task measured the accuracy of rapid perception and recognition of familiar and unfamiliar letters in varying degrees of orthographically nonpermissible and permissible sequences. Children were shown five sets of six stimuli: one set with false fonts (Russian and Hebrew letters were used to build four "letter" words); one set with orthographically nonpermissible four-letter nonwords (e.g., LZYR); one set with orthographically permissible four-letter nonwords (e.g., WIST); one set with familiar, four-letter German words (e.g., WORT); and one set with familiar German words of 5, 6, 7, and 8 letter words (e.g., LICHT). During the task the first two-letter stimulus was exposed for one second. After a 2-second interval, the second four-letter stimuli was exposed for five seconds. The child was asked to respond yes or no depending on whether the second stimulus contained two letters in the exact order found in the preceding stimulus (eg.,

Stimulus 1-XC; Stimulus 2-RXCB; or Stimulus 1-TL; Stimulus 2-ZILT).

Order of letter presentation was controlled, as was number of correct and incorrect second stimuli. Each set was presented discretely as its own unit, with two or more practices before each set presentation to insure that children understood each specific variation of the task. See Table 1.

Rapid Automatized Words (R.A.W). This reading test represented a new measure of reading automaticity. It measures the rate and accuracy of decoding the names of the same five objects, which corresponded to those of the R.A.N. naming test (book, chair, star, hand, dog). Following principles in the original work by Cattell (1886), fluency or automaticity on this task was judged by the *discrepancy* between latencies for naming and reading tasks. That is, when the latency for reading the object-words was clearly faster than for naming the pictured objects, subjects were judged as fluent for this task. The R.A.W. reading task was constructed, administered, and measured according to the R.A.N. test format (Denckla & Rudel, 1976a), where fifty stimulus items or words appear in five rows on a white chart.

Rapid Automatized Pseudowords (R.A.P.). This reading test consisted of a variation of the R.A.W. test, where the real words were replaced with pseudowords. By measuring how rapidly and accurately pseudowords were decoded, knowledge of phoneme-grapheme correspondence rules in the German language in a context-free format was assessed. The pseudowords were monosyllabic, phonologically regular, and followed German phonotactic rules. Modeled in part after Wimmer and Goswami's (in press) pseudoword tasks, stimuli differed from actual words, in that the first letter of a real word was substituted with another letter to create a nonsense word. For example, the word "Brot" (English: "bread"), was changed to "Frot." The R.AP. reading test was also constructed, administered, and measured according to the R.A.N. test format (Denckla & Rudel, 1976a).

Table 1. Battery of Tasks in German Study

Naming-speed Tasks	
Rapid Automatized Naming	(RAN) Letters Numbers Objects Colors
Rapid Alternating Stimulus	(RAS) Patterned 3-Set Random 3-Set
Phonological Tasks	
Phoneme Deletion Phonological Oddity Pseudoword Spelling Phonological Memory	
Reading Tasks	
Orthographic Coding:	False Font (Russian and Hebrew letters)
	Nonpermissible Nonwords (XYBE)
	Permissible Nonwords (PABE)
	Real Words
Rapid Automatized Words (RAW)	
Rapid Automatized Pseudowords (RAP)	
Word Recognition List:	Real Words (Accuracy and Latency) Pseudowords (Accuracy and Latency)
Reading Comprehension	

Word-recognition tasks. Modeled after Näslund and Schneider's (1991) use of Rott and Zielinski's (1985, 1986) original real words and pseudowords, these tests consisted of four individual lists of isolated real words or pseudowords. The first list was composed of 15 high-frequency nouns, the second of 15 high-frequency functor words, the third and fourth of 15 phonologically regular, monosyllabic nonsense words, selected from grade-appropriate phonic workbooks. The nonsense words tested generalization of decoding rules and use of analogies (Goswami, 1986, 1991). The pseudowords also included irregular versions of "sight" words, such as "mien" instead of "mein" (English: "mine"). Such distinctions offer valuable information on patterns of deficit in both developmental and acquired dyslexia cases. Accuracy and latencies were recorded for each list.

The Reading Comprehension test was made up of three parts and based on the Grade 2 comprehension measures designed by Näslund (1987) for the München longitudinal study (Näslund, 1990; Schneider & Näslund, 1992). Because this measure had no Grade 4 extension and because there are no general use, standardized, developmentally sequenced, comprehension tests for German elementary grades, a fourth grade version of the Näslund test was designed. The first two vocabulary sections were extended by adding more sophisticated Grade 4 vocabulary tasks. The comprehension section was comprised of increasingly complex story-passages, with four multiple-choice questions that assessed comprehension of each story. The Comprehension section was changed by incorporating an additional subset of comprehension stories based on Grade 4 vocabulary words, added grammatical complexity (e.g., increased use of varied clause and phrase structure, lengthened sentences, and overall passage length) and increased emphasis on inference in questions following each passage.

RESULTS

Although analyses are not fully completed, we will focus our remarks in this section on two sets of findings that are particularly noteworthy with regard to reading acquisition and disability.

Reading Acquisition Findings

Our major interest in the first aspect of the study was to examine the development of automaticity among German readers. Pivotal to this examination were the results on the Discrepancy Score between the latency for R.A.N. Objects naming task and the latency for the R.A.W. reading task, which, as discussed earlier, was composed of the same words or verbal labels as the objects on the R.A.N. Objects task. This score was conceptualized, sensu Cattell (1886), as a potential marker of evolving automaticity. In Grade 2 children either named objects faster than they read the words, or the scores were approximately equivalent. By Grade 4, all average readers were approximately one standard deviation faster when reading the object word, as opposed to naming the object. Reading latencies by Grade 4 poor readers were in large part the same or slower than object-naming latencies. Thus, this discrepancy measure proved a very good and very simple means of assessing the development of automaticity in word recognition processes.

A fascinating and unexpected finding concerned the Grade 2 R.A.N.- R.A.W Discrepancy score, the unexplained variation present in these scores, and the effects of reading method on developing automaticity. By fortuitous coincidence, our subjects in each grade had acquired reading by two different instructional methods. A comparison of the two Grade 2 classes was performed to examine whether differences might emerge based on method. The class that was taught with traditional German reading methods (i.e., an emphasis on structured, phonic rules in German orthography) was significantly faster on almost all reading tasks than the class taught with the relatively new, less traditional reading methods. In the latter class the teacher emphasized creative writing and the equivalent of whole-language experiences through which the child was expected to infer decoding principles.

A second comparison was performed for Grade 4 classes who had been taught by the same two approaches; no significant differences were found at this time. It appears from these findings that automaticity may be achieved more quickly in the German language through approaches that explicitly teach letter-sound correspondence rules. It also appears that by two years later these differences have largely evaporated in the majority of readers. What remains unresolved in these data are questions of the link between reading method and the effect on reading-disabled children. At an anecdotal level only, it is important to note that the Grade 2 teacher who emphasized language and creative writing was concerned that her approach had proven less successful for the weaker readers in her class. It would be of keen interest to examine in future research (both in Germany and the United States) the link between evolving automaticity (or its lag) and reading method.

Reading Disability Comparisons

Our questions in this aspect of the study concerned 1) the nature of the pervasive speed deficit in German disabled readers; and 2) possible differences in findings that were dependent on how impaired readers were classified. In the first analysis impaired readers were categorized similar to Wimmer's criterion, using a naming-speed deficit (i.e., one standard deviation below on letter-naming latency on R.A.N. letters). As discussed in the previous section, there were significant differences found between the two Grade 2 classes in the development of automaticity. To avoid in the present analyses the possible effects of reading method on development of naming-speed, we have chosen to compare only Grade 4 subjects here. In comparison with average readers, these impaired readers demonstrated: 1) pervasive speed deficits across all RAN and RAS naming tasks; 2) no significant differences on three out of the four phonological tasks (i.e., phoneme deletion, pseudoword spelling, phonological memory), although differences were found on the phonological oddity measure; 3) and in reading, a *mixed* profile with significant differences on orthographic coding tasks, word recognition latency measures (for real and pseudowords), and reading comprehension. No significant differences, however, were found for accuracy in word recognition for real or pseudowords. These results replicate and indeed extend Wimmer's (1993) findings with a German-speaking Austrian sample.

In our second analyses, Grade 4 readers were categorized according to typical American, pseudoword-performance criteria (i.e., one standard deviation below on accuracy for pseudoword-recognition lists). Results were remarkably different from our first analyses. Impaired readers, when compared to average readers, demonstrated: 1) no differences in naming-speed for R.A.N. and R.A.S. naming tasks; 2) significant differences on half of the phonological tasks (i.e., phoneme deletion and phonological oddity); and 3) a different, mixed profile on reading tasks. There were no differences on any orthographic tasks or on the latency for the Rapid Automatized Word task, but significant differences were found on latency and accuracy for all other word recognition tasks (i.e., for pseudowords and real words), and for reading comprehension. These results for German children bear little resemblance to the first analyses' results or to Wimmer's (1993) findings. They do, however, resemble the typical American profile, albeit with less pronounced phonological deficits, due to the lessened emphasis on phonological processing in German orthography. (See group summaries in Tables 2 and 3).

Table 2. German Naming-Speed Deficit Group

			Level of Significance
Naming-speed:			
	All RAN		$p < .001$
	RAS		$p < .001$
Phonological Tasks:			
	Phoneme Deletion		NS
	Pseudoword Spelling		NS
	Phonological Memory		NS
	Phonological Oddity		$p < .02$
Reading Tasks:			
	Orthographic Coding:	Pseudowords	$p < .01$
		Real Words	$p < .01$
	Word Recognition:		
	(Accuracy)	Real Words	NS
		Pseudowords	NS
	(Latency)	Real Words	$p < .001$
		Pseudowords	$p < .001$
		RAP	$p < .001$
		RAW	$p < .05$
	Comprehension		$p < .01$

Table 3. German Decoding-Deficit Group

		Level of Significance
Naming-speed:		
All RAN, RAS		NS
Phonological Tasks:		
Phoneme Deletion		p < .01
Pseudoword Spelling		NS
Phonological Memory		NS
Phonological Oddity		p < .01
Reading Tasks:		
Orthographic Coding (All)		NS
Word Recognition:		
(Accuracy)	Real Words	p < .001
	Pseudowords	p < .001
(Latency)	Real Words	p < .001
	Pseudowords	p < .001
	RAP	p < .01
	RAW	NS
Comprehension		p < .01

A more direct examination of patterns of differences between the two deficit groups is instructive. As shown in Figures 1 and 2, on most naming and reading speed tasks, the decoding-deficit group does not differ from the average readers. Only when the R.A.P.'s pseudoword-decoding requirements are included, do they differ. By contrast, the naming-speed deficit group is predictably slower than both groups on all measures involving timing, beginning at the most basic levels of letter recognition. This pattern of deficit, however, is *not* because of decoding or phonological-based problems, as suggested by some American-based researchers. The naming-speed deficit group of impaired readers is actually better than average readers in accuracy for decoding pseudowords (Figure 1), the major criterion used to classify dyslexic readers in American research, although slower in rapidly naming pseudowords (Figure 2).

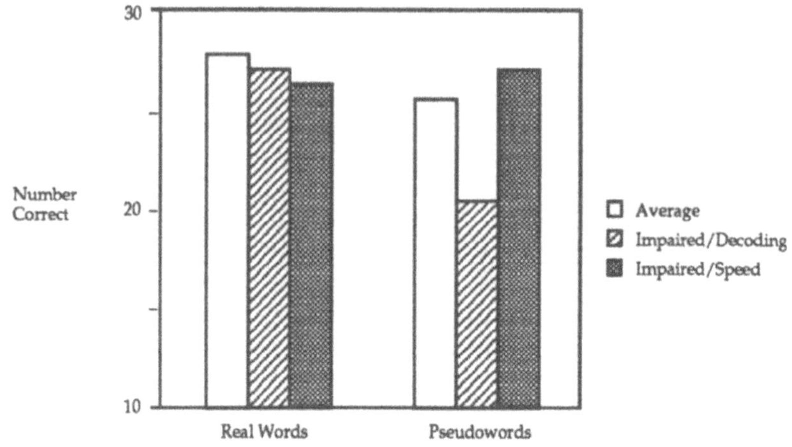

Figure 1. Decoding Accuracy, Grade 4

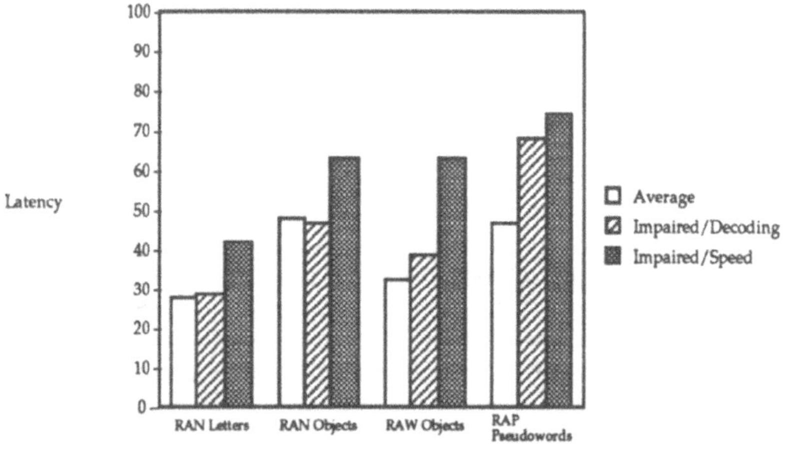

Figure 2. Naming and Reading Speed, Grade 4

The upshot is that we have several possible paths leading to reading comprehension failure among German readers, just as we do among English readers. One path appears based on deficits in the phonological coding system and closely resembles prevalent notions of reading disability among English readers. A second pattern of deficits appears closely associated with naming-speed and timing deficits and may be based on the inability of the individual processes to function in an automatic fashion, thus disrupting the precise interaction required in reading.

This study began with the notion that the regularity of German orthography would result in less pronounced phonological problems. To be sure, the decoding-deficit group was impaired less on these tasks than typical for English speaking readers, reflecting the lowered phonological demands in the learning of written German language. However, our data do not support a view of less prevalent phonological deficits among German readers. Rather, these data in the German orthography indicate that when phonological demands placed on reading are reduced by more regular orthographies, the naming-speed deficit becomes more clearly visible and a core impediment in many impaired readers, alongside a less pronounced but equally present phonological deficit in others. Most importantly, in German as in English, the very worst readers were impaired in both areas (see Bowers & Wolf, 1993a, 1993b).

The central finding is that the double-deficit conceptualization highlighted different deficit patterns of reading failure in German readers. A more universal conceptualization of reading dysfunction, at a minimum, must include both core deficits in our matrix of reading disability factors, if we are not to exclude an entire subgroup of poor readers in our diagnosis and intervention efforts.

CONCLUSIONS

The explicit purpose of this paper was to begin an examination of reading disabilities in several languages with more regular orthographies, with a special focus on the German language. Our implicit purpose was, in fact, to begin the task of going beyond the "implicit, universalist claims" about dyslexia by American researchers.

The consensual view in American research at this time is that phonological deficits are the primary source of reading failure among children. In this chapter we have gathered evidence about reading failure from orthographies whose structure places less phonological demands on the developing reader. Data bases from Dutch, Spanish, and German indicate the presence of a second core deficit, in the *processes underlying the ability* to name visually presented information under speeded conditions. Such a conceptualization, which we have termed the "Double-Deficit Hypothesis" (Bowers & Wolf, 1993a, 1993b; Wolf & Bowers, 1994; see Bowers, *et al.*, chapter 5 in this volume), does not dispute the critical importance of phonological factors in understanding reading problems, but contends that this view is insufficient to portray the heterogeneity of disabled readers and the extensively documented presence of naming-speed deficits among poor readers in various language systems.

There is growing evidence in the German language that poor readers exhibit somewhat less pronounced phonological deficit patterns, and somewhat more pronounced speed deficits in naming and reading (Näslund & Schneider, 1990; Wimmer, 1993; Wolf, 1994). The findings presented in this chapter replicate previous results and extend them. Together, these data in the German orthography indicate that when phonological demands placed on reading are reduced by more regular orthographies, the naming-speed deficit becomes more clearly visible and a core impediment in dyslexic readers. We interpret these data as partial evidence that the particular role forced upon phonological processes by English orthography has obscured the critical role played by processes underlying naming-speed. We also conclude that in the German language, as in English, the most severely impaired readers have deficits in both phonological processes and the processes underlying naming-speed, thus allowing no compensatory mechanisms to operate (Bowers et al., chapter 5, this volume).

Bowers and Wolf (1993a) have suggested that naming-speed deficits may prove to be a marker for the disruption of those automatic processes that underlie the induction of orthographic knowledge and the rapid access to lexical codes. At the very least, the double-deficit hypothesis permits a broader and, we suggest, more universal conceptualization of the dyslexias, that better incorporates the influence of orthographic factors on reading development in different language systems.

Acknowledgements

The authors wish to acknowledge with gratitude the support of the Stratford Foundation, Educational Foundation of America, and Biomedical Support Grants for the first phases of this work, and the Fulbright Research Fellowship Program for research conducted in Germany. Particular thanks is expressed to Professor Patricia Bowers at the University of Waterloo and to the members of the Tufts Developmental Neurolinguistics Laboratory: Denise Segal, Cory Lewkowicz, Mateo Obregon, Haleh Rakni and Cindy Krug.

The cooperation of the principals in Berlin, Frau Bott from Rothenburg Schule and Herr Bellusa from Kronach Schule, and their teachers, Frau Schiller, Frau Heymann, Frau Lüttge, and Frau Döring was extraordinary. They each receive our profound gratitude. Professors Renate Valtin, Heinz Wimmer, and Jan Näslund are thanked for their generous sharing of information and of tasks in designing the German component of the research.

NOTES

1. It should be noted here that in nonalphabetic writing system, such as the Japanese syllabary (Kana) and the Chinese morphemic script, we do not imply that phonologically based processing is largely alleviated. Steadily accumulating data indicates important roles for both phonological mediation and visual coding in the Chinese fluent reader (Leong, 1989; Seidenberg, 1985; Jackson, Lu, & Ju, chapter 2, this volume).
2. Although the process of reading acquisition in German may be simpler, later reading stages pose particular forms of complexity that are not found as frequently in English (e.g., the common use of very lengthy, multisyllabic words based on compounding procedures in German; for example, "Schifffahrtskapitänsmütze" for "a cruise captain's hat").

REFERENCES

Aaron, P.G. & Joshi, R.M. (1989). *Reading and writing disorders in different orthographic systems.* Boston: Luwer Academic Publishers.

Ackerman, P. & Dykman, R.A. (1993). Phonological processes, confrontation naming, and immediate memory in dyslexia. *Journal of Learning Disabilities, 26*, 597-609.

Berninger, V.W. (1990). Multiple orthographic codes: Key to alternative instructional methodologies for developing orthographic-phonological connections underlying word identification. *School Psychology Review, 19*, 518-533.

Berninger, V., Yates, C., & Lester, K. (1991). Multiple orthographic codes in reading and writing acquisition. *Reading and Writing: An Interdisciplinary Journal, 3,* 115-149.

Bishop, D.V.M. (1985). Spelling ability in congenital dysarthria: Evidence against articulatory coding in translating between phonemes and graphemes. *Cognitive Neuropsychology, 2,* 229-251.

Bowers, P.G. (1991). *Implications for reading skills of developing abilities to automatize name retrieval under varied conditions.* Paper presented at a meeting of the Society for Research in Child Development, Seattle, Washington.

Bowers, P.G., Golden, J., Kennedy, A., & Young, A. (1994). Limits upon orthographic knowledge due to processes indexed by naming-speed. In V.W. Berninger (Ed.), *The varieties of orthographic knowledge: Theoretical and developmental issues* (pp. 173-218). Dordrecht, The Netherlands: Kluwer Academic Press.

Bowers, P.G., Steffy, R., & Tate, E. (1988). Comparison of the effects of IQ control methods on memory and naming-speed predictors of reading disability. *Reading Research Quarterly, 23,* 304-309.

Bowers, P.G. & Swanson, L.B. (1991). Naming-speed deficits in reading disability: Multiple measures of a singular process. *Journal of Experimental Child Psychology, 51,* 195-219.

Bowers, P.G. & Wolf, M. (1993a). Theoretical links among naming-speed, precise timing mechanisms and orthographic skill in dyslexia. *Reading and Writing: An Interdisciplinary Journal, 5,* 69-85.

Bowers, P.G. & Wolf, M. (1993b). *A "Double-Deficit Hypothesis" for developmental reading disorders.* Paper presented to SRCD meetings, New Orleans, Louisiana.

Case, R., Kurland, D.M., & Goldberg, J. (1982). Operational efficiency and the growth of short-term memory span. *Journal of Experimental Child Psychology, 33,* 386-404.

Cattell, M. (1886). The time it takes to see and name objects. *Mind, 2,* 63-85.

Chomsky, N. (1972). *Language and Mind.* New York: Hartcourt Brace Jovanovich, Inc.

Chomsky, N. & Halle, M. (1968). *The sound pattern of English.* New York: Harper and Row.

Cornwall, A. (1992). The relationship of phonological awareness, rapid naming, and verbal memory to severe reading and spelling disability. *Journal of Learning Disability, 25*, 532-538.

Cossu, G., Shankweiler, D., Liberman, I.Y., Katz, L., & Tola, G. (1988). Awareness of phonological segments and reading ability in Italian children. *Applied Psycholinguistics, 9*, 1-16.

Daneman, M. & Blennerhassett, A. (1984). How to assess the listening comprehension skills of prereaders. *Journal of Educational Psychology, 76*, 1372-1381.

Denckla, M., & Rudel, R.G. (1974). Rapid automatized naming of pictured objects, colors, letters and numbers by normal children. *Cortex, 10*, 186-202.

Denckla, M.B. & Rudel, R.G. (1976a). Naming of objects by dyslexic and other learning-disabled children. *Brain and Language, 3*, 1-15.

Denckla, M.B. & Rudel, R.G. (1976b). Rapid automatized naming (R.A.N.): Dyslexia differentiated from other learning disabilities. *Neuropsychologia, 14*, 471-479.

Ehri, L.C. & Robbins, C. (1992). Beginners need some decoding skill to read words by analogy. *Reading Research Quarterly, 27*(1), 13-26.

Ehri, L.C. & Wilce, L.S. (1982). Development of word identification speed in skilled and less skilled beginning readers. *Journal of Educational Psychology, 7*, 3-18.

Felton, R. & Brown, I.S. (1990). Phonological processes as predictors of specific reading skills in children at risk for reading failure. *Reading and Writing: An Interdisciplinary Journal, 2*, 39-59.

Felton, R. & Wood, F. (1989). Cognitive deficits in reading deficits in reading disability and attention deficit disorder. *Journal of Learning Disabilities, 22*, 3-13.

Goethe, J.W. (1810). *Das Tagebuch*. Leipzig, Germany: A. Weigel.

Goswami, U. (1986). Children's use of analogy in learning to read: A developmental study. *Journal of Experimental Psychology, 42*, 73-83.

Goswami, U. (1991). Learning about spelling sequences: The role of onsets and rimes in analogies in reading. *Child Development, 62*, 1110-1123.

Jackson, N.E., Lu, W-H., & Ju, D. (1994). Reading Chinese and reading English: Similarities, differences, and second-language reading. In V.W. Berninger (Ed.), *The varieties of orthographic knowledge: Theoretical and developmental issues* (pp. 73-109). Dordrecht, The Netherlands: Kluwer Academic Press.

Leong, C.K. (1989). Reading and reading difficulties in a morphemic script. In P.G. Aaron & R.M. Joshi (Eds.,) *Reading and writing disorders in different orthographic systems*, (pp. 267-282). Boston, MA: Luwer Academic Publishers.

Levy, B.A. & Hinchley, J. (1990). Individual and developmental differences in acquisition of reading skills. In T.H. Carr, & B.A. Levy (Eds.), *Reading and its development: Component skills approaches*. New York: Academic Press.

Liberman, I.Y., Liberman, A.M., Mattingly, I., & Shankweiler, D. (1980). Orthography and the beginning reader. In J.F. Kavanagh & R.L. Venezky (Eds.), *Orthography, reading, and dyslexia*. Baltimore, MD: University Park Press.

Liberman, I.Y., Shankweiler, D., Liberman, A.M., Fowler,C., & Fischer, F.W. (1977). Phonetic segmentation and recoding in the beginning reader. In A.S. Reber & D.L. Scarborough (Eds.), *Toward a psychology of reading*, Hillsdale, NJ: Erlbaum.

Lindgren, S.D., DeRenzi, E., & Richman, L.C. (1985). Cross-national comparison of developmental dyslexia in Italy and the United States. *Child Development, 56*, 1404-1417.

Logan, G. (1988). Toward an instance theory of automatization. *Psychological Review, 95*, 495-527.

Lovett, M. (1993). Developmental dyslexia. In F. Boller & J. Grafman (Eds.), I. Rapin & S. Segalowitz (Section Eds.), *Handbook of neuropsychology, Vol. 7 (pp. 163-185)*. Amsterdam: Elsevier.

Mann, V.A. (1984). Longitudinal prediction and prevention of early reading difficulty. *Annals of Dyslexia, 34*, 117-136.

Morchio, B., Ott, M., & Pesenti, E. (1989). The Italian language: Developmental reading and writing problems. In P.G. Aaron & R.M. Joshi (Eds.), *Reading and writing disorders in different orthographic systems*, (pp. 143-162). Boston, MA: Luwer Academic Publishers.

Näslund, J.C. (1987). *Leseaufgaben (Reading Comprehension test for German Second Graders)*. Munich: Max Planck Institute for Psychological Research.

Näslund, J.C. (1990). The interrelationships among preschool predictors of reading acquisition for German children. *Reading and Writing: An Interdisciplinary Journal, 2,* 327-360.

Näslund, J.C. & Schneider, W. (April, 1990). *Longitudinal effects of verbal ability, memory capacity, phonological encoding and decoding speed on reading comprehension.* Paper presented at the American Education Research Association Meeting. Boston, MA.

Näslund, J.C. & Schneider, W. (1991). Longitudinal effects of verbal ability, memory capacity, and phonological awareness on reading performance. *European Journal of Psychology of Education, 4,* 375-392.

Nicholson, R.I. & Fawcett, A.J. (1994). Reaction times and dyslexia. *Quarterly Journal of Experimental Psychology, 47A* (1), 29-48.

Novoa, L. (1988). *Word-retrieval process and reading acquisition and development in bilingual and monolingual children.* Unpublished doctoral dissertation, Harvard University, Cambridge, MA.

Novoa, L., & Wolf, M. (1984). *Word-retrieval and reading in bilingual children.* Paper presented at Boston University Language Conference, Boston, MA.

Obregón, M. (1994). *Exploring naming timing patterns by dyslexic and normal readers on the serial R.A.N. task.* Unpublished thesis, Tufts University, Boston, MA.

Ojemann, G. (1983). Brain organization for language from the perspective of electrical stimulation mapping. *Behavioral Brain Sciences, 6,* 189-206.

Ojemann, G. (1991). Cortical organization of language. *The Journal of Neuroscience, 11,* 2281-2287.

Olson, R., Forsberg, H., & Wise, B. (1994). Genes, environment and the development of orthographic skills. In V. W. Berninger (Ed.), *The varieties of orthographic knowledge: Theoretical and developmental issues* (pp. 27-71). Dordrecht, The Netherlands: Kluwer Academic Press.

Perfetti, C.A. (1985). *Reading ability.* New York: Oxford University Press.

Perfetti, C.A. (1992). The representation problem in reading acquisition. In P.B. Gough, L.C. Ehri, & R. Treiman (Eds.), *Reading Acquisition* (pp. 145-174). Hillsdale, NJ: Erlbaum.

Perfetti, C.A., Finger, E., & Hogaboam, T. (1978). Sources of vocalization latency differences between skilled and less skilled young readers. *Journal of Educational Psychology, 70,* 730-739.

Petersen, S., Fox, P., Snyder, A., & Raichle, M. (1990). Activation of extrasstriate and frontal cortical areas by visual words and word-like stimuli. *Science, 249,* 1041-1044.

Rack, J.P., Snowling, M.J., & Olson, R.K. (1992). The nonword reading deficit in developmental dyslexia. *Reading Research Quarterly, 27,* 28-53.

Reitsma, P. (1989). Orthographic memory and learning to read. In P.G. Aaron & R.M. Joshi (Eds.), *Reading and writing disorders in different orthographic systems,* (pp. 51-73). Boston, MA: Luwer Academic Publishers.

Rott, C. & Zielinski, W. (1985). Vergleich der Buchstaben-und Wortlesefertigkeit guter und schwacher Leser der 2.-4. Grundschulklasse. *Zeitschrift für Entwicklungspsychologie und Pädagogische Psychologie, 2,* 150-163.

Rott, C. & Zielinski, W. (1986). Entwicklungsstufen der Lesefertigkeit in der Grundschule. *Entwicklungspsychologie und Pädagogische Psychologie, 2,* 165-175.

Rudel, R. (1985). Definition of dyslexia: Language and motor deficits. In F. Duffy & N. Geschwind (Eds.), *Dyslexia: Current status and future directions.* Boston: Little & Brown.

Rutter, M. (1978). Prevalence and type of dyslexia. In A. Benton & D. Pearl (Eds.), *Dyslexia: An Appraisal of Current Knowledge.* New York: Oxford University Press.

Seidenberg, M.S. (1985). The time course of phonological code activation in two writing systems. *Cognition, 19,* 1-30.

Schneider, W. & Näslund, J.C. (1992). Cognitive prerequisites of reading and spelling: A longitudinal approach. In A. Demetriou, M. Shayer, & A. Efklides (Eds.), *Neo-Piagetian theories of cognitive development. Implications and applications for educators* (pp. 256-274). London: Routledge.

Shankweiler, D. & Liberman, I.Y. (1972). Misreading: A search for causes. In J.F. Kavanagh & I.G. Mattingly (Eds.), *Language by ear and by eye* (pp. 293-317). Cambridge, MA: MIT Press.

Skowronek, H. & Marx, H. (1989). Early identification of risks in learning to read and write. In M. Bambring, F. Lösel, & H. Skowronek (Eds.), *Children at risk: Assessment, longitudinal research and intervention,* (pp. 268-294), Berlin: deGruyter.

Spring, C. & Capps, C. (1974). Encoding speed, rehearsal, and probed recall of dyslexic boys. *Journal of Educational Psychology, 66*, 780-786.

Spring, C. & Davis, J. (1988). Relations of digit naming-speed with three components of reading. *Applied Psycholinguistics, 9*, 315-334.

Stanovich, K. (1986). "Matthew effects" in reading: Some consequences of individual differences in acquisition of literacy. *Reading Research Quarterly, 4*, 360-407.

Stanovich, K. (1988). The dyslexic and garden-variety poor reader. The phonological-core variable difference model. *Journal of Learning Disabilities, 21*, 590-604.

Stevenson, H.W., Stigler, J.W., Tucker, G.W., & Lee, S. (1982). Reading disabilities: The case of Chinese, Japanese and English. *Child Development, 53*, 1164-1181.

Swanson, L.B. (1989). *Analyzing naming-speed-reading relationships in children.* Unpublished doctoral dissertation, University of Waterloo, Waterloo, Ontario, Canada.

Torgeson, J.K., Wagner, R.K., Simmons, K., & Laughon, P. (1990). Identifying phonological coding problems in disabled readers: Naming, counting or span measures? *Learning Disabilities Quarterly, 13*, 236-243.

Valtin, R. (1989). Dyslexia in the German language. In P.G. Aaron & R.M. Joshi (Eds.), *Reading and writing disorders in different orthographic systems,* (pp. 119-135). Boston, MA: Luwer Academic Publishers.

Wagner, R.K. & Torgeson, J.K. (1987). The nature of phonological processing and its causal role in the acquisition of reading skills. *Psychological Bulletin, 101*, 192-212.

Wagner, R.K., Torgeson, J.K., & Rashotte, C.A. (1994). The development of reading-related phonological processing abilities: New evidence of bi-directional causality from a latent variable longitudinal study. *Developmental Psychology, 30*, 73-87.

Wimmer, H. (1993). Characteristics of developmental dyslexia in a regular writing system. *Applied Psycholinguistics, 14*, 1-34.

Wimmer, H. & Frith, U. (1991). *Reading development in German and English children.* Paper presented at the developmental Conference of the British Psychological Society. Cambridge, England.

Wimmer, H. & Frith, U. (1992). *Orthographies and learning to read: An English-German comparison.* Unpublished manuscript, University of Salzburg.

Wimmer, H. & Goswami, U. (in press) *The influence of orthographic consistency on reading development: Word recognition in English and German children.*

Wimmer, H., Hartl, M., & Moser, E. (1990). Passen 'englische' Modelle des Schriftspracherwerbs auf 'deutsche' Kinder? Zweifel an der Bedeutsamkeit der logographischen Stufe. *Zeitschrift für Entwicklunfspsychologie und Pädagogische Psychologie, 22,* 136-154.

Wimmer, H., Landerl, K., Linortner, R., & Hummer, P. (1991). The relationship of phonemic awareness to reading acquisition: More consequence than precondition but still important. *Cognition, 40,* 219-249.

Wolf, M. (1982). The word-retrieval process and reading in children and aphasics. In K. Nelson (Ed.), *Children's Language* (Vol. III) (pp. 437-493). Hillsdale, NJ: Erlbaum.

Wolf, M. (1986). Rapid alternating stimulus naming in the developmental dyslexias. *Brain and Language, 27,* 360-379.

Wolf, M. (1991). Naming-speed and reading: The contribution of the cognitive neurosciences. *Reading Research Quarterly, 26,* 123-141.

Wolf, M. (1994). *The Double-Deficit Hypothesis for Developmental Dyslexia in English- and German-Speaking Children.* Unpublished manuscript.

Wolf, M. & Bowers, P.G. (1994). *The Double-Deficit Hypothesis for the developmental dyslexias: Arguments and evidence against a unified phonological theory.* Unpublished manuscript.

Wolf, M. & Obregon, M. (1992). Early naming deficits, developmental dyslexia, and a specific deficit hypothesis. *Brain and Language, 42,* 219-247.

Wolf, M. & Segal, D. (1993). *Retrieval-accuracy and Vocabulary Elaboration (R.A.V.E.): A pilot intervention program for reading disabled children.* Unpublished paper.

Wolff, P.H. (1992, September). *Impaired temporal resolution in developmental dyslexia.* Paper presented at the meeting of the New York Academy of Sciences, Rodin Remediation Academy, New York, NY.

Wolff, P., Michel, G., & Ovrut, M. (1990a). Rate variables and automatized naming in developmental dyslexia. *Brain and Language, 39,* 556-575.

Wolff, P., Michel, G., & Ovrut, M. (1990b). The timing of syllable repetitions in developmental dyslexia. *Journal of Speech and Hearing Research, 33,* 281-289.

Wolff, P., Michel, G., Ovrut, M., & Drake, C. (1990). Rate and timing precision of motor coordination in developmental dyslexia. *Developmental Psychology, 26,* 349-359.

Yap, R. & van der Leij, A. (1991, August). *Rate of elementary symbol processing in dyslexics.* Poster presented at the Rodin Conference. Berne, Switzerland.

Yap, R. & van der Leij, A. (1993). Word processing in dyslexia: An automatic coding deficit? *Reading and Writing: An Interdisciplinary Journal, 5,* 261-279.

Address correspondence to:

Maryanne Wolf
Tufts University
105 College Avenue
Medford, MA 02155-5583
USA

PATRICIA BOWERS, JONATHAN GOLDEN, ALLISON KENNEDY,
& ARLENE YOUNG

LIMITS UPON ORTHOGRAPHIC KNOWLEDGE DUE TO PROCESSES INDEXED BY NAMING SPEED

Research has clearly established the importance of phonemic sensitivity in reading acquisition, as reflected in measures such as the ability to segment words into constituent phonemes. Whether such skill plays as crucial a role in gaining orthographic knowledge, as it does in learning to decode words based on symbol-sound correspondences, is a matter of debate. Some theorists contend that poor development of letter-sound knowledge (Ehri, 1992) and insufficient reading experience or exposure to print (Stanovich, 1992) play the major roles in the orthographic skill deficits of reading disabled (RD) children. We wish to supplement this view by proposing that a largely independent individual difference factor, indexed by speed of naming simple visual symbols such as single digits or letters, has a significant effect upon learning and retrieving orthographic patterns. The reading disabled child typically has difficulties in both phonemic sensitivity and in orthographic processing. We argue that the reading disabled child's failure to abstract orthographic regularity after repeated print exposure and consequent difficulty acquiring automatic word recognition (Venezky & Massaro, 1979) may be due to slow access to letter codes as well as to the spiralling effects of initially poor decoding and restricted reading experience.

Ehri (1992, p. 120) suggests that the two routes to word recognition are distinguished primarily by the "unit that is used to locate a specific word in the lexicon: a blend of phonemes [phonological recoding route] versus a sequence of letters [visual-phonological or sight route]." Phonological recoding of print lays the groundwork for reading, but the need for recoding soon drops out, in favor of specific connections linking spelling to pronunciation and meaning, and retained in memory as orthographic images. "It is this amalgam that is accessed directly when sight words are read and recognized by means of visual-phonological connections" (Ehri, 1992, p. 120).

V.W. Berninger (ed.), The varieties of orthographic knowledge I: Theoretical and developmental issues, 173-218.

Such a systematic representation permits rapid word recognition.

This description of normal reading acquisition is a framework we adopt. However, there are (at least) two points in this description where weaknesses in processing might lead to reading disabilities: poor recoding skill and inadequate development of orthographic images. Ehri highlights the recoding weakness, and suggests that deficits here are sufficient to undermine the orthographic route as well; she does not argue for the existence of another independent individual difference source of variance in orthographic skill. Thus, Ehri's explanation of the slow and inaccurate reading of poor readers is that the recoding which lays the ground for sight words is weak, leading to incomplete analysis and poor recall. "Not only are [poor readers] unable to phonologically recode words very accurately or rapidly, but also their poor recoding skill precludes their learning to read words by sight using the cipher" (Ehri, 1992, p. 139). In a somewhat similar vein, Stanovich (1992) describes a plausible developmental sequence in which poor phonemic sensitivity and letter-sound knowledge, along with a preference for a global rather than analytic strategy of reading words, leads to poor early reading skill and less exposure to print, in or out of school. He argues that the combined effects of these variables might well explain poor orthographic skill and slow reading. While acknowledging the possibility that a problem associated with the "automatic and nonintentional induction of orthographic patterns" (Stanovich, 1988, p. 601) may exist for a small group of dyslexics, he suggests that "overly global processing," with insufficient attention to each letter, rather than some unspecified "hard-wired" process, is a more likely source of impaired ability to form orthographic representations (Stanovich, 1992, p. 321).

Perfetti's (1992) description of the importance of the quality of lexical representation in developing skilled reading is similar in many ways to Ehri's. He stressed that skilled readers have a well developed autonomous lexicon; their word recognition is not affected by context or other influences outside the lexical system, and is therefore fast and reliable. "Autonomy follows naturally from the acquisition of such [fully specified and redundant lexical] representations" (p. 162). The basis for such representations is phonemic and alphabetic knowledge, which develop in tandem. Reading practice affects reading speed mainly because it contributes to a fully specified and redundant system; a fully specified system is thereby an autonomous and fast one. Perfetti (1992) focusses upon the role of phonemic knowledge in interaction with reading in the eventual development of this autonomous lexicon.

Thus, according to Ehri's and Perfetti's models of the emergence of sight words and an autonomous lexicon, when words come to be precisely represented by their letters, they are recalled quickly. One bottleneck to precise representation is that the phonological codes for the letters and words are not adequate for the task. If the child has some difficulty sounding out a word, or recalling the precise phonemic codes, the amalgamation of the sounds to the visual representations of them is impaired or delayed, and the representation cannot be fully specified. The evidence that this is the primary impediment to achieving a precise word representation, given adequate print exposure, is somewhat indirect. Namely, it is known that reading disabled or dyslexic children, while poor in all reading skills, tend to be especially disadvantaged in the reading of nonwords. Almost by definition, decoding nonwords requires good knowledge and use of phonological codes and sound-symbol correspondences, and a willingness to use an analytic strategy to decode rather than to rely on a global (typically guessing) strategy. Furthermore, delayed development of phonological awareness is associated with slow acquisition of reading skill, and there is some evidence that early training in phonological awareness may be helpful in overcoming or preventing reading problems (e.g., Bradley & Bryant, 1985; Torgesen, Morgan, & Davis, 1992). Given the demonstrated importance of phonological awareness to reading acquisition, it has been easy to assume that the primary stumbling block to a precise orthographic representation of words (apart from inadequate levels of exposure to print) is at the sound or phonemic side of the needed correspondence. We have no wish to dispute the reciprocal relationships in the course of reading acquisition of phonological and orthographic knowledge, and thus the cost to the growth in orthographic skill of poor phonemic awareness. We merely argue for another "stumbling block" on the visual or orthographic side of the correspondence, namely processes indexed by naming speed.

Several studies have observed that orthographic skill contributes variance to word recognition above that attributable to phonological skill (Barker, Torgesen & Wagner, 1992; Cunningham & Stanovich, 1990; Manis, Szeszulski, Holt & Graves, 1990; Olson, Wise, Conners, & Rack, 1990). However, we need to learn more about the determinants of such orthographic skill. While it is obvious that some print exposure is necessary to learn orthographic patterns, the impact of extent of exposure on orthographic skill had not been documented until recently. Stanovich and West (1989) and Cunningham and Stanovich (1990) have related variability in out-of-school reading, indexed by indirect measures of print exposure, specifically to orthographic skill. Nevertheless, there remains unexplained variance in orthographic processing skill even after controlling for variables such as IQ, memory, phonological processing and print exposure, in samples of children and adults unselected for reading ability (Barker et al., 1992; Cunningham & Stanovich, 1990; Stanovich & West, 1989; Wagner & Barker, chapter 7, this volume). Perhaps this "unexplained" variance assumes greater importance in reading disabled samples. Such a possibility is supported by the greater independence of phonological and orthographic skills within a sample of disabled readers than within normal readers (Olson et al., 1990), suggesting more "room" for the operation of additional factors affecting orthographic skill in disabled readers.

Rather than accepting the view that the "unexplained" variance may be due to as yet unmeasured practice effects or strategy differences (Barker et al., 1992), we have pursued the hypothesis that a well-known but somewhat isolated literature concerning the relationship between reading and automatized naming (Denckla & Rudel, 1974; 1976; Wolf, 1991) is relevant to understanding the role of orthographic skill in reading. The focus of the research done in our lab over the last several years can be conceptualized as an expansion of the model elaborated by Ehri (1992), an extension designed to better account for the failure of reading disabled children to achieve fluent word recognition, even of well-practiced words. Our hypothesis has been that poor phonological sensitivity is not a sufficient individual difference explanation for reading disabled children's lack of fluency, although it may well be a contributing factor. Along with Wagner and Barker (chapter 7, this volume), we believe that orthographic skill and text fluency are closely related. A number of empirical findings lead us to this revised account of fluent reading. These include the large differences between reading disabled and normally reading children in speed of reading words, even when reading practice is constant across groups (Ehri & Wilce, 1983; Manis, 1985; Reitsma, 1983), the remarkably low level of correlation of phonemic skill with growth in speed of recognition under controlled conditions (Reitsma, 1989; Bowers & Kennedy, 1993), and the commonly reported finding that reading disabled and normally achieving children differ on the speed of naming simple digits, a task not involving phonemic sensitivity. We hypothesize that the processes involved in creating reliable individual differences on a simple digit naming speed test affect equally the speed of recognizing letters; slow symbol recognition might be involved in the slow and limited growth in orthographic skill among very poor readers, and therefore contributes to a nonfluent reading style. We are beginning to develop evidence that supports our view. Given naming speed within a broad "normal" range, the chief "internal" block to skilled sight word reading may well be insufficiently precise phonemic information. However, we will argue that reading disabled children (and some other readers) often have naming speeds slower than this range, indicating the presence of an additional weakness that independently as well as interactively interferes with forming precise orthographic representations of words and accessing them (remembering them) efficiently. (However, see Olson et al., chapter 1, this volume, for an alternative view.)

WHY IS NAMING SPEED FOR VISUAL SYMBOLS CORRELATED WITH READING?

Given our hypothesis of such an important role for the processes indexed by naming speed, we must document some of the reasons for its prominence in our theory. (A more complete review may be found in Wolf, 1991, and Bowers & Wolf, 1993b.) Denckla and Rudel (1974; 1976) demonstrated that reading disabled children differed from normally reading children on the speed with which they named common numbers, letters, color patches and line drawings of objects, arrayed on cards in a continuous list. Denckla and Rudel's task, referred to as Rapid Automatized Naming (R.A.N.), consists of five target items arrayed in five rows of ten items. Spring and Capps (1974) also showed differences in continuous-list digit naming speed between reading disabled and normally achieving students, and presented some evidence that such differences were associated with the dysfunctional rehearsal and memory processes of these children.

Wolf and her colleagues (Wolf, 1984; Wolf, Bally & Morris, 1986) reviewed and extended this work, showing that the power of non-graphological naming speed tests (R.A.N. colors and objects) for predicting reader levels diminished after kindergarten, while R.A.N. numbers and letters continued to predict reading from kindergarten through Grade 2. Spring and Davis (1988) further demonstrated that digit naming speed correlated with accuracy of both irregular-word and nonsense-word reading of older children, despite evidence that these words were processed in different ways. Biemiller (1977-78) and Lovett (1987) showed that continuous-list naming speed was correlated with a variety of reading measures, including speed of identifying printed words. The naming speed deficit associated with reading disability is long lasting. Not only is retest reliability over a two year span about .85 (Bowers & Wolf, 1993b), adults who were reading disabled as children continue to name R.A.N. items more slowly than adults classified as either nondisabled or as borderline disabled in childhood (Felton, Naylor & Wood, 1990).

Of course, correlation with reading skill does not isolate the basis for that correlation. Ellis and Miles (1981) presented evidence that reading disabled children did not differ from normally achieving children on measures of articulation speed, simple visual matching time, or two choice reaction time, even though their lexical access speed was slower. (However, Nicolson & Fawcett [in press] did find differences between dyslexics and controls on choice reaction time, despite there being no difference between groups on a measure of simple reaction time.) Research by Felton, Wood, Brown and Campbell (1987) narrowed further the possible sources of the relationship, by showing that children with Attention Deficit Disorder do not have naming speed deficits unless there is an accompanying reading disability. But the task of identifying what is *not* responsible for the relationship between reading and naming speed is far from complete.

ROLES OF TASK COMPLEXITY AND SAMPLE CHARACTERISTICS IN NAMING - READING CORRELATION

If the crucial variable tapped by naming items on continuous lists is simply speed of retrieving the name of individual items, or lexical access speed (Ellis & Miles, 1981), presenting those items discretely by computer should result in a more refined measurement of retrieval time, or latency to begin pronouncing the name. Yet instead of increasing the power of the discrimination of reader groups, research using this method has had mixed results. Perfetti, Finger and Hogaboam (1978), Stanovich (1981), and Stanovich, Feeman and Cunningham (1983) used a discrete-trial methodology to assess naming speed. They found that latency to correct identification of discretely-presented single digits or letters did not always correlate significantly with reading. In a later study with a similar pattern of data, Stanovich, Nathan, and Zolman (1988) found correlations of only .34 and .36 between letter naming speed on discrete trials and reading comprehension in 3rd and 7th grade children, and no relationship among 5th graders. In subsamples of different grades matched for reading comprehension, discrete-trial letter naming speed correlated with age somewhat better than it did with reading skill, leading the authors to discount its importance to reading disability. Stanovich et al. (1983, p. 200) suggested that naming continuous lists requires more complex responses than naming single items, including "...scanning, sequential response, and motor-production strategies which could differentiate good from poor readers." Hence, they argued that speed of naming such lists should not be considered a good measure of automaticity of name retrieval per se.

Yet, reader group differences using discrete-trial methodology have been documented in some samples. Ehri and Wilce (1983) reported that discrete-trial latencies for digits and pictures of objects as well as words are slower for less skilled readers in Grades 1, 2 and 4. Levy and Hinchley (1990) found poor readers in grades 3 to 6 slower to name discretely-presented object drawings. Among samples of kindergarten and second grade children unselected for reading ability, Walsh, Price and Gillingham (1988) reported that discrete-trial letter naming speed predicted the later reading level of kindergarten but not grade 2 children. They argued for the "transitory" importance of efficient retrieval of letter names per se.

Such varied findings meant we must understand not only differences between results of studies using continuous lists and discrete trials, but also differences among discrete-trial studies. One dimension underlying some of the differences in the strength of the naming speed-reading relationship within the latter studies may be the degree of reading disability of the poorer readers. This dimension may also account for discrepancies between studies using continuous-list and discrete-trial methods, since continuous-list studies tend to sample more severely disabled readers than discrete-trial studies.

Thus, the degree of complexity of the naming task and the nature of the reading groups being discriminated may underlie the differential results obtained in studies employing discrete vs. continuous formats for measuring naming speed. Developing a more precise hypothesis about the nature of the complexity involved on continuous lists, Spring and Davis (1988) suggested that the discrepancy sometimes found between correlations of reading skills with naming speed measured on continuous lists vs. discrete trials might be due to the ability of good readers to overlap different stages in naming items. They argued that good readers named the target while partially processing information to the right of it, while poor readers were restricted to serial processing. Continuous lists gave the opportunity to make use of such parallel processing; discrete trials did not.

Both complexity and subject selection issues were addressed in our lab by Swanson (1989). She compared continuous lists for six digits, six letters and six colors, with the same items presented in several discrete presentation formats on computer. Swanson increased discrete-trial task complexity in two steps. In addition to a standard discrete-trial format of a relatively long interstimulus interval (ISI) between a child's response and the next target, the child named both a single target with no "rest" between items (very brief ISI between response and new target) and also a central target item in a three-item array, also with no rest between items. A hypothesis similar to Spring and Davis' (1988) was explored by including two types of complex, three-item, array. Conditions were devised in which 1) the item to the right of the target (the third item in each array) became a central target item in the next array (relevant condition), and 2) the adjacent item in one array was not the target in the next (irrelevant condition). To discover ages and reader groups in which each format had power to discriminate, poor, average, and good readers in grades 1, 3, and 6 were studied.

The speed of naming digits and letters on both discrete trials and continuous lists discriminated the poor and average reading groups across all grades; average and good readers were discriminated only on the continuous lists, and less strongly than poor and average reader groups. Speed of naming color patches discriminated poor and average readers only in Grade 1. When entered into multiple regression analyses, the speed of naming symbols under the simplest condition (i.e., single symbols presented with a relatively long ISI) accounted for much of the variance in the discrimination of poor and average readers by continuous lists. Both continuous-list and discrete-trial methods appear to tap the single name retrieval automaticity thought to be important to reading. However, the data indicated older (Grade 6) poor readers were better discriminated from average readers by the continuous lists or by the more complex conditions for measuring single item identification speed than by the simplest discrete-trial condition. Contrary to the hypotheses offered by both Spring and Davis (1988) and Swanson (1989), little evidence was obtained that processing of items to the right of the target was involved in reader differences.

Bowers and Swanson (1991) and Bowers (1994) further explored the parameters of naming speed for digits and letters on discrete trials and continuous lists among poor and average readers in a longitudinal study in grades 2, 3, and 4. The level of complexity of discrete presentations was increased and more systematically studied by embedding the target to be named in an array of five items, with the three items to the right of the target being either relevant or irrelevant to the next target, and with ISIs between a child's response and the next array being either long (1.25 sec) or very brief (approximately 3 msec.) Single item presentations with long and brief ISIs were the same as in Swanson (1989). Poor, Moderately Poor and Good Reader groups were defined by children's Grade 4 scores on a test of word identification. Analyses revealed significant effects of reader group not only on speed of naming symbols on continuous lists but also on latency of naming those symbols presented on discrete trials. However, neither type of discrete trial array nor length of ISI interacted with reader group to affect latency of response. Children were faster naming isolated items than naming items embedded in either relevant or irrelevant arrays, but the type of multiple array made no difference to their latencies, confirming Swanson's (1989) study.[1] Brief ISIs tended to impede quick responding in early grades but did not affect responses in Grade 4.

Continuous-list and discrete-trial formats for naming showed similar patterns of response. Scores from the list format correlated highly with the discrete format, for example, in Grade 4, r=.74 for a composite discrete-item measure, and .64 for the commonly used condition of single item presentation with longer ISI. Hierarchical regression analyses predicting five reading measures indicated that the continuous list not only incorporated virtually all the reading-related variance of discrete-trial latencies, but also contributed some unique variance to measures of reading accuracy, although not reading speed. Perhaps there is some additional role for the coordination of naming processes (tapped by list format) in decoding words and nonwords.

It is the most disabled readers, however, who are particularly slow to name symbols. On all formats tapping naming speed, the poor readers (below the 25th percentile on Word Identification scores) were slower than both the moderately poor (between the 26th and 35th percentiles) and good readers (above the 35th percentile), while the latter groups did not differ from one another. Figure 1 portrays the latencies for discrete-trial digit naming for each group, under two ISI conditions. Note that the latencies are reported for groups defined by their Grade 4 scores, when these children were in Grades 2, 3, and 4. In samples with very few poor readers, slow naming may lose its predictive ability.

There is additional evidence that reading disabled children's slow speed of naming symbols is not restricted to continuous-list performances. Yap and Van der Leij (1991) presented digits under varying conditions of discrete trials to dyslexics and chronological age and reading age controls matched on number of words read correctly in one minute on a standardized test. Dyslexics were less accurate than controls when two stimuli had to be processed within a 200 msec frame. Yap and Van der Leij (1993) presented subjects with words and pseudowords on discrete trials under either speeded (stimuli masked after 200 msec) or unspeeded (stimuli available until response made) conditions. Accuracy of responses of reading age control groups, whether consisting of normally achieving readers or moderately poor readers, were affected similarly by the restriction of time for processing targets, while dyslexic readers' pseudoword naming was much more affected by the time restriction. Interestingly, speeded processing adversely affected dyslexics more than it did some of the control groups on audio-visual matching and lexical decision tasks as well as

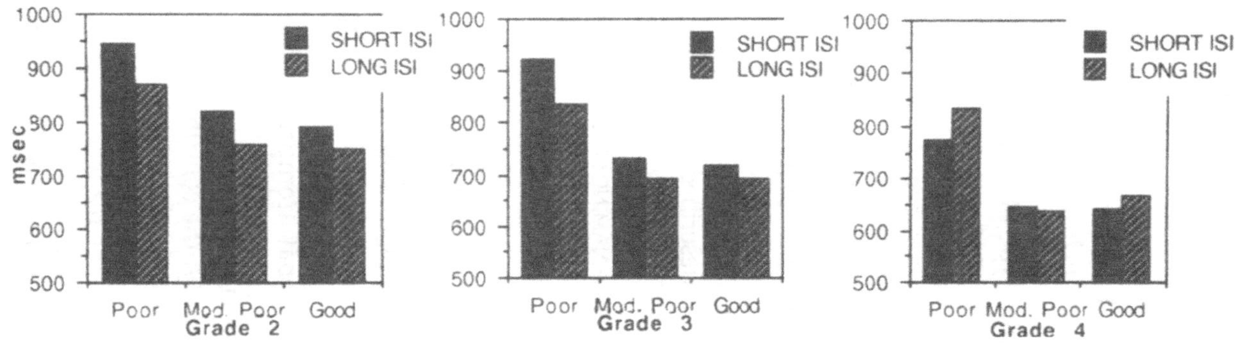

Figure 1
Latencies for discrete-trial naming of digits for each ISI length across type of array, for each year of longitudinal study. Reader groups are defined by Grade 4 reading scores.

naming tasks. This pattern led the authors to suggest cautiously the presence of both phonological and automatization deficits. Wolff, Michel, and Ovrut (1990) studied dyslexic adolescents and showed that R.A.N. continuous-list object and color speed was highly correlated (.79 for adolescents; .81 for adults) with errors made on the same stimuli when they were presented discretely on a film, with either exposure duration limited or speed of film presentation increased. When the stimuli were presented at slow speeds *and* with long exposure durations, neither dyslexics nor controls made many errors and therefore did not differ, but when either type of speeded presentation occurred, the number of errors made was correlated with speed of naming items on R.A.N. continuous lists, a condition in which typically few errors occur presumably because the subject adjusts his/her time to avoid errors.

In short, our favored hypothesis asserts that tests of rapid naming of symbols are associated with reading largely because slow speed on such tests marks an inability to identify graphemes sufficiently quickly to support efficient word recognition. While this hypothesis has survived some of the challenges against it, as described above, there are several other plausible alternative explanations of the relationship.

ALTERNATE ACCOUNTS OF NAMING SPEED-READING RELATIONSHIPS

Role of IQ

Is it possible that IQ plays some role in the naming speed deficits of reading disabled children? Results in ours and others' laboratories strongly suggest this is not the case. For example, in a clinic sample of children aged 8 to 11 (Bowers, Steffy & Tate, 1988), continuous-list naming speed predicted reading skill controlling for variance in reading contributed by Kaufman's (1979) Verbal Comprehension and Perceptual Organization factor scores for the Wechsler Intelligence Scale for Children-Revised (WISC-R) (Wechsler, 1974). In Bowers' (1994) longitudinal study, the contribution of naming speed to reading is independent of the contribution of WISC-R Vocabulary (which correlates highly with Verbal IQ) within a sample of poor and average readers in a public school. In fact, Wolf (1991) reported that her normal IQ sample of specific dyslexics had slower naming speed than "garden-variety" poor readers, with lower IQs than the dyslexics.

Role of Word Finding

A more difficult question to answer is whether the simple symbol naming *speed* measure is tapping a broader word finding problem, one that shows itself on tests of confrontation naming such as the Boston Naming Test. On such tests, children are shown line drawings of common objects and their task is to provide the name of the object. Accuracy rather than speed is required, whereas on tests of digit or letter naming, accuracy is at ceiling levels and only speed differentiates good and poor readers. Wolf (1984) describes a pattern of data in which dyslexics often have both naming speed and confrontation naming deficits; however, the measures are correlated differentially to reading subskills, with naming speed contributing more to lower level reading skill while the ability to retrieve a specific name accurately is more strongly related to reading comprehension. Badian (1993) studied a sample of children evaluated for possible reading difficulties but who were classified as adequate vs. poor readers. While these groups differed markedly on R.A.N. speed to name letters and objects, they did not differ significantly on the Boston Naming Test. Felton and Brown (1990) report insignificant relationships between Boston Naming Test scores in Kindergarten and reading scores one year later, in a sample thought in Kindergarten to be at some risk for poor reading; R.A.N. scores in kindergarten for these same children did predict later reading.

However, a study with a different design yielded contrasting results. Murphy, Pollatsek and Well (1988) chose dyslexics with especially slow R.A.N. scores and found that they also had other oral language dysfunctions, including more errors on the Boston Naming Test and fewer words used to retell a story they had heard. In addition, they describe the children as having particular difficulty using a direct, sight word route to reading (as indicated by lexical decision tests) and being more reliant on an indirect, phonological assembly route, a pattern conceptualized as due to a deficit in the visual input logogen system. Murphy et al. suggest that the deficits in an output logogen may be associated with both R.A.N. and the expressive language difficulties. An alternative explanation of their data, however, in keeping with the theoretical story being developed here, is that the R.A.N. is implicated in the other deficit shown by their sample, the inadequate development of the direct route. Unfortunately, there is no way to disentangle the several deficits in children in this study, since no comparison group of poor readers with higher R.A.N. scores was included. As well, the poorest readers may well be those children with independent and additive difficulties in these areas. Our current view is that children with word finding difficulties may well be poor readers and slow on R.A.N., but the converse may not be true. If a child has word finding problems, he or she may be slow in retrieving names that are correct, and therefore may also be slow on R.A.N. However, other children are slower to name the most common symbols, without errors of retrieval on confrontation naming tasks; when this occurs, the slower R.A.N. may reflect a quite different problem.

Role of Phonological Abilities

Finally, is there reason to believe that naming speed is part of a phonological weakness that shows itself in *both* poor phonemic sensitivity and slow retrieval of names for visual material? Wagner and Torgesen (1987) categorize phonological skill into phonological awareness, phonological recoding in lexical access, and phonetic recoding in working memory. Tests of rapid naming are classified as tapping phonological recoding in lexical access. Findings reviewed below underline the independence of these categories, and argue against the usefulness of focussing on the phonological aspects of symbol naming speed to the exclusion of its visual and speed components. (See Wolf et al., Chapter 4, this volume, for a more complete presentation of this argument.) We believe that differences between kinds of phonological tasks may be more important than their similarities, a possibility obscured by focussing on naming speed's phonological properties. Our work has instead spoken to task *differences* and the independence of rapid naming from either phonemic sensitivity or verbal short term memory, rather than focussing on the fact that some sort of phonological representation is no doubt involved in all three tasks.

Phonemic Awareness. In reference to reading acquisition and reading disability, it is sensitivity to individual phonemes in words that has been associated with precise representation of orthographic information. Only by studying both phonemic sensitivity and naming speed in the same sample can we learn whether individual differences in phonemic sensitivity account for naming speed-reading relationships. That these tasks contribute independent variance to reading was first shown by Blachman (1984) and Mann (1984). Felton and Brown (1990), Badian (1993), Bowers (1994), Bowers and Swanson (1991), Cornwall (1992) and Wimmer (1993) are among others documenting this independence using various tasks. In our work, we have typically measured both naming speed for digits and letters and several kinds of phonological awareness skill, such as sound categorization and phoneme deletion (Bowers, 1994). Among the tests of phonological awareness, phoneme deletion (Auditory Analysis Test, Rosner & Simon, 1971) has correlated more strongly than other tests with reading, perhaps because ceiling effects on easier tests appear to attenuate relationships. We have found phoneme deletion and rapid naming skills to be modestly related, in the .3 range, and to be related differentially to various reading skills.

Fewer than half the children categorized as poor readers when in Grade 2 retained their poor reader status when in Grade 4, making Grade 4 reading scores the better criterion for evaluating the role of earlier skills. Analyses were conducted to explore how well phonemic and naming speed skills assessed in early Grade 2 predicted reading in Grade 4. Table 1 presents results of commonality analyses (Pedhazur, 1982) based on hierarchical regression analyses for a sample of 38 children in Grade 4 who were originally chosen as poor and average readers in the same six classes in Grade 2. Presented are the estimates of variance (R^2 change) contributing to several Grade 4 reading tests by Grade 2 predictors. A variable's unique contribution represents the additional variance accounted for when it is entered at Step 3.

Typically, naming speed is related least strongly to nonword reading accuracy and most strongly to word reading latency, while the opposite pattern is present for phonemic awareness, as indicated by the Auditory Analysis Test. Phonological awareness skill is implicated very little in latency for correct recognition of easy, highly frequent words. Moreover, these contributions to reading skills are reasonably independent. This pattern of results is found at each grade level in the longitudinal sample, as well as in predicting from Grade 2 naming speed and phoneme deletion to Grade 4 reading. In some analyses, there is an interaction of naming speed and phoneme deletion in predicting latency for recognizing moderately frequent words, such that when naming speed is fast, word recognition is fast, regardless of phoneme deletion score, but when naming speed is slow, phoneme deletion skill contributes to faster word recognition. Thus, children low on both skills are particularly slow to identify these words.

Table 1.

Hierarchical regression analyses predicting Grade 4 reading from Grade 2 variables: Total Variance contributed to Grade 4 reading by Grade 2 WISC-R Vocabulary; Common and unique variance contributed to Grade 4 reading by Grade 2 Digit Naming Speed (DNS) and Auditory Analysis Test (AAT).

Variable	Word Ident.[a]	Word Attack[a]	Pas. Comp.[b]	Easy Word lat.[c]	Harder Word lat.[d]
Vocab: Total	.18	.10	.25	.00	.05
DNS and AAT:					
Common	.10	.10	.06	.11	.10
DNS: Unique	.06+	.04	.10*	.28***	.29***
AAT: Unique	.11*	.22**	.03	.04	.03
Interaction of DNS X AAT	.06+	.02	.05+	.04	.09*

[a] Subtest of Woodcock Reading Mastery Test (Woodcock, 1973). [b] Subtest of Woodcock Reading Mastery Test-Revised (Woodcock, 1987). [c] Words taken from Olson et al. (1985). [d] Words taken from list of moderately frequent words (Lovett, Ransby & Barron, 1988).
+ $p < .1$, *$p < .05$, **$p < .01$; ***$p < .001$, indicating significance level of the unique contribution of DNS, AAT, and their interaction.

A similar differential pattern occurred with respect to several measures of text reading proficiency in the same sample (Bowers, 1993). Although phoneme deletion was related to the number of errors made on a given passage, it was not strongly related to the number of words read per minute on that passage. Conversely, naming speed contributed to errors less strongly than did phoneme deletion, but was related much more strongly to words read per minute. More intriguing still, naming speed was related to words/minute even when a child's score on a standardized test of word identification was controlled. Moreover, when children practiced reading the text several times, text speed after practice was a function not only of speed before practice (as expected, a very strong effect) but also of naming speed to a small but significant extent. This finding was especially true for children whose reading speeds were slower initially, suggesting that among slower readers, the child with slower speed to name symbols benefitted slightly less than faster naming peers from each additional practice with text. Phoneme deletion scores were not related to gains in text speed.

Young and Bowers (1994) also looked at the role of naming speed in fluent, expressive reading of fifth grade children who were poor or average readers. A major question addressed in this study was the role of the difficulty level of the text in determining the expressiveness of reading it. If poor readers read sufficiently easy text, will their reading style be similar to that of average readers reading much more difficult text? Raters assigned scores for each child's oral readings according to Allington's (1983) Fluency Scale. Scores ranged from 1 (word by word reading) to 6 (read in phrases...expression approximates normal speech). Results showed that average readers performed significantly better than poor readers in terms of accuracy, reading rate, and fluency over all levels of text difficulty (i.e., readability levels of text estimated at grades 2, 3 and 5). Even when poor readers were given prior practice reading words (in isolation) on the easiest text, so that accuracy of poor readers on Grade 2 text and average readers on Grade 5 text was equally high, the poor reader group read their easy text more slowly than average readers read their harder text. Controlling statistically for these speed differences, the poor readers were still significantly less expressive and fluent when reading the easiest text than the average readers were on grade appropriate text. Digit naming speed was strongly associated with text speed and ratings of fluency independently of Word Identification and phoneme deletion skill. Phoneme deletion's contribution to fluency was common to that contributed by word identification. The poor readers in this sample also took part in a training study to explore the impact of different treatment conditions on fluency (Young, 1993). In a fashion similar to Bowers (1993a), naming speed but not phoneme deletion predicted additional variance to posttest reading speed and fluency, even after controlling for pretest values on these measures.

Verbal Memory. Wagner and Torgesen (1987) also list phonetic recoding in working memory as a third type of phonological skill. Does rapid naming reflect or affect skills involved in verbal short term memory? The results of studies of this topic are mixed. Spring and Capps (1974) and Spring and Perry (1983) suggested these were closely related processes, as did the review by Dempster (1981) indicating that item identification speed is related to short term memory skill. However, studies by Bowers (1994), Bowers et al. (1988), Cornwall (1992), Felton and Brown (1990) and Wimmer (1993) did not find significant relationships between rapid naming and verbal digit span and/or sentence memory in their samples selected to study reading disability. In fact, in Bowers et al. (1988) and Cornwall (1992), digit span was more highly related to word attack skills than other reading measures, a pattern of relationship quite different from that found for rapid naming tests.

Conclusion of Search for Alternate Account

This review of the literature on the relationships among various predictors of reading skill has persuaded us that rapid naming tests are related to reading independently of other well-established predictors. We have concluded that the continuous-list task discriminates the poorest readers from somewhat better readers for largely similar reasons as do discrete-item tasks; they both appear to tap the speed to access names of highly automatized printed symbols. Moreover, speed on both formats is more highly correlated with measures of reading speed than with other reading skills (Bowers & Swanson, 1991; Bowers, 1994). The continuous-list naming speed tasks tend to correlate somewhat more strongly with word identification accuracy measures than do discrete trial measures, especially in older readers. Perhaps this difference is related to the fact that occasional errors on continuous lists are considered "process indicative" (Rudel, as cited in Wolf, 1991) and may add to the sensitivity of the continuous list in its discrimination of reader groups. In contrast, discrete trials with errors or self corrections are dropped from analyses. Consequently, we have been content to employ the very easily administered continuous-list task in our studies of naming speed.

WHAT ARE THE IMPLICATIONS OF SLOW READING?

As indicated above, digit or letter naming speed correlates with many measures of reading proficiency using both accuracy and speed criteria (Spring & Davis, 1988; Wolf et al., 1986). However, digit or letter naming speed is especially strongly correlated with the speed of identifying isolated words (Bowers & Swanson, 1991; Bowers, 1994; Levy & Hinchley, 1990; Lovett, 1987) or speed of reading text (Biemiller, 1977-78; Bowers, 1993; Cornwall, 1992). For example, Bowers (1994) reported that Grade 4 correlations of digit naming speed and latency for correct recognition of highly frequent and moderately frequent words presented in isolation by computer were .69 and .63, respectively. Indeed, evidence from our lab suggests that naming speed's relationship to untimed reading comprehension is accounted for by variance in speed of naming isolated words, whether they follow regular symbol-sound correspondence rules or are exception words. Given the strong relationship between speed of identifying isolated words and text reading speed, it is not surprising that digit naming speed and speed of reading text of an appropriate difficulty level for each child, correlated about .7 (Bowers, 1994). Naming speed is related to text speed even when the substantial variance attributable to a standardized test of word recognition accuracy is controlled. Note that very quick access to the name of a word suggests that it has become a "sight" word and has been remembered on the basis of its orthographic image (Ehri, 1992) rather than reconstructed by decoding it. Wagner and Barker (chapter 7, this volume) offer a similar rationale.

While speed of reading familiar words is one measure (associated with rapid naming tests but not phoneme deletion in our studies) indicating use of an orthographic route, we do not wish to argue that phonological information does not participate in the recognition of words via an orthographic route. Perfetti's (1992) description of how redundant information contributes to an autonomous lexicon is pertinent here. However, the distinction between addressed (orthographic) and assembled (phonological) routes is viable even when it is recognized that these processes are not independent and that information about both graphemes and phonemes interact in contributing to both.

Other Reading Behaviors Associated With Slow Reading

While reading speed taps orthographic skill, such skill is more commonly assessed by other measures of letter pattern knowledge, including tests of exception word accuracy. (Since exception words cannot be recognized solely by decoding rules, letter pattern knowledge contributes to accuracy of their identification.) Yet speed of reading words, text, letters and numbers has rarely been examined along with a variety of letter pattern skill measures. Examination of the reading behaviors associated with slow reading, as distinct from those behaviors associated with poor decoding skill, might help us learn if slow reading is in fact associated strongly with other aspects of orthographic processing. Alternatively, speed of reading might be so imperfect a correlate of orthographic skill that when children are selected on this basis, they might be characterized by a very narrow pattern of deficits confined to speed of reading words, text, and perhaps graphemic symbols. To learn the implications of slow reading as distinct from poor decoding, Bowers and Wolf (1993a) reanalyzed data from two longitudinal samples. The first sample was described above and consisted of 38 poor and average readers tested in Grades 2, 3 and 4; the other sample traced children, unselected for reading ability, from kindergarten to Grade 4 (Wolf, 1991). On the basis of Grade 4 scores, children were divided into four groups based on nonword decoding and speed of recognizing easy regular words. We will describe the results from the Bowers study, which were presented in a different framework earlier in this chapter. Wolf's data presented a very similar picture.

The Grade 4 children in the longitudinal sample were divided into four groups based upon Woodcock Reading Mastery Test (WRMT) (Woodcock, 1973) Word Attack scores above and below the 35th percentile for grade, and average speed (above and below 750 msec) of correctly reading easy regular words. These words, taken from a list of words estimated to be at the Grade 2 level (Olson, Kliegl, Davidson, & Foltz, 1985) were read with ceiling accuracy. Representative words are "home," "did," and "but." Using these criteria, 15 of the children had no deficits, 8 were both poor decoders and slow readers, 8 were just slow readers and 7 were just poor decoders. The two slow reader groups were similar in word speed but differed in Word Attack scores, and the two poor decoder groups were similar in Word Attack but differed in speed. (See Table 2.)

Table 2.

Means for nonword decoding and easy word latency for each of the groups formed on the basis of these variables.

	Nonword Decoding	
Latency for words	**High** **above 35th percentile**	**Low** **below 35th percentile**
Fast (below 750 ms)	n = 15 Decoding: 66 %ile Latency: 611 ms	n = 7 Decoding: 26 %ile Latency: 634 ms
Slow (above 750 ms)	n = 8 Decoding: 58 %ile Latency: 911 ms	n = 8 Decoding: 20 %ile Latency: 1136 ms

MANOVAs were performed on reading and reading related variables listed in Table 3 to examine the effects of two levels of each of two factors on the various tests. The results demonstrated that each factor had a strong main effect on some variables and a tendency to affect other variables. There were few interactions of factors. However, each factor affected most strongly a different subset of variables. Good vs. poor nonword reading (across levels of speed) was significantly associated with good and poor WRMT Word Identification accuracy, Vocabulary knowledge, WRMT and WRMT-R untimed reading comprehension and Auditory Analysis Test scores, in a clear demonstration of the importance of decoding skills. However, slow vs. fast reading of simple words (across levels of decoding accuracy) was significantly associated with the untimed test of reading comprehension, number of correct identifications of both exception words and less frequent words, story reading speed and errors on those stories, and digit naming speed. Thus, the good decoders who differed on speed of naming easy regular words also differed on reading comprehension. Despite being similarly accurate on a standardized test of word identification, they nevertheless differed on accuracy of reading exception words (whose letter patterns are, by definition, encountered relatively infrequently) and less frequent words. While their story reading speeds differed in expected ways, errors while reading those stories also differed. (A somewhat similar pattern of deficits was found for the rate-disabled children studied by Lovett, 1987.) Similarly, poor decoders who were fast vs. slow on these easy words also differed from each other on the same variables. Those who had double deficits (with both poor decoding *and* slow reading) were clearly the worst readers in the study, differing from each single deficit group as well as from the no deficit group on some or all reading measures. The *double deficit* children were especially poor readers, and the children with single deficits in the present study, while poorer readers on some skills than the "no deficit" group, could compensate for their weaknesses to some extent. The single deficit groups were similar to one another on many variables, including interestingly, the Auditory Analysis Test.

Table 3.

Measures in longitudinal study.

1. Word Identification and Word Attack from Woodcock Reading Mastery Test (WRMT) (Woodcock, 1973) in Grades 2, 3 and 4.
2. Passage Comprehension from WRMT (Woodcock, 1973) in Grade 3, and from WRMT-R (Woodcock, 1987) in Grade 4.
3. Number of isolated words presented on computer read accurately, and latency for correctly read words, for the following word types:
   a) High frequency regular and exception words in Grade 4 (Olson et al. 1985)
   b) Moderate frequency regular and exception words in Grade 4 (Lovett et al., 1988)
4. Speed of naming single digits on a continuous list (Swanson, 1989), measured in items per second in Grades 2, 3, and 4.
5. Auditory Analysis Test (Rosner & Simon, 1971): deletion of the first or second consonant of a consonant blend, or of the last consonant, Grades 2, 3 and 4.
6. Vocabulary subtest from WISC-R in Grades 2 and 4.
7. Story reading measures: Children read 100 word passages adapted from SRA stories at a level of difficulty appropriate for each child. Analyzed are:
   a) Story difficulty level
   b) Number of errors
   c) Words read per minute for first reading of one story

However, they differed on the naming speed test. Since the worst readers in the study had "double deficits," it is perhaps unsurprising that these problems have been thought to be part of the same core (phonological) deficit rather than symptoms of two coexisting problems—one in phonological decoding and the other in lexical access speed.

The emergence of a pattern of deficits somewhat independent of phonological decoding, consisting of slow naming of digits, letters, and words, as well as more errors for exception words and less frequent words, pointed to the involvement of the orthographic system and supported our further exploration of the hypothesis that processes indexed by naming speed were involved specifically in the development of orthographic codes and ease of access to them.

THE DEVELOPMENT OF ORTHOGRAPHIC REPRESENTATIONS

Orthographic codes refer to the mental representation of all letters in words and subwords in proper sequence; when such codes are accessed, words or word parts are remembered rather than sounded out. It has been difficult to devise good measurements of the quality and extent of orthographic representations and their use in reading. Since the orthographic route is a "direct" rather than "sounding out" route to word recognition, it is typically fast. However, such speed is based on processing *all* the letters of a word or subword. An adult can read a word at least as fast as an individual letter, yet knowledge of the word is not vague or global, since s/he can notice small variations in letters. In order to tap these characteristics, researchers use measures of reading accuracy and speed for exception words, and decision tasks in which a person must choose which word of a pair is a real word rather than a similarly sounding nonword (eg., peece vs. peace; salmon vs sammon). Someone with good orthographic skill is familiar with the specific letter patterns in the real word which permits him/her to decide more quickly that, for example, "salmon" is a word and "sammon" is not a word, without pondering the decision.

Factors Affecting Differential Growth in Orthographic Knowledge

Symbol naming speed's strong relationship to speed of reading words and text, and significant association with accurate identification of words, especially exception words, suggested it might fit into a model of reading as an index of facility in using orthographic (or letter pattern) information. However, a more comprehensive understanding of factors governing orthographic skill development was needed to refine the hypothesis that rapid naming ability had something to do with growth in the formation of orthographic representations as well as their use. A review of the literature suggested the following conclusions about factors associated with orthographic skill; each of them will be discussed below.

a) Exposure to print from "out of school" reading (Cunningham & Stanovich, 1990) is related to speed of distinguishing familiar words from nonwords.

b) With brief practice, normal beginning readers recognize a specific letter pattern faster than they sound out a new pattern, whereas brief practice does not lead to this difference in reading-age matched (but older) reading disabled children (Reitsma, 1983). Word and text reading practice in controlled settings affects reading speed differentially for good and poor readers (Bowers, 1993; Ehri & Wilce, 1983; Manis, 1985).

c) Ability to detect letter clusters in words is related to better reading (Berninger, 1987; Berninger, Yates, & Lester, 1991).

d) Beginning readers find that certain letter clusters are easier to use to recognize new words, namely, those related to the rime patterns of words. There is a developmental pattern to which letter clusters are used to read "by analogy" (Goswami, in press).

Print Exposure. Stanovich and his colleagues (Stanovich & West, 1989; Cunningham & Stanovich, 1990) have demonstrated how, controlling for phonological decoding skill, measures of print exposure, presumably reflecting "out of school" reading experience, have an important and specific impact upon the orthographic knowledge of several samples of adults and children. Those who read more have greater knowledge of orthographic patterns, such that they can very quickly discriminate real words from sound-alike nonword foils, or homonym foils. Manis (1993) also showed that accuracy in choosing correct orthographic patterns either from nonword or homonym foils, was related to word identification skill both among reading disabled (RD) children, and among their chronological age (CA) controls, even after controlling variance in phonemic skill. Print exposure measures contributed variance to word identification, overlapping slightly more with orthographic than phonological measures. Although the RD children's orthographic skills increased relatively more than their phonological skills during a one-year period, their orthographic skills increased less during that period than did the skills of their reading level controls.

Differential Effects of Practice on Orthographic Knowledge. Research suggests that practice or print exposure does not have equal effects on the orthographic skill of all readers. Reitsma (1983) observed the effects of practice in identifying a new word on the orthographic knowledge gained about that word by young beginning readers and older reading disabled children. The design of the study was complex; for simplicity, we will describe only part of it. The disabled and normal readers were matched in reading skill despite their age differences. If amount of practice led to different effects on letter pattern knowledge for these groups, some undefined factor associated with reading disabled status must moderate the effect of practice. Over two days, children practiced reading 12 words, unfamiliar in written form, in short sentences, reading some of the words 2 times, some 4 times, and some 6 times. Three days later, Reitsma presented to them on computer screens, in mixed order, both the practiced words and nonwords pronounced like these words, and measured the time to begin naming both types of targets. The beginning readers' time to name the words previously practiced four or more times was significantly faster than the time to name their paired nonword; for the dyslexic children, *there was no difference between the speed of practiced words and unpracticed nonwords even after six practices.* He concluded that unlike the normal readers, the reading disabled children had failed to make any progress in representing these new words orthographically. Reitsma (1989) replicated these results using even more extensive practice. Although he speculated that it was the poorer phonological skills of the dyslexics that kept them from making orthographic progress, his particular measure of phonological awareness (nonword repetition) was correlated with growth of the orthographic route only minimally.

Similar results were found in studies comparing disabled readers with their CA controls. Ehri and Wilce (1983) and Manis (1985) demonstrated the differential effects of practice on reading speed for reading disabled vs. normally reading children. Ehri and Wilce (1983) had reading disabled and normally achieving readers practice words and nonwords up to 18 times. They wished to learn the course of progress toward unitization of targets in the two groups, that is, the degree to which practiced items would be pronounced as fast as simple digits. Results indicated that unlike normally achieving children, disabled readers did not unitize their recognition of any practiced word or nonword. Manis (1985) showed that the differential effects of practice were most evident for words of certain types. The reading disabled children showed much slower and less effective learning as a result of practice with complex regular words and exception words than with simpler regular words, while the normally achieving children readily learned to read all types of words.

Reitsma (1984; 1989) also explored phonological concomitants of differential rates of growth in orthography. Normal beginning readers showed a shift in their use of phonemic cues with practice of particular orthographic patterns. Deciding whether a practiced word was in a particular category or not (e.g., Is it an animal?) was facilitated by prior presentation of a speech sound similar vs. dissimilar to the last part of the word only for briefly practiced words. (An English language example is that /ni/ would prime "bunny.") Four or more practices made the priming sound irrelevant to performance. This finding was not true for older disabled readers matched with the beginning readers on reading age (RA) for whom the priming sound cue was always facilitative, even after 18 practices. Thus the practice-induced shift from relatively stronger reliance on phonemic codes toward reliance on orthographic codes, was much more pronounced for normal readers. Manis et al. (1990) also showed that most dyslexics showed a normal regularity effect, despite poorer phonological decoding ability than normally achieving children. Thus they continued to rely on phonological information despite less accurate phonemic knowledge, perhaps because they could not rely on good orthographic memory for words. This interpretation is bolstered by the data from a subgroup of dyslexics who had special difficulties using orthographic information. Despite their weaker phonological skills than CA controls, they tended to have a greater regularity effect than the other dyslexics or normally achieving children. It appeared these children compensated somewhat for their poor orthographic knowledge by heavier than normal reliance on whatever phonological knowledge they possessed. The pattern seems similar to Reitsma's finding that dyslexics continued to rely on phonemic cues long after RA matched younger readers no longer used them.

Letter-Cluster Orthographic Codes. Another study that caught our attention was reported by Berninger (1987). She suggested that the letter cluster was an insufficiently studied type of orthographic unit. Most researchers discussed only orthographic representation of whole words. Berninger showed that a kindergarten or first grade (Berninger, 1987) or first, second, or third grade (Berninger et al., 1991) child's ability to detect whether a letter cluster was present or absent in a given word was a good predictor of reading ability. Likewise, reproduction of letter clusters in a word was a good predictor of nonword reading in fourth, fifth, and sixth graders (Berninger, Cartwright, Yates, Swanson, & Abbott, in press). For example, Berninger et al. (1991) showed the children a word for one second (e.g., "clock"), and then a letter cluster actually in the word ("cl") or a letter cluster that had not appeared in the word, "co." Recognition memory for the cluster was associated with more proficient reading. She argued that skill in recognizing subword orthographic patterns could help identify nonwords as well as words.

A more extensive literature on subword letter clusters exists for older children and adults. For example, Frederiksen (1981) explored the facility of high school students with differing reading ability for reporting more vs. less frequent bigrams presented both in isolation and in words, pseudowords, and nonwords. The less skilled readers were slower to recognize bigrams overall, but were also more affected by the frequency of bigrams, taking longer to report less frequent ones, while frequency did not affect high skilled readers. High skilled readers were also better able to make use of more familiar orthographic patterns in decoding pseudowords than were lower skilled readers. It appeared that the less skilled readers needed to decode pseudowords letter by letter, unlike the more skilled who could use multiletter orthographic units.

Reading by Analogy. Goswami's research (eg., Goswami, 1991; Goswami, in press) suggests that normal beginning readers learn letter clusters corresponding to the rhyming part of a word more easily than other clusters. Thus, if they are taught to read "peak," they may be able to read by analogy "beak," without direct instruction, since they share the same rime pattern. They may not be able to read "bean," even though beak and bean share the same series of letters, since the rime differs. As children gained more experience with print, they used knowledge of other parts of the word to read new words by *analogy* rather than by a strictly "sounding out graphemes" route.

Is reading by orthographic analogy also seen in dyslexics? Lovett, Warren-Chaplin, Ransby, and Borden (1990) found that even when extensive practice with particular words resulted in severely dyslexic children learning those patterns, the children did not transfer their knowledge to new words. Thus, even learning "part" did not result in learning "cart," suggesting that the induction of orthographic subword patterns, in a form suitable for transfer, did not occur automatically for these children. Lemoine, Levy, and Hutchinson (1993) reported similar results. Their study showed that poor readers could retain speed gains for overlearned words and located the effects of extensive whole word practice in the direct visual route rather than in the more efficient use of rime segments to assemble phonology.

Here we summarize what these and other studies tell us about orthographic skill development. One index of orthographic knowledge is how quickly a word is recognized compared to a nonword foil, since the word is directly remembered rather than sounded out. Secondly, orthographic skill is affected by practice or experience, but this effect interacts with whether a child is a normal beginning reader or a reading disabled child, even when the latter child is older and matched on reading skill. Thirdly, subword as well as word units are represented orthographically, presumably on the basis of these units having been seen together often and because they correspond to a sound pattern the child can easily discriminate. Yet severely reading disabled children, unlike normal beginners, do not spontaneously use orthographic analogies to read even new words that share a rime pattern.

Role of Rapid Naming in Gaining Orthographic Knowledge

Measures of naming speed have rarely been used in investigations of orthography. (However, see Olson et al,, this volume.) In our data, the pattern of relationships of naming speed to reading measures was very similar to that of orthographic skill and reading. In fact, Barker et al.'s (1992) study of Grade 3 children's orthographic skill as measured by lexical decision, showed a pattern of relationships to various reading skills remarkably similar to that between digit naming speed and reading in the Bowers' (1994) study. Thus, independent of phoneme deletion skill, lexical decision in the Barker et al. study and naming speed in the Bowers' study were strongly related to speed of reading, especially of connected text, and less strongly to accuracy of word and nonword reading. Furthermore, Bowers (1994) demonstrated that naming speed is related to *gaining* speed after practice rereading text, even when level of reading skill is controlled, a finding analogous to that of Reitsma (1983).

Moderating the Effects of Practice. To test the hypothesis that the similarity in pattern of correlation was more than coincidental, several studies were conducted using digit naming speed and phoneme deletion to predict the effects of practice. Kennedy and Bowers (1991) studied the effect of 10 practices on latency to identify regular and exception words and nonwords. Using 18 very easy targets and analyzing data only for items which the children identified on first exposure, children categorized as poor, average and above average readers in Grades 2 and 3 practiced items in mixed order ten times. For Grade 2 children, naming speed not only correlated with initial latency to pronounce targets, but also predicted gains in reading latency, even controlling for both initial latency and phoneme deletion scores. The results were not replicated in the Grade 3 sample, perhaps because the targets were too simple for this group of children. This pattern of results suggested to us that processes tapped by naming speed moderated the effectiveness of each practice in moving a child along a dimension of reading from low to high dependence on orthographic coding processes, a dimension which at the "high" end is represented by "sight" words and an autonomous lexicon.

Letter Cluster Codes. Recently, Golden and Bowers (1993) have focussed upon the letter cluster identification skill of children. The orthographic redundancy model of Adams (1981) has guided our thinking in this area. Based on exposure to English text, normally achieving readers begin to recognize letters no longer as independent units, but as units of letter patterns. The strength with which various letters are associated with one another is dependent upon the frequency with which these letters have co-occurred in the individual's own reading experience. Letters that have been seen together in print often will tend to facilitate each other's recognition. The greater the history of co-occurrence, the greater the facilitation. Conversely, letters that have infrequently co-occurred in text, will tend to inhibit or slow each other's recognition. The greater the rarity of the co-occurrence, the greater the degree of inhibition (Adams, 1981; 1990; Seidenberg & McClelland, 1989). For example, the perception of d might be slightly inhibited following z, while the perception of u might be slightly facilitated following q, for a person who has been exposed to a sufficient number of real words. To explore the idea that even in the early grades, naming speed differences between readers are associated with the formation and use of orthographic codes, the tests of multiple orthographic codes designed by Berninger et al. (1991) were employed. Each of 43 children from Grades 1, 2, and 3 (unselected for reading ability) was administered three orthographic coding tasks. Each of the three tasks began with the presentation of a whole word for one second. What differed by coding task condition was the type of stimulus which followed: whole word, single letter, or letter-cluster. Within each task, each word was paired with both a subsequent stimulus that was "correct" and a reasonably similar "foil." The child's task was to indicate by a "yes" or "no" response whether the word, letter, or letter cluster presented was identical to or contained in the word seen previously.

Consistent with the theory that recognition of letter *patterns* is an important correlate of skilled reading, only individual differences in accuracy of letter-cluster performance accounted for significant variance in standardized reading measures for Grades 2 and 3, even controlling for age and its associated difference in reading experience. (In Grade 1, only detecting a letter in a word correlated with reading.) The question of course is what accounts for one child's ability to detect clusters better than another. A child's ability to rapidly name digits on the R.A.N. was significantly correlated with both reading skill and letter-cluster recognition. Individual differences in R.A.N. added no unique variance to reading after controlling for the significant contribution of letter cluster performance. The extremely high correlation between letter and digit naming speed in previous research (.9 in each grade of Bowers', 1994, longitudinal study) suggests the interpretation that skillful readers become quick and accurate in recognizing individual letters before being able to respond to letter clusters in words. We speculate that if a beginning reader is slow in identifying individual letters (as indexed by rapid naming tests), then single letters in a word will not be activated in sufficiently close temporal proximity to allow the child to become sensitive to letter patterns that frequently co-occur in print (Adams, 1990). Conversely, being able to quickly identify letters allows readers to forge meaningful associations between frequently seen letters. It is the already developed associations within a letter-cluster which enable quick and accurate cluster recognition, and are predictive of standardized reading performance. (We recognize that alternative conceptualizations of these findings, such as working memory accounts, have not been ruled out in this particular study, although results of other studies using memory and rapid naming tasks make this a less likely interpretation.) The phoneme deletion ability of children in Grades 2 and 3 also correlated with letter cluster ability and word identification, but a significant part of its contribution to letter cluster ability was independent of naming speed's contribution.

The orthographic redundancy interpretation of naming speed's relationship to letter cluster knowledge suggests that Spring and Davis' (1988) and Swanson's (1989) hypothesis about why good readers are faster on continuous-list tests of rapid naming bears reexamination. Recall that they speculated that poor readers might be restricted to serial processing of items on a continuous list, while good readers could overlap stages in processing, partially processing items to the right of focal attention, and thus naming them more quickly. This hypothesis was not confirmed in two studies. However, the hypothesis may apply only to frequently seen orthographic patterns, the very patterns researchers eliminate from formats for rapid naming tests. Good readers may overlap processing of letters for which there is high associative strength or learned connections; if the connections are weak for the poor readers, they are restricted to serial processing of that material. Adams discusses the word superiority effect (e.g., identifying a letter in a word more quickly than an isolated letter) as dependent upon the association strengths between letters in frequent letter patterns. If the ability to strengthen associations between letters seen in words is dependent upon rapid letter recognition, the relationship between reading facility and naming speed may well be due to continued use of serial processing by poor readers who name symbols slowly, and for whom associations between letters in common patterns are weak. Golden (1993) is investigating this possibility.

CORRELATES OF ADULT READING ABILITY

While our primary goal has been to understand whether slow naming speed marks an important bottleneck to the development of the orthographic route for reading disabled children, we recognize that a great deal of work has been done studying adult orthographic skill. Is it possible that less developed orthographic skill in university students might still show a trace of the hypothesized roots of those deficits in slower symbol naming speed? Several studies of individual differences among adult readers have included measures of speed to name numbers and letters, or related measures, but have not attempted to distinguish between correlates of orthographic processing as distinct from other reading skills.

Jackson and McClelland (1979) chose university students in the highest and lowest quartile of "effective reading speed," that is, speed of reading text multiplied by degree of comprehension of this text. Although listening comprehension was the single best predictor of effective reading speed, stepwise multiple regression analyses indicated that an additional contribution was made by the time to decide that two letters had the same name (e.g., A a). They interpret the relationship between several similar reaction time measures and reading as a function of better readers having quicker access from print to letter codes stored in long term memory. Jackson (1980) replicated and extended this work. While Jackson and McClelland (1979) did not focus upon orthographic skill per se, their reading measure included the text speed variable which was associated in the child literature with both orthographic skill (Barker et al., 1992) and digit and letter naming speed (Bowers & Wolf, 1993a).

Jackson and McClelland's (1979) measure of letter name matching speed was also employed in a study of university students (unselected for reading ability) conducted by Cunningham, Stanovich and Wilson (1990). Using measures of various reading and listening skills, they tested the hypothesis that for adults as well as children, word recognition contributed variance to reading comprehension, controlling for verbal comprehension. In addition, they explored the impact upon reading skill not only of letter name matching speed, but also of discrete-trial symbol, letter and number naming speed. (Unlike the naming speed items typically used in child studies, the letter set included 25 letters, and the numbers were 20 two-digit numbers.) Cunningham et al. (1990) concluded that word decoding indeed contributed variance in addition to verbal comprehension, to reading comprehension. Letter name matching was not significantly associated with reading comprehension in this sample, although a small but significant association was seen with easy word reaction time. While the number and letter naming time correlations with reading comprehension were modest, it is of interest that even in this unselected sample, number and letter naming speed correlated about .4 both with a combined score of accuracy and speed of isolated word recognition and with a similar score for pseudoword decoding. The correlation with speed of easy word naming was about .5 While the authors emphasize that the relationship of pseudoword or word facility to reading comprehension did not depend upon the naming speed variance or a general speed factor, it is certainly notable that a relationship between naming speed and word recognition persists in this sample.

Orthographic Processing in Adult Readers

Orthographic skill in adult readers has usually been studied with the aim of learning about basic processes in reading rather than determinants of individual differences in reading ability. We focussed above on the naming speed correlates of some aspects of word recognition ability in university samples; other correlates of reading ability include listening comprehension (Palmer, MacLeod, Hunt, & Davidson, 1985), working memory (Daneman & Carpenter, 1980), print exposure (Stanovich & West, 1989), and phonological and orthographic skill (Cunningham et al., 1990; Stanovich & West, 1989). Stanovich and West (1989) developed the Author Recognition Test (ART) to measure print exposure in a fashion relatively unaffected by social desirability factors. Using subjects from two universities, ART as well as phonological and orthographic ability were significantly correlated with word identification skill. Their studies demonstrated that even controlling for phonological skill, the ART was significantly related to several measures of orthographic skill, such as spelling ability for exception segments and orthographic and homophone choice tasks.[2] However, print exposure did not exhaust all reliable orthographic variance, and the authors speculated that factors such as nonanalytic style of reading might account for additional orthographic variance.

Early in this chapter, we argued that samples of children with naming speed in a broad normal range might show the pattern of effects sketched by Ehri, namely, strong effects of phonemic skill upon orthographic knowledge; effects of naming speed on orthographic skill might be confined to those with especially slow speed. However, the results of the Jackson and McClelland (1979) and Cunningham et al. (1990) studies in which speed of letter identification was associated with faster reading, even in university students, encouraged us to pursue the hypothesis that speed of access to letter names would contribute uniquely to orthographic skill in this sample.

Since it appeared that orthographic ability was a separable component of individual differences in adults, Kennedy and Bowers (1992) hypothesized that naming speed would be more highly predictive of adults' orthographic skill than their phonological skill. The role of sample characteristics in the relationship between naming speed and reading was highlighted in our review of studies of naming speed; samples with insufficient numbers of poorer readers sometimes failed to find relationships apparent in more selected samples. To gather a sufficient sample of less orthographically skilled university students, we used the ART (Stanovich & West, 1989) to screen several hundred students, and selected 72 of them to represent a rectangular distribution of the full range of reading ability (especially orthographic skill) available in the university population. Phonological skills were assessed by nonword decoding and a pseudohomophone decision task, and orthographic skills by lexical decision and homophone decision measures similar to those used by Stanovich and West (1989).

We asked whether tests of phonemic awareness (tapped by phoneme deletion and phoneme reversal measures) and continuous-list digit naming speed would be differentially related to accuracy and latency measures of phonological and orthographic skill. This hypothesis received only limited support. Phonemic awareness was related to accuracy on phonological and orthographic measures, and naming speed was related to orthographic speed only in interaction with phonemic awareness. The pattern of interaction was such that when naming speed was fast, phonemic awareness made a strong contribution to orthographic speed; with slower naming speed, phonemic awareness did not contribute additional variance. Those students with "double assets" were particularly fast orthographic processors, considerably faster than any other group.[3] Perhaps the pattern of a strong contribution to orthographic knowledge from phonemic skill in this sample is consistent with the developmental model described by Ehri (1992), and there is only a limited role for variance in symbol recognition speed among relatively competent readers. Not surprisingly, the relationships between naming speed and components of word recognition become more complex as the subskills of reading become increasingly integrated in more skilled readers. Indeed, naming speed was more directly related to speed of decoding nonwords in this sample than to the whole word tests of orthography. It is possible that the letter cluster knowledge required to decode these more complex nonwords accounted for the relationship, but such an interpretation is made tentatively. That naming speed of simple digits continues to have some (albeit complex) association with fast recognition of the appropriate real word letter pattern lends some support to the hypothesis that speed on a very simple task may share variance with complex letter pattern recognition.

A SPECULATIVE ACCOUNT OF THE ROUTE BY WHICH RAPID NAMING AFFECTS ORTHOGRAPHIC DEVELOPMENT

We theorize that relatively brief practice enables children with letter naming speeds in the normal range to progress rapidly along the dimension of word recognition characterized by slow construction of a word vs. fast remembering of it. Slow naming speeds indicate that processes that typically support the learning of associations between letters that frequently occur together and their amalgamation with corresponding phonological codes, are not working efficiently. At the least, much more practice is needed to achieve sufficient strength of letter associations and amalgamation of codes such that words are remembered directly from their orthographic patterns. There is ample room for the effects of poor phonemic codes on the eventual development of orthographic codes, but their role is not exclusive. Certainly if phonological codes and letter-sound correspondence knowledge are poor, few words may be identified accurately, and so practice is not helpful. As well, if phonological codes are of poor quality, perhaps the phonological and visual code connections cannot be made precisely enough for good orthographic representations. But it would appear that another major bottleneck for developing sight words is indexed by slow recognition of single letters. As Wolf et al. (chapter 4, this volume) suggest, the role of this letter deficit may be highlighted in an orthography with regular grapheme-phoneme correspondences, and obscured in complex orthographies such as English.

The mechanisms underlying individual differences in speed of letter recognition are not yet known. Wolf (1991) suggests that very slow naming speed for letters and numbers may reflect disruption in precise timing mechanisms, and cites neuropsychological data concerning these mechanisms in various systems subserving reading and speech. Bowers and Wolf (1993b) also speculate that dyslexics' precise timing difficulties in visual and motor domains have some relationship to their deficits on tests of rapid naming, although the nature of the relationship is unclear and may not be causal. Whatever the status of such arguments for the underlying *basis* of slow naming, the *effect* of slow letter recognition may well be the disruption of the optimal timing between the excitation of two or more letter codes, and between such codes and their corresponding phonological codes. A connectionist framework for word learning similar to that sketched by Adams (1990) (a framework adapted from Seidenberg & McClelland, 1989), is congenial to the view that building orthographic patterns depends on the close connection in time of the excitation of letter codes for bigram and trigram patterns. Using the phonological code for subword parts (such as the rhyming part of a word) while inspecting the corresponding letter pattern (e.g., the rime) may well be sufficient exposure to learn that orthographic pattern, for children with normal speed of letter recognition. For example, most beginning readers have sufficiently fast letter recognition to learn rime letter patterns which they can then use to read other words by analogy. But without that letter recognition speed, it would be difficult to learn the corresponding letter patterns without extensive practice.

Reitsma (1989) also notes the usefulness of a connectionist

lexical model with multiple interacting units of differing sizes. His suggestion that dyslexics may have a system of connections such that the weights between units are slower to stabilize and/or there are fewer connections, seems consonant with possible effects of slower recognition of letter units.[4] To become a fluent reader, specific connections between "orthographic input patterns and phonological output patterns" may be more influential than knowing abstract rules of phonics, although learning the rules "may be extremely important as organizing principles or mnemonic devices until lexical activation becomes an automatic consequence of word recognition." (p. 70). A similar point is made by Adams (1990). In a sense, learning the rules may be more important for the child with deficits in letter recognition speed; the rules may act as a prosthesis for the weaker ability to induce the orthographic pattern from exposure to words.

Perfetti (1985) alerted us to the unfortunate effects of slow word recognition processes on reading comprehension. However, speed of word recognition has been thought to be inextricably bound up with the phonological processes used in nonword as well as word decoding. The current perspective argues instead that letter recognition speed can play a partially independent role in determining not only speed of reading but also the development of orthographic skill more generally. As an independent contributor, strengths and weakness in naming speed can be a boon or a bane to a child with a given level of phonemic decoding skill. Educators may have mistakenly blamed a good decoder's reading comprehension failures on poor vocabulary knowledge or comprehension monitoring skill, when instead, they may be the result of orthographic processing deficits. Similarly, the failure of some aspects of oral reading fluency and comprehension to respond to training in phonics may also be a result of lack of attention to individual differences in a child's ability to induce orthographic knowledge from the kind of exposure to print that is usually sufficient for it. As amply demonstrated, frequent and varied exposure to print is a primary condition for the growth of orthographic skill, but some poor readers, despite equivalent letter and word practice, have such slow letter recognition processes that conditions for their learning of orthography must be altered. Research documenting what conditions are most helpful for children with slow naming speed is of vital importance.

NOTES

1. Note that the target and its neighbor are not previously practiced patterns. The hypothesis that results would be quite different if the letter neighbors were highly frequent associates of target letters (and thus common orthographic patterns) is discussed later in this text.
2. The orthographic choice task requires subjects to choose a real word from a set consisting of a word and its pseudohomophone (break braik). The homophone choice task requires subjects to choose the correct written form of a word from a set of sound-alike words, eg., Which is an animal: hair hare)
3. In contrast, in a sample of Grade 4 poor and average readers, recall that naming speed was related to faster word reading both directly and in interaction with phonemic awareness. However the nature of the small but significant interaction was such that among *slower* namers, phonemic awareness contributed additional variance to reading speed, while among faster namers, reading speed was faster without regard to level of phonemic awareness. If such differential patterns were replicated, the need to take into account reading level when discussing effects of phonemic awareness and naming speed is highlighted.
4. Seidenberg's (1992) simulations of dyslexias, by limiting either precision of orthographic input or amount of resources (hidden units), may be pertinent to this argument. Either simulation produced a pattern of results similar in some ways to the pattern associated with slow naming speed in our data. While this is far from conclusive evidence of similarity of processes, it is suggestive that pursuing this line of theorizing may be productive.

REFERENCES

Adams, M.J. (1981). What good is orthographic redundancy? In O.J.L. Tzeng and H. Singer (Eds.), *Perception of print: Reading research in experimental psychology,* (pp. 197-221). Hillsdale, NJ: Erlbaum Associates.

Adams, M.J. (1990). *Beginning to Read: Thinking and Learning about Print.* Cambridge, MA: MIT Press.

Allington, R.L. (1983). Fluency: The neglected reading goal. *The Reading Teacher, 36,* 556-561.

Badian, N.A. (1993). Phonemic awareness, naming, visual symbol processing, and reading. *Reading and Writing: An Interdisciplinary Journal, 5,* 87-100.

Barker, T.A., Torgesen, J.K., & Wagner, R.K. (1992). The role of orthographic processing skills on five different reading tasks. *Reading Research Quarterly, 27,* 334-345.

Berninger, V.W. (1987). Global, component, and serial processing of printed words in beginning reading. *Journal of Experimental Child Psychology, 43,* 387-418.

Berninger, V.W., Cartwright , A.C., Yates, C.M., Swanson, H.L., & Abbott, R.D. (in press). Developmental skills related to writing and reading acquisition in the intermediate grades: Shared and unique functional systems. *Reading and Writing: An Interdisciplinary Journal.*

Berninger, V.W., Yates, C., & Lester, K. (1991). Multiple orthographic codes in reading and writing acquisition. *Reading and Writing: An Interdisciplinary Journal, 3,* 115-149.

Biemiller, A. (1977-1978). Relationships between oral reading rates for letters, words, and simple text in the development of reading achievement. *Reading Research Quarterly, 13,* 223-253.

Blachman, B.A. (1984). Relationship of rapid naming ability and language analysis skills to kindergarten and first-grade reading achievement. *Journal of Educational Psychology, 76,* 610-622.

Bowers, P.G. (1993). Text reading and rereading: Predictors of fluency beyond word recognition. *Journal of Reading Behavior, 25,* 133-153.

Bowers, P.G. (1994). *Tracing symbol naming speed's unique contribution to reading disabilities over time.* Paper submitted for publication.

Bowers, P.G., & Kennedy, A. (1993). Effects of naming speed differences on fluency of reading after practice. *Annals of the New York Academy of Sciences, 682,* 318-320.

Bowers, P.G., Steffy, R.A., & Tate, E. (1988). Comparison of the effects of IQ control methods on memory and naming speed predictors of reading disability. *Reading Research Quarterly, 23,* 304-319.

Bowers, P.G., & Swanson, L.B. (1991). Naming speed deficits in reading disability: Multiple measures of a singular process. *Journal of Experimental Child Psychology, 51,* 195-219.

Bowers, P.G., & Wolf, M. (1993a, March). *A double-deficit hypothesis for developmental reading disability.* Paper presented to the meetings of the Society for Research in Child Development, New Orleans.

Bowers, P.G., & Wolf, M. (1993b). Theoretical links between naming speed, precise timing mechanisms and orthographic skill in dyslexia. *Reading and Writing: An Interdisciplinary Journal, 5,* 69-85.

Bradley, L., & Bryant, P. (1985). *Rhyme and Reason in Reading and Spelling.* Ann Arbor: University of Michigan Press.

Cornwall, A. (1992). The relationship of phonological awareness, rapid naming, and verbal memory to severe reading and spelling disability. *Journal of Learning Disabilities, 25*, 532-538.

Cunningham, A.E., & Stanovich, K.E. (1990). Assessing print exposure and orthographic processing skill in children: A quick measure of reading experience. *Journal of Educational Psychology, 82*, 733-740.

Cunningham, A.E., Stanovich, K.E., & Wilson, M.R. (1990). Cognitive variation in adult college students differing in reading ability. In T.H. Carr & B A. Levy (Eds.), *Reading and its development: Component skills approaches*. New York: Academic Press.

Daneman, M., & Carpenter, P.A. (1980). Individual differences in working memory and reading. *Journal of Verbal Learning and Verbal Behavior, 19*, 450-466.

Dempster, F.N. (1981). Memory span: Sources of individual and developmental differences. *Psychological Bulletin, 89*, 63-100.

Denckla, M., & Rudel, R.G. (1974). Rapid "automatized" naming of pictured objects, colors, letters and numbers by normal children. *Cortex, 10*, 186-202.

Denckla, M., & Rudel, R.G. (1976). Rapid "automatized" naming (R.A.N.): Dyslexia differentiated from other learning disabilities. *Neuropsychologia, 14*, 471-479.

Ehri, L.C. (1992). Reconceptualizing the development of sight word reading and its relationship to recoding. In P.B. Gough, L.C. Ehri, & R. Treiman (Eds.), *Reading acquisition* (pp. 107-143). Hillsdale, NJ: Lawrence Erlbaum Associates, Inc.

Ehri, L.C., & Wilce, L.S. (1983). Development of word identification speed in skilled and less skilled beginning readers. *Journal of Educational Psychology, 75*, 3-18.

Ellis, N.C., & Miles, T.R. (1981). A lexical encoding deficiency I:Experimental evidence. In G.Th. Pavlidis, & T.R. Miles (Eds.), *Dyslexia Research and its Applications*, (pp. 177-215). John Wiley & Sons Ltd.

Felton, R., & Brown, I.S. (1990). Phonological processes as predictors of specific reading skills in children at risk for reading failure. *Reading and Writing: An Interdisciplinary Journal, 2*, 39-59.

Felton, R.H., Naylor, C.E., & Wood, F.B. (1990). Neuropsychological profile of adult dyslexics. *Brain and Language, 39*, 485-497.

Felton, R.H., Wood, F.B., Brown, I.S., & Campbell, S.K. (1987). Separate verbal memory and naming deficits in attention deficit disorder and reading disability. *Brain and Language, 31*, 171-184.

Frederiksen, J.R. (1981). Sources of process interactions in reading. In A.M Lesgold, & C.A. Perfetti (Eds.), *Interactive processes in reading*, (pp. 361-386). Hillsdale, NJ: Lawrence Erlbaum Associates.

Golden, J. (1993). *Analysis of orthographic processing skill and its relationship to rapid naming*. Unpublished manuscript.

Golden, J., & Bowers, P.G. (1993, July). *Knowledge of letter patterns and its relationship to reading skill*. Poster presented to Meetings of the Canadian Society for Brain, Behavior and Cognitive Science, Toronto.

Goswami, U. (1991). Learning about spelling sequences: The role of onsets and rimes in analogies in reading. *Child Development, 62*, 1110-1123.

Goswami, U. (in press). Towards an orthographic analogy model of reading development: Decoding vowel graphemes in beginning reading. *Journal of Experimental Child Psychology*.

Jackson, M.D. (1980). Further evidence for a relationship between memory access and reading ability. *Journal of verbal learning and verbal behavior, 19*, 683-694.

Jackson, M.D., & McClelland, J.L. (1979). Processing determinants of reading speed. *Journal of Experimental Psychology: General, 108*, 151-181.

Kaufman, A.S. (1979). *Intelligent testing with the WISC-R*. NY: John Wiley & Sons.

Kennedy, A., & Bowers, P.G. (1991, August). *The effect of practice on word identification speed in children*. Poster presented to the Meetings of the American Psychological Association, San Francisco.

Kennedy, A. & Bowers, P.G. (1992, August). *Individual differences in reading ability amongst university students*. Poster presented to the Meetings of the Canadian Society for Brain, Behavior and Cognitive Science, Quebec City.

Lemoine, H.E., Levy, B.A., & Hutchinson, A. (1993). Increasing the naming speed of poor readers: Representations formed across repetitions. *Journal of Experimental Child Psychology, 55*, 297-328.

Levy, B.A., & Hinchley, J. (1990). Individual and developmental differences in the acquisition of reading skills. In T.H. Carr & B.A. Levy (Eds.), *Reading and its development: Component skills approaches* (pp. 81-128). NY:Academic Press.

Lovett, M.W. (1987). A developmental approach to reading disability: Accuracy and speed criteria of normal and deficient reading skill. *Child Development, 58*, 234-260.

Lovett, M., Ransby, M., & Barron, R. (1988). Treatment, subtype, and word type effects in dyslexic children's response to remediation. *Brain and Language, 34*, 328-349.

Lovett, M.W., Warren-Chaplin, P.M., Ransby, M.J., & Borden, S.L. (1990). Training the word recognition skills of reading disabled children: Treatment and transfer effects. *Journal of Educational Psychology, 82*, 769-780.

Manis, F.R. (1985). Acquisition of word identification skills in normal and disabled readers. *Journal of Educational Psychology, 77*, 78-90.

Manis, F.R. (1993, March). *A longitudinal study of print exposure, phonological skill and orthographic skill in normal and disabled readers.* Paper presented at the Meetings of the Society for Research in Child Development, New Orleans.

Manis, F.R., Szeszulski, P.A., Holt, L.K., & Graves. L. (1990). In T.H. Carr, & B.A. Levy (Eds.), *Reading and its development: Component skills approaches* (pp. 207-259). New York: Academic Press.

Mann, V. (1984). Review: Reading skill and language skill. *Developmental Review, 4*, 1-15.

Murphy, L.A., Pollatsek, A., & Well, A.D. (1988). Developmental dyslexia and word retrieval deficits. *Brain and Language, 35*, 11-23.

Nicolson, R.I., & Fawcett, A.J. (in press). Towards the origins of dyslexia. In R. Groner, R. Kaufmann-Hayoz, and S.F. Wright (Eds.), *Reading and Reading Disorders: International Perspectives.* North Holland: Elsevier.

Olson, R., Forsberg, H., & Wise, B. (1994). Genes, environment, and the development of orthographic skills. In V.W. Berninger (Ed.), *The varieties of orthographic knowledge I: Theoretical and developmental issues* (pp. 27-71). Dordrecht, The Netherlands: Kluwer Academic Press.

Olson, R.K., Kliegl, R., Davidson, B.J., & Foltz, G. (1985). Individual and developmental differences in reading disability. In G.E. MacKinnon, & T.G. Waller (Eds.), *Reading Research: Advances in Theory and Practice: Vol. 4*. Orlando, FL: Academic Press.

Olson, R., Wise, B., Conners, F., & Rack, J. (1990). Organization, heritability, and remediation of component word recognition and language skills in disabled readers. In T H. Carr, & B.A. Levy (Eds.), *Reading and its development: Component skills approaches* (pp. 261-322). New York: Academic Press.

Palmer, J., MacLeod, C.M., Hunt, E., & Davidson, J.E. (1985). Information processing correlates of reading. *Journal of Memory and Language, 24*, 59-88.

Pedhazur, E.J. (1982). *Multiple regression in behavioral research: Explanation and prediction*. New York: CBS College Publishing.

Perfetti, C.A. (1985). *Reading Ability*. New York: Oxford University Press.

Perfetti, C.A. (1992). The representation problem in reading acquisition. In P.B. Gough, L.C. Ehri, & R. Treiman (Eds.), *Reading Acquisition* (pp. 145-174). Hillsdale, NJ: Lawrence Erlbaum Associates, Inc.

Perfetti, C.A., Finger, E., & Hogaboam, T. (1978). Sources of vocalization latency differences between skilled and less skilled young readers. *Journal of Educational Psychology, 710*, 730-739.

Reitsma, P. (1983). Printed word learning in beginning readers. *Journal of Experimental Child Psychology, 36*, 321-339.

Reitsma, P. (1984). Sound priming in beginning readers. *Child Development, 55*, 406-423

Reitsma, P. (1989). Orthographic memory and learning to read. In P.G. Aaron, & R.M. Joshi (Eds.), *Reading and Writing Disorders in Different Orthographic Systems*. The Netherlands: Kluwer Academic Publishers.

Rosner, J., & Simon, D.P. (1971). The auditory analysis test: An initial report. *Journal of Learning Disabilities, 4*, 1-15.

Seidenberg, M.S. (1992). Dyslexia in a computational model of word recognition in reading. In P.B. Gough, L.C. Ehri, and R. Treiman (Eds.), *Reading acquisition* (pp. 243-273). Hillsdale, NJ: Lawrence Erlbaum Associates.

Seidenberg, M.S., & McClelland, J.L. (1989). A distributed, developmental model of word recognition and naming. *Psychological Review, 96*, 523-568.

Spring, C., & Capps, C. (1974). Encoding speed, rehearsal, and probed recall of dyslexic boys. *Journal of Educational Psychology, 66,* 780-786.

Spring, C., & Davis, J.M. (1988). Relations of digit naming speed with three components of reading. *Applied Psycholinguistics, 9,* 315-334.

Spring, C., & Perry, L. (1983). Naming speed and serial recall in poor and adequate readers. *Contemporary Educational Psychology, 8,* 141-145.

Stanovich, K.E. (1981). Relationships between word decoding speed, general name-retrieval ability, and reading progress in first-grade children. *Journal of Educational Psychology, 73,* 809-815.

Stanovich, K.E. (1988). The dyslexic and the garden-variety poor reader: The phonological-core variable-difference model. *Journal of Learning Disabilities, 21,* 590-604.

Stanovich, K.E. (1992). Speculations on the causes and consequences of individual differences in early reading acquisition. In P.B. Gough, L.C. Ehri, & R. Treiman (Eds.), *Reading acquisition* (pp. 307-342), Hillsdale, NJ: Erlbaum.

Stanovich, K.E., Feeman, D.J., & Cunningham, A.E. (1983). The development of the relation between letter-naming speed and reading ability. *Bulletin of the Psychonomic Society, 21,* 199-202.

Stanovich, K.E., Nathan, R.G., & Zolman, J.E. (1988). The developmental lag hypothesis in reading: Longitudinal and matched reading-level comparisons. *Child Development, 59,* 71-86.

Stanovich, K.E., & West, R.F. (1989). Exposure to print and orthographic processing. *Reading Research Quarterly, 24,* 402-433.

Swanson, L.B. (1989). *Analyzing naming speed-reading relationships in children.* Unpublished doctoral dissertation, University of Waterloo, Waterloo, Ontario, Canada.

Torgesen, J.K., Morgan, S.T., & Davis, C. (1992). Effects of two types of phonological awareness training on word learning in kindergarten children. *Journal of Educational Psychology, 84,* 364-370.

Venezky, R., & Massaro, D. (1979). The role of orthographic regularity in word recognition. In L. Resnick, & P. Weaver (Eds.), *Theory and practice of early reading: Vol. 1,* (pp. 85-108). Hillsdale, NJ: Erlbaum.

Wagner, R. K., & Barker, T. (1994). The development of orthographic processing ability. In V.W. Berninger (Ed.), *The varieties of orthographic knowledge I: Theoretical and developmental issues* (pp. 243-276). Dordrecht, The Netherlands: Kluwer Academic Publishers.

Wagner, R.K., & Torgesen, J.K. (1987). The nature of phonological processing and its causal role in the acquisition of reading skills. *Psychological Bulletin.*, *101*, 192-212.

Walsh, D.J., Price, G.G., & Gillingham, M.G. (1988). The critical but transitory importance of letter naming. *Reading Research Quarterly*, *23*, 108-122.

Wechsler, D. (1974). *Wechsler Intelligence Scale for Children: Revised*. New York: Psychological Corporation.

Wimmer, H. (1993). Characteristics of developmental dyslexia in a regular writing system. *Applied Psycholinguistics*, *14*, 1-33.

Wolf, M. (1984). Naming, reading, and the dyslexias: A longitudinal overview. *Annals of Dyslexia*, *34*, 87-115.

Wolf, M. (1991). Naming speed and reading: The contribution of the cognitive neurosciences. *Reading Research Quarterly*, *26*, 123-141.

Wolf, M., Pfeil, C., Lotz, R., & Biddle, K. (1994). Towards a more universal understanding of the developmental dyslexias: The contribution of orthographic factors. In V.W. Berninger (Ed.), *The varieties of orthographic knowledge I: Theoretical and developmental issues* (pp. 137-171). Dordrecht, The Netherlands: Kluwer Academic Press.

Wolf, M., Bally, H., & Morris, R. (1986). Automaticity, retrieval processes and reading: A longitudinal study in average and impaired readers. *Child Development*, *57*, 988-1005.

Wolff, P.H., Michel, G.F., & Ovrut, M. (1990). Rate variables and automatized naming in developmental dyslexia. *Brain and Language*, *39*, 556-575.

Woodcock, R. (1973). *Woodcock Reading Mastery Test*. Circle Pines, MN: American Guidance Service.

Woodcock, R. (1987). *Woodcock Reading Mastery Test-Revised.* Circle Pines, MN: American Guidance Service.

Yap, R., & van der Leij, A. (1991, August). *Rate of elementary symbol processing in dyslexics*. Poster presented at the Rodin Conference, Berne, Switzerland.

Yap, R., & van der Leij, A. (1993). Word processing in dyslexics: An automatic decoding deficit? *Reading and Writing: An Interdisciplinary Journal*, *5*, 261-279.

Young, A. (1993). *Determinants of oral reading fluency and expressiveness in poor and average readers.* Unpublished doctoral dissertation, University of Waterloo, Waterloo, Ontario, Canada.

Young, A. R., & Bowers, P.G. (1994). *Individual differences and text difficulty determinants of reading fluency and expressiveness.* Paper submitted for publication.

Address correspondence to:

Patricia Bowers
University of Waterloo
Waterloo, Ontario
Canada N2L 3G1

RODERICK W. BARRON

THE SOUND-TO-SPELLING CONNECTION: ORTHOGRAPHIC ACTIVATION IN AUDITORY WORD RECOGNITION AND ITS IMPLICATIONS FOR THE ACQUISITION OF PHONOLOGICAL AWARENESS AND LITERACY SKILLS

Documented cases of individuals who are fluent in the acarne skill of talking backwards can be divided into two groups (Cowan, Braine & Leavitt, 1985; Cowan & Leavitt, 1982; Cowan, Leavitt, Massaro & Kent, 1982). One group appears to activate the orthographic representation of the word and then pronounce it by reversing the spelling (e.g., "bomb" is reversed as /bəmɑb/) while a second group pronounces the word by reversing the phonemes (e.g., "bomb" is reversed as /mɑb/). The second group, however, is not completely immune from the effects of activating and using orthographic information during the process of reversing speech because the spelling of the word can influence choice of the units to be reversed. The two phonemes /k/ and /s/, for example, which are typically represented by the single letter x in words such as FOX, are treated as a single phoneme in about one third of their backward utterances. Like backwards talkers, I intend to take a backwards approach to orthographic knowledge because this chapter will be concerned with the phenomenon, interpretation, and significance of the activation of orthographic information during the process of auditory word recognition.

I will begin this chapter by proposing that traditional definitions of literacy need to be reconsidered because of what is known about the effects of print exposure on the development of literacy, language, and cognition and because of what is known about prereaders' knowledge of orthography. This will be followed by a review of evidence for orthographic activation in auditory word recognition among fluent adult readers, dyslexic readers, prereaders and beginning and developing readers. Finally, I will consider the implications of this evidence for understanding the interplay between

V.W. Berninger (ed.), The varieties of orthographic knowlesge I: Theoretical and developmental issues, 219-242.

orthographic and phonological knowledge in the development of phonological awareness and literacy.

REDEFINING THE ONSET OF LITERACY

Stanovich and his colleagues have shown that measures of print exposure in literate children and adults are powerful, independent predictors of individual differences in literacy skills as well as verbal intelligence, general knowledge, and specific content knowledge (e.g., Stanovich, 1993; Cunningham & Stanovich, 1990, 1991; Stanovich & Cunningham, 1992, 1993; Stanovich & West, 1989). One question that arises from their findings is when does literacy first have an impact on the development of language and cognition? Answering this question may require a reconsideration of the definition of literacy.

The onset of literacy has typically been defined as the point in time when children can read single words aloud and spell them to dictation. Adams (1990), however, estimates that activities such as being read to aloud, watching pre-school educational television programs like Sesame Street, and playing word and letter games provide middle class children with several thousand hours of exposure to printed words and their corresponding phonological representations well before they are able to read or spell any words. Furthermore, research on children's emergent literacy suggests that literacy skills and forms of literacy related knowledge are gradually acquired during the course of language development before formal schooling and are fostered by environments that offer many opportunities to interact with printed information (e.g., Clay, 1976; Hiebert, 1993; Mason, 1992; Teale, 1986; Teale & Sulzby, 1986; Wells, 1985).

Although much of their interaction with print is passive, children acquire considerable knowledge about the relationships between print and sound, including the sub-syllabic units that are involved in phonological awareness (see note 1), well before they are able to satisfy the conventional definition of literacy—accurately reading individual words aloud that are presented out of context and accurately spelling them to dictation. Read (1986) has shown that prereaders can use strings of letter-name and letter-sound associations to represent the phonetic structure of spoken words (e.g., WTR for the word WATER). Ehri and Wilce (1985) found that prereaders with high letter-name and letter-sound association knowledge were able to learn and remember more easily nonsense words made up of letters whose sounds and names correspond to real words (e.g., SZRS = scissors) than items which were visually distinctive but did not correspond phonologically (e.g., qDjK) to real words. Byrne and Fielding-Barnsley (1989, 1990) have described a similar advantage for high letter-sound knowledge among prereaders who were taught a small set of words (e.g., MAT, SAT) and then required to transfer their knowledge to the reading of unknown words (e.g., MOW, SOW). Finally, Stuart (1990) has shown that prereaders with high letter-sound knowledge perform above chance in choosing between a correctly spelled printed word (PAN) corresponding to a picture (picture of a pan) and a printed distracter word (CUT), whereas children with low letter-sound knowledge perform at chance on this task.

Taken together, these results suggest that the conventional definition of literacy may need to be expanded to include proto-literacy—knowledge of letter-name and letter-sound associations that are learned before children can read words aloud or spell them to dictation (Barron, 1986; Barron, 1991; Barron, Golden, Seldon, Tait, Marmurek & Haines, 1992). Proto-literate knowledge arises from prereaders' exposure to print and may represent one of the earliest instances in which specific, print-based information directly influences linguistic and cognitive processing. It is possible that this initial connection between print and sound, which is made before literacy is acquired, may signal the beginning of an important but ignored change in the development of language—activation of orthographic information during the process of auditory word recognition. Evidence will be presented suggesting that this activation of sound-to-spelling information is not just an irrelevant epiphenomenon accompanying the process of recognizing spoken words. Instead, orthographic activation may play an important and possibly causal role in the acquisition of literacy. One possibility that will be examined in this chapter is that orthographic activation is involved in the acquisition of phonological awareness (specifically awareness of phoneme and onset subsyllabic units of spoken words); a prerequisite skill for acquiring literacy (e.g. Goswami & Bryant, 1990; Stanovich, 1986; Wagner & Torgesen, 1987).

ACTIVATION OF ORTHOGRAPHIC INFORMATION DURING AUDITORY WORD RECOGNITION: FLUENT READERS

In order to develop the argument that orthographic activation influences the acquisition of literacy skills it is important to review the evidence for such activation in the auditory word recognition performance of fluent readers. Seidenberg and Tanenhaus (1979) were the first to report that auditory word recognition can be influenced by a word's spelling. They required their subjects to decide whether or not two spoken words rhymed. In their task, subjects heard two words, such as "dune" and "tune," and then indicated their rhyme decision by pressing a button labelled YES or a button labelled NO. Response time was recorded from the onset of the second spoken word until the subject pressed either of the response buttons. Seidenberg and Tanenhaus (1979, experiment 3) found that subjects made 99 millisecond faster YES responses on pairs of words that rhymed and had the same spelling (e.g., "tune," "dune"; mean response time = 779 milliseconds) than on pairs of word that rhymed, but had different spellings (e.g., "moon," "dune"; mean response time = 878 milliseconds). Similarly, they made 58 millisecond slower NO responses on pairs of words that were spelled the same but did not rhyme (e.g., "tough," "cough"; mean response time = 961 milliseconds) than on pairs of words that did not rhyme and were not spelled the same (e.g., "stuff," "cough"; mean response time = 903 milliseconds). These results were similar in magnitude and pattern to those obtained with printed words in visual word recognition tasks (e.g., Meyer, Schvaneveldt & Ruddy, 1974; Seidenberg & Tanenhaus, 1979, experiment 1).

Nelson and McEvoy (1979) have reported that subjects rate pairs of rhyming words that are similar in both spelling and sound as being more familiar than pairs that are similar in sound alone, possibly because of more frequent experience with rhyming pairs that are similar in both spelling and sound. If familiarity rather than spelling similarity was the critical variable in producing the results reported by Seidenberg and Tanenhaus (1979), then their auditory orthographic activation effect would be limited to the pairs of items that rhymed (i.e., pairs requiring a YES response). Auditory orthographic activation would not be predicted by a familiarity interpretation for the pairs of items that do not rhyme (i.e., pairs requiring a NO response) because items that are similar in spelling (e.g., "tease," "lease") would be unlikely to be any more familiar as word pairs than items that are dissimilar (e.g., "piece," "lease").

Auditory orthographic activation effects have been reported by these investigators in several other tasks (e.g., Tanenhaus, Flanigan & Seidenberg, 1980; Donnenwerth-Nolan, Tanenhaus & Seidenberg, 1981; Zecker, Tanenhaus, Alderman, & Siqueland, 1986) and by other investigators (e.g., Jakimik, Cole & Rudnicky, 1985). Tanenhaus, Flanigan and Seidenberg (1980, experiment 2), for example, used a Stroop paradigm in which their subjects heard two words and then were required to name the color of ink in which a third word was printed. Color naming time was slower when the two auditorially presented words were spelled the same as the Stroop target word (e.g., auditory presentation of "light" and "fight" followed by the word EIGHT printed in color) than when the spelling was different (auditory presentation of "bite" and "kite" or "moon" and "soon" followed by the word EIGHT printed in color). Similar auditory orthographic effects involving cross-modal priming have been obtained in lexical decision tasks (Hillinger, 1980) and sentence comprehension tasks (Hudson & Tanenhaus, 1985). These data are consistent with the view that orthographic information is activated automatically during the time course of auditory word recognition.

Beach and Jakimik (1986) showed that an orthographic activation effect can also be obtained when subjects are required to make explicit judgments about the spelling of spoken word pairs. In making decisions about whether or not the words were spelled the same after the initial consonant cluster, subjects made faster "yes" responses when the similarly spelled pairs rhymed ("most" "post") than when they did not ("frost" "post") and slower "no" responses when the dissimilarly spelled pairs rhymed ("boast" "post") then when they did not ("drab" "post").

Finally, Jakimik et al. (1985) have also obtained evidence of orthographic activation in auditory word recognition. Using a priming task, they found that subjects were faster at making lexical (i.e., word, nonword) decisions about spoken words when the priming word was related to the target word in both the spelling and sound of the initial syllable (e.g., "nap," "napkin") than when the items were unrelated (e.g., "blanket," "pill"). Contrary to their expectations, however, the prime-target pairs that were related only in the sound (e.g., "definite," "deaf") or only in the spelling (e.g., "legislate," "leg") of the first syllable were not significantly different from the unrelated condition. These latter results suggest that lexical decision tasks and manipulations of syllable similarity may be less likely to produce orthographic activation effects than rhyming tasks and manipulations of sub-syllabic similarity.

Taken together, these results provide evidence that fluent readers activate orthographic information during the process of recognizing spoken words and that this activation is automatic. They are also consistent with the assumption made in both network (e.g., Collins & Loftus, 1975) and connectionist (e.g., Seidenberg & McClelland, 1989; Van Orden, Pennington & Stone, 1990) models of the word recognition that all of the information associated with a word is activated when it is presented either visually or auditorially. Although these classes of models do not make explicit assumptions about bi-directional activation between spelling and sound, examination of the architecture of these models suggests that phonology can activate orthography as readily as the orthography can activate phonology (e.g., see Seidenberg & McClelland, 1989; Figure 1, p. 526).

Evidence consistent with the possibility of bi-directional activation between orthography and phonology has recently been reported at the level of individual graphemes and phonemes by Dijkstra, Frauenfelder and Schreuder (1993) with Dutch speakers. These investigators used a GO/NO GO task in which a letter or a non-alphabetic symbol was presented in close temporal proximity with a vowel phoneme. In the NO GO part of the task, the subjects were instructed not to respond to the letter E or its corresponding phoneme /e/. In the GO part of the task, they presented the letter A 100 milliseconds before the onset of its corresponding phoneme /a/ and recorded subjects' response time to the letter. They found that subjects responded faster in this A before /a/ experimental condition than in control conditions in which the letter was replaced by a non-alphabetic symbol (e.g., * before /a/) or by a different letter (e.g., U before /a/) suggesting that the phoneme activated its corresponding letter and facilitated letter processing through phoneme-to-grapheme activation. Importantly, the letter and its corresponding phoneme did not differ in response time when each was presented alone. They also obtained evidence for grapheme-to-phoneme activation when the letter-phoneme order was reversed (the phoneme /a/ preceded the letter A by 100 milliseconds) and subjects' response time to the phoneme was recorded.

The Dijkstra et al. (1993) results suggest that both phoneme-to-grapheme and grapheme-to-phoneme activation is very rapid and automatic because the stimulus onset asynchronies in their experiments were short (100 milliseconds), the subjects' response times were quick (300 - 400 milliseconds), and their results were obtained for both blocked and mixed presentations under different instructions and stimuli. Rapid and automatic phoneme-to-grapheme activation is consistent, for example, with the fluent performance of backward talkers who employ orthographic information when reversing their speech (e.g., Cowan et al, 1985) and with the evidence presented above for the auditory orthographic activation effect. Rapid and automatic grapheme-to-phoneme activation is consistent with reports of pre-lexical phonological activation occurring early in the process of visual word recognition (e.g., Perfetti & Bell, 1991; Perfetti, Bell & Delaney, 1988; Van Orden et al., 1990).

ACTIVATION OF ORTHOGRAPHIC INFORMATION DURING AUDITORY WORD RECOGNITION: DYSLEXIC READERS

Although the auditory orthographic activation effects are consistently obtained for fluent adult readers, it is possible that such effects would not be obtained for dyslexic readers. The primary basis for this expectation is that these individuals tend to have persistent deficiencies in phoneme awareness (e.g., Bradley & Bryant, 1978) and spelling-to-sound correspondence knowledge (e.g., Rack, Snowling & Olson, 1992) so that they perform at levels that are below that of normal readers of the same age and normal readers that are several years younger. Bruck (1992) compared the performance of normal readers with developmentally dyslexic readers and with adult dyslexic readers who were diagnosed with developmental dyslexia as children. These subjects performed a phoneme counting task in which they heard nonwords and were required to count the number of phonemes they contained. One half of the items had the same number of letters as phonemes (e.g., "tisk") while the remaining items contained diagraphs that had more letters than phonemes (e.g., "leem"). In addition to higher overall levels of performance than the dyslexic subjects, the normal subjects made more "overshoot" errors—reporting that the digraph words had extra phonemes (e.g., that "leem" has four phonemes). These results suggest that the normal subjects were more likely to activate the spelling of the word in performing the task and then mistakenly count the number of letters rather than the number of phonemes. In contrast, all of the dyslexic subjects were less able to analyze the individual phonemes and to activate and use orthographic representations of the words. The normal subjects' greater use of orthographic information was further supported in a phoneme deletion task where they were much more likely than dyslexic subjects to report, for example, "hoace" rather than "oace" when asked to delete the first sound (i.e., /θ/ = th) of the nonword "thoace."

Bruck's (1992) findings that normal readers are more likely to use orthographic information than dyslexic readers has not been uniformly supported (also see Olson et al., and Assink & Kattenberg, and Bowers et al.,Volume I and Lennox & Siegel, Vol. II of this series). Rack (1985, experiment 2), for example, found that disabled readers produced a larger auditory orthographic effect than normal readers on the Seidenberg and Tanenhaus (1979) rhyming task and Zecker (1991) found that older dyslexics and normal readers produced an equivalent sized auditory orthographic effect. Younger dyslexic readers in Zecker's (1991) experiment, however, produced a smaller auditory orthographic activation effect compared to normals. Finally, Martin (1984) examined the relationship between spelling skill and the ability to activate orthographic information. Based on work by Frith (1980), she identified grade six children who were good readers but poor spellers and compared their performance to a group of good readers and spellers in the same grade and to a group of younger (grade four) good readers and spellers on the Seidenberg and Tanenhaus (1979) rhyme task. Martin (1984) found that all three groups of spellers produced a significant and equivalent sized auditory orthographic effect indicating that the tendency to activate orthographic information in auditory word recognition was not related to spelling ability, at least within the range of skill that was examined.

Bruck (1992) has pointed out that orthographic effects in phoneme counting and phoneme deletion tasks may require both automatic activation of orthographic information in auditory word recognition and the deliberate and conscious use of that information to perform the demanding tasks of counting and deletion. In contrast, orthographic effects in the Seidenberg and Tanenhaus (1979) rhyming tasks may be based solely on automatic activation. Perhaps dyslexic and normal readers differ primarily in their ability to use orthographic information in resource demanding tasks rather than in the ability to activate that information initially.

One exception to this conclusion, however, comes from Campbell and Butterworth (1985) who reported a case study of a developmental dyslexic whose disability was identified in early adulthood. Their subject had very poor phonological awareness skills and had considerable difficulty reading and spelling nonwords, but was classified as a good reader and speller based on literacy assessments involving real words. This individual appeared to perform phonological awareness tasks by activating and using orthographic information because overshoot errors were very frequent in a phoneme counting task. In addition, considerably more orthographic responses were made compared to a normal control group in an auditory acronym task in which taking the first sound of each word in an orally presented sequence such as "hold ache toes" will yield "hate" if performed phonemically as required, and "hat" if performed orthographically. Campbell and Butterworth's (1985) results indicate that their subject had learned to compensate for severe impairments in phonological processing and awareness skill by forming print-to-sound associations at the whole word level and using them to read and spell. Apparently, this lexical level orthographic knowledge was used in performing phonological awareness tasks.

ACTIVATION OF ORTHOGRAPHIC INFORMATION DURING AUDITORY WORD RECOGNITION: PREREADERS AND BEGINNING AND DEVELOPING READERS

Auditory orthographic activation effects have also been obtained with normally developing children. Ehri and Wilce (1980) found that children use "silent" letters (a letter that does not have a unique corresponding phonemic representation in a word) in performing auditory phoneme counting tasks. They reported that grade four children tended to produce overshoot errors as they counted five phonemes in a word like "pitch" or a nonsense word like "tadge" and four phonemes in "rich" or "taj" even though the two corresponding words ("pitch" and "rich"; "tadge" and "taj") had the same pronunciation and contained the same number of phonemes. These results are consistent with the overshoot errors produced by the young normal subjects in Bruck (1992). Tumner and Nesdale (1982) also used a phoneme counting task very similar to that of Bruck (1992) and Ehri and Wilce (1980). They found, however, that even children in Kindergarten and grade one tended to make overshoot errors (e.g., the children gave four rather than three taps to items like THEM and THEB) despite the fact that they were not exposed to the word's spelling and were just learning to read. Finally, Nichols, Donnerwerth-Nolan, Tanenhaus and Carlson (1984) used the Seidenberg and Tanenhaus (1979) rhyming task with adults and good and poor readers in grades one through six. They found that poor readers in grades four through six, good readers in grades two through six, and adults were faster and more accurate at making yes responses to orthographically similar rhyming pairs (e.g., "pie," "tie") than on rhyming pairs that were spelled differently ("guy," "tie"). Waters and Seidenberg (1983) have reported a similar pattern of results.

Considered together, the Bruck (1992, young normal reader results), Ehri and Wilce (1980), Nichols et al, (1984), Tumner and Nesdale (1982), and Waters and Seidenberg (1983) results all suggest that beginning readers can activate and use orthographic information in auditory word recognition. One question arising from these findings is whether or not prereaders might also show some influence of orthographic knowledge in their auditory word recognition performance before they are able to express that knowledge in the conventional production tasks of reading aloud and spelling to dictation. The Seidenberg and Tanenhaus (1979) rhyming task might be particularly useful for examining this possibility. One advantage of this task is that it is a relatively "natural" language task which can executed with sufficient fluency by five and six year-old prereaders that it is possible to obtain a reliable response time measure of automatic activation of orthographic information during the course of auditory word recognition. In addition, rhyming does not appear to make the same cognitive demands that are associated with other possible tasks, such as phoneme counting and phoneme deletion, which tend to have more substantial memory and production requirements. Accordingly, rhyming tasks may be more likely than other tasks to reveal what, if any, orthographic knowledge prereaders may have acquired.

In response to these considerations, Pearson and Barron (1986) investigated the auditory orthographic effect in children who were in the very early stages of learning to read. We identified two groups of children who, following the definitions proposed by Ehri and Wilce (1985), were referred to as Novices and Veterans. The Novices (N = 18) were all in grade one, averaged six years, four months of age, could produce 73 percent of the sounds and 94 percent of the letters of the alphabet, but could only read six percent and spell seven percent of the words used in the rhyming task. In contrast, the Veterans (N = 20) were all in grade two, averaged seven years five months of age, could produce 95 percent of the sounds and 100 percent of the names of the alphabet and could read aloud 85 percent of the words used in the rhyming task and spell to dictation 61 percent. Both groups of subjects were faster on orthographically similar ("far" "car") than dissimilar ("tea" "key") rhyming pairs and slower on orthographically similar ("low" "cow") than dissimilar ("face" "ring") nonrhyming pairs. Furthermore, the size of this auditory orthographic effect was the same for both groups of subjects and the errors (average less than five percent) and response times were positively correlated.

Pearson and Barron (1989; in preparation) attempted to replicate these results with different words and subjects, including a group of adult subjects. In addition, pictures rather than spoken words were used as the second item in each rhyming pair (the first item was always a spoken word) in order to see if the phenomenon could be generalized and the likelihood reduced that the effect could be attributed to some unidentified acoustic property of the words that triggered the onset of our timer upon the presentation of the second word in the pair. In the picture version of the task, the subjects heard the first word and then saw a picture. They were instructed to decide whether or not the word and the name of the picture rhymed. The Novices (N = 20) were all in grade one and averaged six years, four months of age. They could produce 76 percent of the sounds and 91 percent of the names of the letters of the alphabet, but they could only read three percent of the words used in the rhyming tasks. The Veterans (N = 20) were all in grade two and averaged seven years, two months of age. They could produce 96 percent of the sounds and 100 percent of the names of the letters of the alphabet and could read 92 percent of the words. The adults (N = 35) were all university students and fluent readers.

Our earlier pattern of results was replicated when both of the words making up the rhyme were presented auditorially; the Novices and the Veterans showed an auditory orthographic effect that was the same size for both groups. When the second word in the rhyming pair was a picture (e.g., similar rhyme = "cook," picture of a hook; dissimilar rhyme = "chew," picture of a shoe; similar nonrhyme = "gone," picture of a bone; dissimilar nonrhyme = "rule," picture of a bell) the earlier pattern of results was also replicated. In fact, the word-picture condition produced virtually the same pattern of results as the word-word condition. Finally, the adult sample also produced an auditory orthographic activation effect in both the word-word and word-picture conditions. Considered together, these results indicate that the orthographic representations of words are activated by children (Novice readers) who were only able to read aloud and spell about five percent of the words used in the rhyming tasks (range = three to seven percent). Furthermore, the pattern of the Novice readers' performance was very similar to that of the Veteran readers (who could read and spell most of the words) and fluent adult readers. Finally, these auditory orthographic activation effects were obtained in two different experiments which involved different subjects, words, and experimental procedures (e.g., word-word and word-picture rhyme tasks).

The presence of an auditory orthographic effect among prereaders is surprising unless consideration is given to the fact that the Novice readers had high letter-sound knowledge (it is assumed that they also had high sound-letter knowledge although this was not measured directly). Unlike Bruck's (1992) dyslexic readers, it is also likely that they had good phonological awareness skills as both Stuart and Coltheart (1988) and Vellutino and Scanlon (1987) have reported that letter-sound knowledge and measures of phonological awareness are highly correlated (r = .60 to .80). In order to decide whether or not two words rhyme, these subjects were required to segment each of the words into onset and rime units and compare the rime units. Phonologically identical rime units yield a YES response and phonologically different rime units yield a "NO" response. The rimes, however, consist of phonemes and at least some of these phonemes are associated with letters. It is assumed that some of these associated letters are activated rapidly and automatically as the rime and onset units are segmented and compared and that they influence the rhyme (YES)-nonrhyme (NO) decision process by activating orthographic information that is either consistent or inconsistent with the phonological information.

It is not clear from the Pearson and Barron (1986, 1989, in

preparation) results whether consistent orthographic and phonological information facilitates the decision and inconsistent information has no influence on performance or whether inconsistent orthographic and phonological information inhibits the decision and/or initiates a re-checking process. Regardless of the precise comparison and decision mechanisms, this interpretation does not require that the complete lexical spelling of the word be represented in order to obtain an auditory orthographic activation effect; a partial representation may be sufficient. On the other hand, letter-sound knowledge itself may not be sufficient to account for the auditory orthographic activation effect because some of the words, particularly among the orthographically similar nonrhyming pairs (e.g., "cough," "tough"), have irregular spellings.

Regardless of whether the Novice readers' orthographic representations are incomplete or complete (i.e., represents all of the letters in the word) or are prelexical or lexical, the representations are not yet sufficiently developed to be used effectively in producing accurate reading aloud or spelling-to-dictation responses. There is, however, some suggestion from Tumner and Nesdale's (1982) research with kindergarten children that the orthographic representations activated by Novice readers in auditory word recognition may be able to support the use of orthographic information in phoneme counting tasks (as evidenced by overshoot errors). Such a possibility would implicate these representations in the initial acquisition of phonological awareness skill as well as later in acquisition where Bruck (1992) has shown that the use of orthographic strategies in phonological awareness tasks increases with level of reading skill in normal readers.

RECIPROCAL ACTIVATION BETWEEN LETTERS AND SOUNDS AND THE ACQUISITION OF PHONOLOGICAL AWARENESS

Barron (1991, Barron et al., 1992) proposed that proto-literate knowledge (letter-name and letter-sound associations) may influence the acquisition of phonological awareness through a mechanism of reciprocal activation between letters or letter clusters (e.g., t, th) and their corresponding sounds (/t/, /θ/). These proposals about the role of proto-literate knowledge in phonological awareness draw upon Ehri's theoretical framework, particularly the idea that letters come to symbolize sound during the course of the acquisition of reading and spelling skills (e.g., Ehri, 1978, 1979, 1983, 1984, 1993). Isolated speech sounds that are generated in letter-sound association tasks only approximate the individual phonemes that are represented in the context of a spoken syllable or word. In fact, generating a consonant sound in isolation may involve two phonemes (e.g., the response "buh" to the letter B consists of the stop consonant /b/ and a following neutral vowel /ə/). Nevertheless, these embedded, contextualized phonemes may be sufficiently similar to isolated speech sounds that they activate their corresponding letters during the process of auditory word recognition. Conversely, letters that appear in printed words have the potential of activating their corresponding phonemic representations. Accordingly, each letter and each phoneme encounter has the potential of strengthening letter-sound associations. The fluent, bi-directional phoneme-grapheme activation effects obtained in the experiments reported by Dijkstra et al. (1993) are one potential consequence of this learning in the longer-term.

In the shorter-term, however, this bi-directional activation may be implicated in the development of phonological awareness in the following manner. Although rhyming skill appears quite early in language development (e.g., MacLean, Bryant & Bradley, 1987; Bryant, Bradley, MacLean & Crossland, 1989; Bryant, Maclean, Bradley & Crossland, 1990), possession of this skill does not imply awareness of phonemic units because rhyming may be carried out using wholistic, undifferentiated representations of rime units (Bertelson & deGelder, 1989; Stanovich, 1986). In fact, evidence from data collected on children and illiterate adults suggest that awareness of phonemes requires literacy whereas awareness of rimes does not (e.g., Morais, Cary, Alegria & Bertelson, 1979; Bertelson, deGelder, Tfouni & Morais, 1989; Morais, Alegria & Content, 1987).

The rime units involved in the auditory orthographic activation effect with prereaders (i.e., novice readers) are unlikely to be represented wholistically. Instead, it is assumed that they are differentiated into phonemes. Even though the phonemes are embedded within a rime, the fact that they are associated with letters may allow them to be more accessible to conscious awareness and available in phonological awareness tasks that specifically require the isolation and manipulation of onsets and individual phonemes. Barron (1991) has argued that proto-literacy, in the form of letter-sound knowledge, may represent the minimal level of "literacy" necessary for the awareness of onsets and phonemes. Barron et al. (1992), reporting evidence from a training experiment with kindergarten children who could not yet read or spell, found that children with high letter-sound knowledge showed significant pre-test to post-test gains in performance on a phoneme deletion task relative to an alternative training control group when they were given printed as well as computer generated speech feedback. In contrast, only children with low letter-sound knowledge showed gains relative to the control group in a task involving rime units and their performance was not influenced by print feedback. Barron, et al. (1992) also showed that letter-sound knowledge did not influence oddity task performance involving rime units (e.g., identify the word "tap" containing the odd sound /p/ in the final position of the word in the series—"cat," "tap," "fat") during the acquisition phase of their training experiment. Children with high letter-sound knowledge, however, performed at a significantly higher level and above chance compared to children with low letter-sound knowledge on oddity tasks involving onset units (e.g., identify the word "cow" containing the odd sound /k/ in the initial position of the word in the series—"bet," "bag," "cow"). In addition, Barron, Seldon, Golden, Marmurek and Haines (1991, in preparation) used fixed order regression analyses on 112 non-reading Kindergarten children to show that letter-sound knowledge accounted for significant variance in onset and phoneme awareness performance after the deletion of variance attributable to WPSSI I.Q., WRAT-R MATH, memory skill, and task specific performance. In contrast, letter-sound knowledge did not account for any variance in task performance involving rime units following the removal of the above variables.

Further evidence that proto-literacy, in the form of letter-name and letter-sound association knowledge, influences the acquisition of phonological awareness comes from a recent longitudinal study of the relationship between phonological awareness and literacy reported by Wagner, Torgesen and Rashotte (1994); see Wagner and Barker, chapter 7 of this volume. Using latent variable causal modelling procedures, these investigators found that letter-name and letter-sound knowledge in Kindergarten exerted a causal influence upon the children's phonological awareness performance in grade one. Furthermore, this pattern was repeated the following year with letter-name and letter-sound knowledge in grade one having a causal influence on phonological awareness in grade two.

Considered together, the Barron et al., (1991, 1992) and Wagner et al. (1994) results are consistent with bi-directional causal models of the relationship between phonological awareness and literacy (e.g., Bertelson & deGelder, 1989). They also indicate that the level of the phonological unit and the definition of literacy are important factors in specifying the complex set of interactive relationships that are involved. Overall, the evidence indicates that neither proto-literacy or literacy influence the acquisition of rhyming skill, but evidence from Bradley and Bryant (1983); Bryant, Bradley, MacLean and Crossland (1989); Bryant, MacLean, Bradley and Crossland (1990); and MacLean, Bryant and Bradley (1987) indicates that rhyming skill influences the acquisition of literacy. The Barron et al. (1991, 1992) evidence indicates that proto-literacy influences the acquisition of phoneme awareness and onset awareness among nonreaders and nonspellers while the Wagner et al. (1994) evidence indicates proto-literate knowledge also influences the acquisition of phonological awareness skills of beginning readers. Other evidence from research with adult illiterates (e.g., Morais, Carey, Alegria & Bertelson, 1979; Morais, Alegria & Content, 1987) and children (e.g., Foorman, Novy, Francis, & Liberman, 1991; Kirtley, Bryant, MacLean & Bradley, 1989; Perfetti, Beck, Bell & Hughes, 1987) indicates that reading and spelling skill influences the acquisition of onset and phoneme awareness. Finally, onset and phoneme awareness also influences the acquisition of literacy directly (e.g., Bradley & Bryant, 1983; Stanovich, 1986; Wagner & Torgesen, 1987; Wagner et al., 1994).

SUMMARY AND CONCLUSIONS

The acquisition of proto-literate knowledge, in the form of letter-name and letter(s)-sound associations, may provide a basis for the subsequent development of the awareness of onsets and phonemes embedded in spoken words by providing a representation of phonological information that is integrated with the orthographic structure of words. Once initially formed, these representations may become more firmly established through a mechanism of reciprocal activation between graphemes and phonemes, as well as between larger orthographic and phonological units at both the pre-lexical and lexical levels. Although these representations may not be sufficiently well formed to support accurate reading or spelling responses, they may be relatively accessible consciously and, therefore, they may facilitate performance in phonological awareness tasks by making orthographic information available for use in the process of segmenting and manipulating onsets and phonemes (Bruck, 1992; Tumner & Nesdale, 1982). In addition, these representations may provide a basis for constructing an orthographic lexicon for use in reading and spelling (e.g., Ehri, 1993). The auditory orthographic activation effect with Novice prereaders can be regarded as an early indication that such integrated representations have been formed and are potentially available for use in enhancing phonological awareness skills and in acquiring literacy.

NOTE

1. Onsets, rimes, and phonemes constitute the basic phonological units of a syllable and recent evidence indicates that they are organized hierarchically within a syllable (e.g., "top" "stop"). Onsets, which consist of a consonant (e.g., /t/) or consonant cluster (e.g., /st/), occupy an intermediate position in the hierarchy along with rimes, which consist of a vowel (e.g., /ɑ/) plus any following consonants (e.g., /p/). Phonemes (e.g., /s/, /t/, /ɑ/, /p/) are at the bottom level of the hierarchy (see Treiman, 1992, for a review).

REFERENCES

Adams, M.J. (1990). *Beginning to read: Thinking and learning about print*. Cambridge, MA: M.I.T. Press.

Assink, E., & Kattenberg, G. (1994). Higher-order linguistic influences on development of orthographic knowledge: Illustrations from spelling problems in Dutch and assessment tools. In V.W. Berninger (Ed.), *The varieties of orthographic knowledge I: Theoretical and developmental issues* (pp. 111-136). Dordrecht, The Netherlands: Kluwer Academic Publishers.

Barron, R.W. (1986). Word recognition in early reading: A review of the direct and indirect access hypotheses. *Cognition, 24*, 93-119.

Barron, R.W. (1991). Proto-literacy, literacy, and the acquisition of phonological awareness. *Learning and Individual Differences, 3*, 243-255.

Barron, R.W., Golden, J.O., Seldon, D.M., Tait, C.F., Marmurek, H.H.C. & Haines, L.C. (1992). Teaching prereading skills with a talking computer: Letter-sound knowledge and print feedback facilitate nonreaders' phonological awareness training. *Reading and Writing: An Interdisciplinary Journal, 4,* 179-204.

Barron, R.W., Seldon, D.M., Golden, J.O., Marmurek, H.H.C. & Haines, L.P. (1991, April). *Proto-literacy and nonreaders' acquisition of phonological awareness.* Society for Research in Child Development, Seattle, Washington.

Barron, R.W., Seldon, D.M., Golden, J.O., Marmurek, H.H.C. & Haines, L.P. (in preparation). The effects of proto-literate knowledge upon the acquisition of phonological awareness and literacy skill.

Beach, C. & Jakimik, J. (1986, May). *Interactions between orthographic and phonological properties of words.* Paper read at the Midwestern Psychological Association, Chicago, Illinois.

Bertelson, P. & deGelder, B. (1989). Learning about reading from illiterates. In A.M. Galaburda (Ed.), *From neurons to reading* (pp. 1-23). Cambridge, MA: M.I.T. Press.

Bertelson, P., deGelder, B., Tfouni, L.V. & Morais, J. (1989). Metaphonological abilities of adult illiterates: New evidence of heterogeneity. *European Journal of Cognitive Psychology, 1,* 239-250.

Bowers, P., Golden, J., Kennedy, A., & Young, A. (1994). Limits upon orthographic knowledge due to processes indexed by naming speed. In V. W. Berninger (Ed.), *The varieties of orthographic knowledge I: Theoretical and developmental issues* (pp. 173-218). Dordrecht, The Netherlands: Kluwer Academic Press.

Bradley, L. & Bryant, P.E. (1978). Difficulties in auditory organization as a possible cause of reading backwardness. *Nature, 271,* 746-747.

Bradley, L. & Bryant, P.E. (1983). Categorizing sounds and learning to read: A causal connection. *Nature, 301,* 419-421.

Bruck, M. (1992). Persistence of dyslexics' phonological awareness deficits. *Developmental Psychology, 28,* 874-886.

Bryant, P.E., Bradley, L., MacLean, M. & Crossland, J. (1989). Nursery rhymes, phonological skills, and reading. *Journal of Child Language. 16,* 407-428.

Bryant, P.E., MacLean, M., Bradley, L. & Crossland, J. (1990). Rhyme and alliteration, phoneme detection, and learning to read. *Developmental Psychology, 26,* 429-438.

Byrne, B. & Fielding-Barnsley, R. (1989). Phonemic awareness and letter knowledge in the child's acquisition of the alphabetic principle. *Journal of Educational Psychology, 81,* 313-321.

Byrne, B. & Fielding-Barnsley, R. (1990). Acquiring the alphabetic principle: A case for teaching recognition of phoneme identity. *Journal of Educational Psychology, 82,* 805-812.

Campbell, R. & Butterworth, B. (1985). Phonological dyslexia and dysgraphia in a highly literate subject: A developmental case with associated deficits in phonemic processing and awareness. *Quarterly Journal of Experimental Psychology, 37A,* 435-475.

Clay, M.M. (1976). Early childhood and cultural diversity in New Zealand. *Reading Teacher, 29,* 333-342.

Collins, A.M. & Loftus, E.F. (1975). A spreading activation theory of cognitive processing. *Psychological Review, 82,* 407-428.

Cowan, N., Braine, M.D.S. & Leavitt, L.A. (1985). The phonological and metaphonological representation of speech: Evidence from fluent backward talkers. *Journal of Memory & Language, 24,* 679-698.

Cowan, N. & Leavitt, L.A. (1982). Talking backwards: Exceptional speech play in late childhood. *Journal of Child Language, 9,* 481-495.

Cowan, N., Leavitt, L.A., Massaro, D. & Kent. R. (1982). A fluent backward talker. *Journal of Speech & Hearing Research, 25,* 48-53.

Cunningham, A.E. & Stanovich, K.E. (1990). Assessing print exposure and orthographic processing skill in children: A quick measure of reading experience. *Journal of Educational Psychology, 82,* 733-740.

Cunningham, A.E. & Stanovich, K.E. (1991). Tracking the unique effects of print exposure in children: Associations with vocabulary, general knowledge, and spelling. *Journal of Educational Psychology, 83,* 264-274.

Dijkstra, T, Frauenfelder, U.H. & Schreuder, R. (1993). Bidirectional grapheme-phoneme activation in a bimodal detection task. *Journal of Experimental Psychology: Human Perception and Performance, 19,* 931-950.

Donnenwerth-Nolan, S., Tanenhaus, M.K. & Seidenberg, M.S. (1981). Multiple code activation in word recognition: Evidence from rhyme monitoring. *Journal of Experimental Psychology: Human Learning and Memory, 7,* 170-180.

Ehri, L.C. (1978). Beginning reading from a psycholinguistic perspective: Amalgamation of word identities. In F.B. Murray (Ed.), *The recognition of words: IRA series on the development of the reading process* (pp. 1-33). Newark, DE: International Reading Association.

Ehri, L.C. (1979). Linguistic insight: Threshold of reading acquisition. In T. G. Waller & G. E. MacKinnon (Eds.), *Reading research: Advances in theory and practice* Vol. 1, (pp. 63-114). New york: Academic Press.

Ehri, L.C. (1983). A critique of five studies related to letter-name knowledge and learning to read. In L. Gentile, M. Kamil & J. Blanchard (Eds.), *Reading research revisited* (pp. 143-153). Columbus, OH: C. E. Merrill.

Ehri, L.C. (1984). How orthography alters spoken language competencies in children learning to read and spell. In J. Downing & R. Valtin (Eds.), *Language awareness and learning to read* (pp. 119-147). New York: Springer-Verlag.

Ehri, L.C. (1993). How English orthography influences phonological knowledge as children learn to read and spell. In R.J. Scholes (Ed.), *Literacy and language analysis.* Hillsdale, NJ: Lawrence Erlbaum Associates.

Ehri, L.C. & Wilce, L.S. (1980). The influence of orthography on readers' conceptualization of the phonemic structure of words. *Applied Psycholinguistics, 1,* 371-385.

Ehri, L.C. & Wilce, L.S. (1985). Movement into reading: Is the first stage of printed word learning visual or phonetic? *Reading Research Quarterly, 20,* 163-179.

Frith, U. (1980). Unexpected spelling problems. In U. Frith (Ed.), *Cognitive processes in spelling* (pp. 495-515). London: Academic Press.

Foorman, B.R., Novy, D.M., Francis, D.J. & Liberman, D. (1991). How letter-sound instruction mediates progress in first-grade reading and spelling. *Journal of Educational Psychology, 83,* 456-459.

Goswami, U. & Bryant, P. (1990). *Phonological skills and learning to read.* East Sussex, United Kingdom: Lawrence Erlbaum Associates.

Hiebert, E.H. (1993). Young children's literacy experiences in home and in school. In S.R. Yussen & M.C. Smith (Eds.). *Reading across the life span* (pp. 33-55).

Hillinger, M.I. (1980). Priming effects with phonemically similar words: The encoding-bias hypothesis reconsidered. *Memory & Cognition, 8*, 115-124.

Hudson, S.B. & Tanenhaus, M.K. (1985). Phonological code activation during listening. *Journal of Psycholinguistic Research, 14*, 557-567.

Jakimik, J., Cole, R.A. & Rudnicky, A.I. (1985). Sound and spelling in spoken word recognition. *Journal of Memory and Language, 24*, 165-178.

Kirtley, C., Bryant, P.E., MacLean, M. & Bradley, L. (1989). Rhyme, rime, and the onset of reading. *Journal of Experimental Child Psychology, 48*, 224-245.

Lennox, C., & Siegel, L. (in press). Development of orthographic and phonological proceses in normal and disabled reading. In V.W. Berninger (Ed.), *The varieties of orthographic knowledge II: Relationships to phonology, reading, and writing*. Dordrecht, The Netherlands: Kluwer Academic Publishers.

MacLean, M., Bryant, P.E. & Bradley, L. (1987). Rhymes, nursery rhymes, and reading in early childhood. *Merrill Palmer Quarterly, 33*, 255-281.

Mason, J.M. (1992). Reading stories to preliterate children. In P.B. Gough, L.C. Ehri & R. Treiman (Eds.), *Reading Acquisition* (pp. 215-241). Hillsdale, NJ: Lawrence Erlbaum Associates.

Martin, V.L (1984). *The influence of orthography on auditory word recognition for good and poor spellers.* Unpublished Masters Thesis, University of Guelph.

Meyer, D.E., Schvaneveldt, R.W. & Ruddy, M. (1974). Functions of graphemic and phonemic codes in visual word recognition. *Memory & Cognition, 2*, 309-321.

Morais, J., Alegria, J. & Content, A. (1987). The relationships between segmental analysis and alphabetic literacy: an interactive view. *Cahiers de Psychologie Cognitive, 7*, 415-438.

Morais, J., Cary, L., Alegria, J. & Bertelson, P. (1979). Does awareness of speech as a series of phones arise spontaneously? *Cognition, 7*, 323-331.

Nelson, D.L. & McEvoy, C.L. (1979). Encoding context and set size. *Journal of Experimental Psychology: Human Learning and Memory, 5*, 292-314.

Nichols, C., Donnerwerth-Nolan, S., Tanenhaus, M.K. & Carlson, G.N. (1984, May). *Development of orthographic effects in rhyming*. Paper presented at the Midwestern Psychological Association, Chicago, Illinois.

Olson, R., Forsberg, H., Wise, R. (1994). Genes, environment, and the development of orthographic skills. In V.W. Berninger (Ed.), *The varieties of orthographic knowledge I: Theoretical and developmental issues* (pp. 27-71). Dordrecht, The Netherlands: Kluwer Academic Publishers.

Pearson , L.L. & Barron, R.W. (1986, June). *Activation of orthography by beginning readers in an auditory rhyme task.* Canadian Psychological Association meetings, Toronto, Ontario, Canada

Pearson, L.L. & Barron, R.W. (1989, March). *Orthography influences beginning readers' auditory rhyme judgments.* American Educational Research Association meetings, San Francisco, California.

Pearson, L.L. & Barron, R.W. (in preparation). Interactions between spelling and sound before literacy: Evidence for an orthographic activation effect with prereaders.

Perfetti, C.A., Beck, I., Bell, L. & Hughes, C. (1987). Phonemic knowledge and learning to read are reciprocal: A longitudinal study. *Merrill-Palmer Quarterly, 33*, 283-319.

Perfetti, C.A. & Bell, L.C. (1991). Phonemic activation during the first 40ms of word identification: Evidence from backward masking. *Journal of Memory and Language, 30*, 473-485.

Perfetti, C.A., Bell, L.C. & Delaney, S.M. (1988). Automatic (prelexical) phonetic activation in silent word reading. *Journal of Reading and Language, 27*, 59-70.

Rack, J.P. (1985). Orthographic and phonetic coding in developmental dyslexia. *British Journal of Psychology, 76*, 325-340.

Rack, J.P., Snowling, M.J. & Olson, R.K. (1992). The nonword reading deficit in developmental dyslexia: A review. *Reading Research Quarterly, 27*, 29-53.

Read, C. (1986). *Children's creative spelling*. London: Routledge & Kegan Paul.

Seidenberg, M.S. & McClelland, J.L. (1989). A distributed, developmental model of word recognition and naming. *Psychological Review, 96*, 523-568.

Seidenberg, M.S. & Tanenhaus, M.K. (1979). Orthographic effects of rhyme monitoring. *Journal of Experimental Psychology, 5,* 546-554.

Stanovich, K.E. (1986). Matthew effects in reading: Some consequences of individual differences in the acquisition of literacy. *Reading Research Quarterly, 21,* 360-407.

Stanovich, K.E. (1993). Does reading make you smarter? Literacy and the development of verbal intelligence. In H. W. Reese (ED.), *Advances in child development and behavior* (Vol. 24, pp. 133-180). San Diego, CA: Academic press.

Stanovich, K.E. & Cunningham, A.E. (1992). Studying the consequences of literacy within a literate society: The cognitive correlates of print exposure. *Memory and Cognition, 20,* 51-68.

Stanovich, K.E. & Cunningham, A.E. (1993). Where does knowledge come from? Specific associations between print exposure and information acquisition. *Journal of Educational Psychology, 85,* 211-229.

Stanovich, K.E. & West, R.F. (1989). Exposure to print and orthographic processing. *Reading Research Quarterly, 24,* 402-433.

Stuart, M. (1990). Factors influencing word recognition strategies in prereading children. *British Journal of Psychology, 81,* 135-146.

Stuart, M. & Coltheart, M. (1988). Does reading develop in a sequence of stages? *Cognition, 30,* 139-181.

Tanenhaus, M.K., Flanigan, H.P., & Seidenberg, M.K. (1980). Orthographic and phonological activation in auditory and visual word recognition. *Memory and Cognition, 8,* 513-520.

Teale, W.H. (1986). Home background and young children's literacy development. In W.H. Teale & E. Sulzby (Eds.), *Emergent literacy: writing and reading.* Norwood, NJ: Ablex Publishing Corporation.

Teale, W. & Sulzby, E. (1986). *Emergent literacy: writing and reading.* Norwood, NJ: Ablex.

Treiman, R. (1992). The role of intrasyllabic units in learning to read and spell. In P.B. Gough, L.C. Ehri & R. Treiman, (Eds.), *Reading acquisition* (pp. 65-106). Hillsdale, NJ: Lawrence Erlbaum Associates.

Tumner, W.E. & Nesdale, A.R. (1982). The effects of digraphs and pseudowords on phoneme segmentation in young children. *Applied Psycholinguistics, 3,* 299-311.

Van Orden, G.C., Pennington, B.F. & Stone, G.O. (1990). Word identification in reading and the promise of subsymbolic psycholinguistics. *Psychological Review, 97,* 488-552.

Vellutino, F. & Scanlon, D.M. (1987). Phonological coding, phonological awareness, and reading ability. *Merrill-Palmer Quarterly, 33,* 321-364.

Wagner, R., & Barker, T. (1994). The development of orthographic processing ability. In V. W. Berninger (Ed.), *The varieties of orthographic knowledge I: Theoretical and developmental issues* (pp. 243-276). Dordrecht, The Netherlands: Kluwer Academic Publishers.

Wagner, R.K. & Torgesen, J.K. (1987). The nature of phonological processing and its causal role in the acquisition of reading skill. *Psychological Bulletin, 101,* 192-212.

Wagner, R.K., Torgesen, J.K. & Rashotte, C.A. (1994). The development of reading-related phonological processing abilities: New evidence of bi-directional causality from a latent variable longitudinal study. *Developmental Psychology, 30,* 73-87.

Waters, G. & Seidenberg, M.S. (1983, April). *Orthographic and phonological code activation in auditory and visual word recognition in good and poor readers.* American Educational Research Association meetings, Montreal, Quebec, Canada.

Wells, G. (1985). Preschool literacy-related activities and success in school. In D.R. Olson, N. Torrance, N. & A. Hildyard (Eds.), *Literacy, language, and learning* (pp. 229-255). New York: Cambridge University Press.

Zecker, S. (1991). The orthographic code: Developmental trends in reading-disabled and normal children. *Annals of Dyslexia, 41,* 178-192..

Zecker, S., Tanenhaus, M.K., Alderman, L., & Siqueland, L. (1986). Lateralization of lexical codes in auditory word recognition. *Brain and Language, 29,* 372-389.

Address Correspondence to:

Roderick W. Barron
Department of Psychology
University of Guelph
Guelph, Ontario
Canada N1G 2W1

RICHARD K. WAGNER & THEODORE A. BARKER

THE DEVELOPMENT OF ORTHOGRAPHIC PROCESSING ABILITY

When children learn to read, their success is determined by a number of factors. Some determinants of success are found in the environment, including the intensity, duration, and quality of the reading instruction provided, and the nature of the oral and written language the child must attempt to master. Other determinants of success are found within the child. Examples include maturational readiness (the majority of 6-year-olds can learn to read whereas few 2-year-olds can), fluency in oral language, and an interest in reading (for summaries of the reading literature, see Adams, 1990; Crowder & Wagner, 1991; Rayner & Pollatsek, 1989). During the past decade, a great deal of progress has been made in our understanding of beginning reading in general, and in the areas of phonological and orthographic knowledge and processing in particular.

Phonological processing refers to making use of the phonological or sound structure of oral language when processing written or oral language (Wagner & Torgesen, 1987). The focus of much of the research on phonological processing in the context of beginning reading has been on causal relations between the development of various phonological processing abilities and the development of reading ability and reading disability.

In a research program that has involved cross-sectional and longitudinal studies of preschool and primary-school children, we have found that young children's phonological processing abilities are well-described by five, correlated abilities (Wagner, Balthazor, Hurley, Morgan, Rashotte, Shaner, Simmons, & Stage, 1987; Wagner, Torgesen Laughon, Simmons, & Rashotte, 1992; Wagner, Torgesen, & Rashotte, 1994). *Phonological analysis* refers to the ability to break whole words into constituent parts, as when counting or segmenting the three basic sounds or phonemes in the spoken word "cat" represented by the letters c, a, and t. *Phonological synthesis* refers to the ability to combine

V.W. Berninger (ed.), The varieties of orthographic knowledge I: Theoretical and developmental issues, 243-276.

isolated sound segments into whole spoken words, as when blending three phonemes together to form the spoken word"cat." The common term phonological awareness subsumes both phonological analysis and synthesis. *Phonological coding in working memory* refers to the ability to use phonological information or codes to represent speech-based information for short-term storage. The common digit span task is a good measure of this phonological processing ability, especially when the digit presentation rate is relatively rapid (e.g., 2 per second) and the children are young (e.g., third grade or under), both of which discourage other more elaborate or strategic kinds of processing. *Isolated naming* refers to retrieving phonological codes to name objects or symbols presented one at a time, as when a voice key is used to time how long it takes to begin to pronounce the name of an object depicted on a computer screen. *Serial naming* refers to retrieving phonological codes to name series of objects or symbols presented simultaneously, as when being asked to name several rows of drawings of common objects as quickly and accurately as possible. The two kinds of naming, isolated and serial, obviously have much in common, but appear to involve somewhat different processing as well.

Individual and developmental differences in young children's phonological processing abilities appear to be causally related to the acquisition of beginning reading skills, although questions remain about possible causal mechanisms and even predominant causal directions (Ball & Blachman, 1988; Bradley & Bryant, 1985; Bryant, Bradley, MacLean, & Crossland, 1989; Ehri, 1987; Stanovich, 1986; Lundberg, Frost, Petersen, 1988; Perfetti, Beck, Bell, & Hughes, 1987; Treiman, 1991; Tunmer & Nesdale, 1985; Wagner, 1988; Wagner & Torgesen, 1987; Wagner, Torgesen, & Rashotte, 1994). In addition, a severe deficit in some aspect of phonological processing is viewed as a likely contributor to the development of reading disability or dyslexia (Bradley & Bryant, 1978; Bruck, 1990; Bruck & Treiman, 1990; Felton & Wood, 1990; Manis, Szeszulski, Holt, & Graves, 1990; Olson, Wise, Conners, & Rack, 1990; Olson, Wise, Conners, Rack, & Fulker, 1989; Rack, Snowling, & Olson, 1992; Siegel & Ryan, 1988; Shankweiler & Liberman, 1989; Stanovich, 1988, in press; Torgesen, 1991, in press; Tunmer, 1989; Wagner, 1986).

In a recent longitudinal study of approximately 250 children from kindergarten through second grade, we found evidence of causal relations between each of the five kinds of phonological processing abilities and subsequent decoding when each phonological processing ability was considered individually; however when considered simultaneously, their causal roles appeared to be redundant for the most part (Wagner, Torgesen, & Rashotte, 1994). This finding means that an aspect of phonological processing that is common to these different kinds of phonological processing abilities is at the core of their causal relations with the acquisition of beginning reading skills.

Orthographic processing refers to making use of orthographic information when processing written or oral language. An orthography refers to the system of marks that make up a printed language. For the English language, orthography includes upper and lower case letters, numerals, and punctuation marks. We will consider alternative working definitions of orthographic processing abilities shortly, but for purposes of introduction, consider an everyday example. Think about what you do when you are not sure how to spell a word and a dictionary is not at hand. The most common strategy in such a situation is to write out the word and look at it to determine whether the spelling looks correct. If you use this strategy, what you are doing at some level is comparing a visual image of the word you have written with a stored orthographic image that you have built up from previous encounters with the word in question.

Compared to our knowledge about young children's phonological processing abilities, knowledge about young children's orthographic processing abilities is somewhat sketchy. Whereas there is an emerging consensus about the nature of phonological processing abilities and suitable tasks for measuring them, there is more disagreement about what orthographic processing abilities are—and even whether they exist at all! In addition, little agreement exists about suitable tasks for measuring orthographic processing abilities. And whereas there is an emerging consensus that phonological processing abilities are causally related to the acquisition of beginning reading skills, relations between orthographic processing abilities and reading are a bit more confusing. In fact, it can be difficult to distinguish orthographic processing tasks from word recognition and spelling tasks (Vellutino, Scanlon, & Tanzman, 1994).

With this as a back-drop, we are ready to consider the development of orthographic processing ability. We have divided our chapter into three parts. In the first part, we briefly consider alternative conceptualizations of orthographic processing abilities, and present our working conceptualization. In the second part, we consider the initial development of rudimentary orthographic processing abilities of children who are not yet fluent readers. In the third part, we consider the further development of orthographic processing abilities as children become fluent readers.

CONCEPTUALIZING ORTHOGRAPHIC PROCESSING ABILITIES

As mentioned, there is as yet little consensus about the construct of orthographic processing abilities. Thus it should not be surprising that a standard approach for assessing orthographic processing abilities has yet to emerge (Berninger & Lester, 1990; Olson, Forsberg, Wise, & Rack, 1994; Vellutino, Scanlon, & Tanzman, 1994).

A sampling of recent conceptualizations of orthographic processing is presented in Table 1. A comparison of these conceptualizations reveals informative differences and issues that have yet to be resolved. One difference is whether orthographic processing is conceptualized within the context of a decoding model such as Coltheart's dual-route model (e.g., Leslie & Thimke, 1986; Olson et al., in press; Stanovich, in press) or is conceptualized in more "stand alone" fashion (e.g., Ehri, 1980; Perfetti, 1984; Vellutino et al., 1994). The advantage of viewing orthographic processing within the context of a decoding model is that one begins with relatively well-worked out relations between orthographic processing and decoding that result from viewing both within the confines of a single model. A corresponding disadvantage is that growing discontent with the decoding model that provides a contextual background, as has recently characterized dual-route models, can spill over onto one's conceptualization of orthographic processing abilities. Related to this difference is whether orthographic processing ability is considered to be an individual differences variable of interest in its own right, as opposed to just one of several parts of a theoretical reading model.

A second difference obvious in the conceptualizations presented in Table 1 is whether phonological coding is viewed to be an integral and perhaps inseparable aspect of orthographic processing. Thus, Ehri (1980) considers a word's

Table 1

Definitions of Orthographic Knowledge and Processing

1. "Orthographic coding may be defined as the ability to represent the unique array of letters that defines a printed word, as well as general attributes of the writing system such as sequential dependencies, structural redundancies, letter position frequencies, and so forth." (Vellutino, Scanlon, & Tanzman, 1994).

2. "...variance in the ability to form, store, and access orthographic representation..." (Stanovich & West, 1989, p. 404).

3. "Orthographic skills refer to immediate analysis of words into orthographic units with optional phonological recoding." (Foorman & Liberman, 1989, p. 350).

4. "...orthographic coding allows direct access to a mental lexicon for familiar words based on their unique orthography..." (Szezulski & Manis, 1990, p. 182.).

5. Orthographic ability refers to "the knowledge a reader has about permissible letter patterns" (Perfetti, 1984, p. 47).

6. "...word's orthographic form...is thought to be incorporated not as a rotely memorized geometric figure but rather as a sequence of letters bearing systematic relationships to phonological properties of the word." (Ehri, 1980, p. 313).

7. "Thus an orthographic form is not simply a visually-similar sequence of letters: it is the identity of the letters in the sentence and their systematic relationship to sound which is important." (Goswami, 1990, p. 324).

8. "...knowledge of orthographic structure affects letter or word recognition in the feature analysis process." (Leslie & Thimke, 1986, p. 230).

9. "...orthographic syllabication; that is, whole words are represented in the lexicon as syllables constructed not within articulatory or purely morphemic constraints (although morphological consideration is an intrinsic component of the BOSS hypothesis), but within the constraints of English orthography." (Jordan, 1986, p. 523).

10. the ability to "...use familiar orthographic sequences to access the lexicon without phonological mediation." (Stanovich, in press).

11. Using orthographic sequences to access the lexicon "where phonological processing may occur but the output of the phonological processor is not sufficient to make a decision about the lexical identity of a letter string." (Olson, Forsberg, Wise, & Rack, 1994).

orthographic form not to be merely a geometric figure but rather a "sequence of letters bearing systematic relationships to phonological properties of the word." Similarly, Goswami (1990) dismisses mere visual sequences of letters as an adequate conceptualization of orthographic knowledge, in favor of the alternative view that it is the letters' "systematic relationship to sound which is important."

Our view is that it is premature to close in on any one conceptualization or task. We are particularly doubtful about the feasibility of constructing "pure" measures of orthographic processing ability, just as we doubt whether tasks such as decoding nonwords provide as pure a measure of phonological coding as most of us once thought that they did (Treiman, Goswami, & Bruck, 1990). Perhaps the best we can do is to construct tasks that differ in the degree to which they elicit or at least encourage orthographic or phonological coding. Consequently, we have tended to use a wide variety of tasks to sample orthographic knowledge and processing in our studies, ranging from letter knowledge to analyses of invented spellings to orthographic choice tasks in which the child is asked either to identify the correctly spelled word (e.g., RAIN - RANE) or the homophone that is consistent with the context (e.g., "The insect that buzzes and makes honey is the honey ...BE - BEE."). And we routinely incorporate measures of orthographic processing and phonological processing in the same studies, and favor analyses that allow us to examine the simultaneous influences of both kinds of processing. Finally, although we are keenly interested in models of decoding, we also are interested in examining orthographic processing abilities from an individual differences standpoint, and we do not embed our conceptualization of orthographic processing abilities in any particular model of decoding.

EARLY DEVELOPMENT OF ORTHOGRAPHIC PROCESSING ABILITIES

In studies of the orthographic and phonological processing abilities of very young children, an important consideration is whether or not the children can read. In studies of kindergarten children, bimodal distributions are common, with a small number of readers performing remarkably well on oral and written language tasks, and a larger number of prereaders who provide a second distribution of scores well below that of the readers.

The problem with categorizing young children as readers or prereaders is that the criterion to be used must be somewhat arbitrary (e.g., no alphabetic reading ability as demonstrated by an inability to pronounce any simple nonwords; no knowledge of sight words as demonstrated by a score of 0 on Word Identification), and it ignores the fact that children may have acquired a good deal of rudimentary knowledge about print even though they are unable to read or spell whole words. Barron (1991) terms this rudimentary knowledge "proto-literacy." It consists of such things as knowledge of letter names, possible knowledge of several letter sounds, and perhaps some highly familiar logos such as McDonald's. With programs such as Sesame Street, and with the increasing prevalence of parents and preschool teachers reading to young children, many children accumulate several thousand hours of exposure to written language before formal instruction in reading or spelling is initiated (Adams, 1990).

We have taken two approaches to studying young children's rudimentary orthographic knowledge. The first is to study young children's invented spellings, and the second is to study the causal role of letter knowledge on subsequent development of decoding and of phonological processing abilities.

Young Children's Invented Spellings

Young children's spellings provide a much needed window through which we can observe the development of their orthographic and phonological knowledge, especially for children whose reading skills are so rudimentary that having them attempt to decode words provides little or no information. Nevertheless, such children gamely will produce invented spellings when asked to spell common words in their spoken vocabularies.

Read's (1971, 1986) early studies of young children's invented spellings uncovered three common and systematic spelling errors. The first was a tendency to confuse letter names with their sounds, as when spelling the word BOAT as BOT and BITE as BIT. Although the letter O is named "oh," it does not make that sound without a second vowel to complete a digraph or a final E. The second systematic error was a tendency to confuse letters associated with phonemes that are similar in how they are articulated, as when the letter I in the word BIT is replaced with an E. These short vowel sounds are quite similar in how they are produced by the articulatory apparatus. The third systematic error was to omit nasals (i.e., the sounds made by m, n, and ng) from consonant clusters, as when spelling WENT as WET. Treiman (1985) carried out a massive examination of over 5,000 spellings produced by a class of first-grade children that has provided a wealth of information about additional systematic errors. For example, she noted that young children routinely omit the second consonant in consonant clusters, as when spelling STOP as SOP.

Obviously, producing written spellings is a complex cognitive task. Making inferences about young children's developing knowledge of their orthography from their spellings would seem to require a better understanding of the complex and multiple determinants of performance. As a first step in this process, we carried out an investigation of the nonword spellings produced by a total of 187 children—45 each from kindergarten, first, and second grade, and 52 from third grade (Stage & Wagner, 1992).

We set out to address three specific questions. First, how does knowledge of orthography and phonology vary as a function of phonemic category (e.g., stop consonant, fricative, nasal) and position within syllable (e.g., initial, medial, or final position)? Differences in the accuracy with which phonemes are represented by graphemes as a function of phonemic category and position might reflect (a) characteristics of the mapping between orthography and phonology such as the number of sounds associated with a particular orthographic symbol, (b) isolated characteristics of the phoneme category members such as how easy they are to articulate or to discriminate auditorially, or (c) contextual characteristics such as coarticulation, the fact that the specific sound of a phoneme depends on the identity of the preceding and following phonemes because the pronunciations overlap to some degree. Coarticulation tends to affect vowel sounds to a greater degree than other phonemes. The second question we set out to answer was that of the origin of individual differences in early spelling performance, and whether the answer to this question varies developmentally. Plausible origins of individual differences in spelling performance include individual differences in (a) letter knowledge, (b) phonological awareness, (c) knowledge of grapheme-to-phoneme correspondences, (d) phonological memory, and (e) more general aspects of cognitive functioning such as general verbal ability. The third question that we set out to answer was that of which of the potential origins of individual differences in spelling performance account for the substantial correlations between spelling performance and beginning word-decoding, and whether the answer to this question also varies developmentally. Any of the potential origins of individual differences in spelling might also be origins of individual differences in word decoding skills, and consequently, might be responsible for the observed correlations between measures of spelling and word decoding.

Regarding the question of how knowledge of orthography and phonology vary as a function of phonemic category (e.g., stop consonant, fricative, nasal) and position within syllable (e.g., initial, medial, or final position), one must deal with the fact that in natural language samples, phoneme category and position are confounded. For example, vowels are over represented in the medial position and underrepresented in the initial and final positions, whereas the opposite is the case for consonants. To handle this naturally occurring confound, we examined the effects of position while statistically controlling for the effects of phoneme category, and we examined the effects of phoneme category while statistically controlling for the effects of phoneme position.

We found reliable differences in accuracy of spellings as a function of phoneme category, ranging from a proportion correct of .68 for stop consonants to a low of .35 for medial vowels. Reliable differences in accuracy of spelling also were found as a function of position, with best performance for the initial position, poorest performance for the medial position, and an intermediate level of performance for the final position. Thus, by controlling for the naturally occurring confound of phoneme category and position, we found that both exerted independent effects on spelling performance. One interesting effect of controlling for phoneme position in our analyses of the effects of phoneme category was the degree to which it attenuated the ubiquitous finding of vowels being much more difficult to read and spell than are consonants. Before controlling for the effect of phoneme position, we found that the average proportion of correctly represented vowels (.42) was about a third lower than that for consonants (.61), which is a typical result. But when position was controlled, the average proportion correct for vowels (.50) was much more comparable to that of consonants (.57).

Regarding the question of the origins of individual differences in early spelling performance, and whether they vary developmentally, an origin of individual differences in spelling performance that was relatively constant across developmental level was phonological awareness. A second origin of individual differences in spelling performance was phonological memory, but its relation to spelling performance varied developmentally: The magnitude of the relation diminished with advancing grade levels, as evidenced by correlations between phonological memory and spelling performance of .46, .27, and .10 for first, second, and third grade, respectively. This decreasing trend in correlations was significant at the .05 level.

Regarding the question of which of the potential origins of individual differences in early spelling performance account for the substantial correlations between spelling performance and beginning word-decoding, we again found developmental differences. For young children, observed correlations between spelling and decoding performance can be explained by the fact that both require phonological awareness and phonological memory. As children become more fluent in written language, phonological awareness and phonological memory no longer account for the extent of the observed correlation between spelling and decoding performance. The most likely additional factor that is implicated is individual differences in developing orthographic processing ability.

Overall, we found that young children's nonword spellings reflected the joint influences of linguistic knowledge (orthographic and phonological) and psychological processes (phonological memory limitations), and that these influences varied developmentally. Limited phonological memory constrained the spelling performance of younger children but not of older children. For younger children, individual differences in phonological awareness and phonological memory account for nearly all of the shared variance between spelling and word decoding. For older children, additional factors also are implicated.

The lesson that we have learned from this study and from similar studies by others is that whereas it is possible and important to study the development of rudimentary orthographic knowledge using tasks such as invented spelling, one must not lose sight of the fact that performance is affected by a variety of factors including such things as phonological awareness and phonological memory.

Causal Influences of Letter Knowledge

A common measure of prereaders' and beginning readers' rudimental orthographic knowledge is their knowledge of letter names (Berninger & Alsdorf, 1988; Barron, 1991; Ehri, 1989). In our longitudinal correlational study of relations between the development of phonological processing abilities and the acquisition of beginning reading skills, we also included a measure of letter name knowledge administered in kindergarten (Wagner, Torgesen, & Rashotte, 1994).

In a structural equation model of these causal relations, we did not find a direct causal influence of early letter name knowledge on subsequent decoding, when phonological processing measures and the autoregressive effect of previous decoding were included as additional causes. However, we did find an indirect causal influence of letter name knowledge on subsequent decoding through phonological processing abilities. In other words, letter name knowledge played a causal role in the acquisition of subsequent phonological processing abilities that, in turn, played a causal role in the further development of decoding. The causal influences of letter name knowledge in kindergarten on phonological analysis and phonological synthesis in first grade are depicted in Figure 1. In this figure, the phonological analysis and phonological synthesis are represented by oval shaped latent variables (i.e., factors defined in terms of multiple observable indicators). Letter name knowledge and a measure of verbal ability, Stanford-Binet Vocabulary, are observed variables represented by rectangles. The autoregressive effects of prior phonological analysis and synthesis are included to allow for the fact that a plausible cause of level of performance of future behavior is level of previous performance, and that it is a mistake to omit such known plausible causes (Gollub & Reichardt, 1987). The important thing to note is the standardized path coefficients of .19 and .27 from letter name knowledge to phonological analysis and synthesis, respectively, which represent a causal influence of letter name on subsequent phonological analysis and synthesis. Although we have not included the additional figures here (see Wagner, Torgesen, & Rashotte, 1994, Figures 2 and 3), the results showed that phonological analysis and synthesis in turn played a causal role in the subsequent development of decoding. This, then completes an indirect causal path in which letter knowledge influences subsequent decoding through phonological processing abilities.

In our previously described study of young children's invented spellings, we remarked on the lesson that phonological processing played an integral role in performance. In the present study of causal influences of letter knowledge, we once again see phonological processing playing an integral role, which is one of facilitating an indirect causal influence between letter knowledge and subsequent decoding.

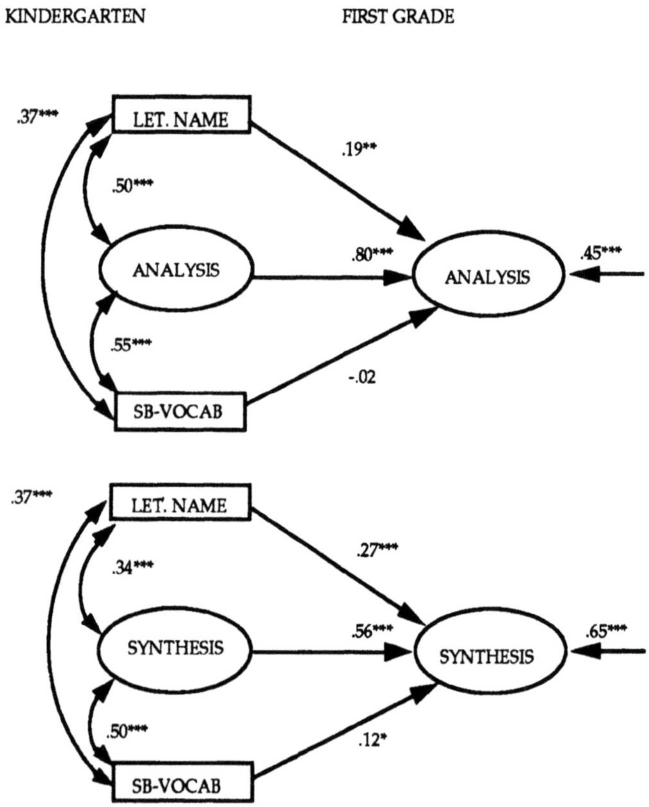

Figure 1. Causal influences of kindergarten letter name knowledge on first grade phonological analysis and synthesis.

SUBSEQUENT DEVELOPMENT OF ORTHOGRAPHIC PROCESSING ABILITIES

The results considered in the previous section concerned the development and role of rudimentary orthographic knowledge, and its relation to phonological processing abilities and decoding. We turn now to a consideration of the orthographic processing ability of older, more fluent readers.

Studies of Orthographic Processing Skill, Print Exposure, And Phonological Processing

Stanovich, West, and Cunningham (1992) describe results from several studies that inform about individual differences in orthographic processing abilities. These studies make three important points.

First, individual differences in orthographic processing skill predict word-level decoding independently of individual differences in phonological processing skill. In one reported study, 180 adult readers were given measures of word decoding, phonological processing (pseudoword naming: "henk," "kanth," "vilp"; phonological choice: "bape-baik," "leeve-meave"), and orthographic processing (orthographic choice: "snoe-snow," "turtle-tertle"; homophone choice: "Which is a number" ate-eight") (Stanovich & West, 1989, Study 2). Hierarchical multiple regression was used to analyze the data. In the first step, the two phonological processing measures were used as predictors of decoding, accounting for 49 percent of the variance. In a second step, the two orthographic processing measures were added to the prediction equation. Because the phonological processing predictors are already in the prediction equation at this point, any additional variance accounted for by adding the orthographic processing measures is independent of phonological processing ability. The results were that an additional 7 percent of the variance in decoding was accounted for by the orthographic processing measures. In a second study, 98 third- and fourth-grade children were given phonological processing measures (phonological choice, and a phoneme deletion task: "Say spark without the /s/ sound"—correct reply is "park") and orthographic processing measures (orthographic choice and homophone choice) (Cunningham & Stanovich, 1990). For predicting performance on the Woodcock Word Identification subtest, the phonological processing measures accounted for 26 percent of the variance, and the orthographic processing measures added an additional 12 percent of variance that was independent of that accounted for by the phonological processing measures.

The second important point made by these studies is that individual differences in print exposure account for some individual differences in orthographic processing skill. In these studies, print exposure was measured using a novel approach. An Author Recognition Test (ART) has an adult subject scan a list of names and check those that they know to be authors. The list is comprised of the names of well-known authors and writers and foils—additional names that are not the names of authors and writers. Subjects are informed of the existence of the foils to discourage guessing, and performance is scored by adding up the number of authors and writers checked and then subtracting the number of foils checked. An analogous measure they constructed to assess children's print exposure is the Title Recognition Test (TRT). This list contains the names of popular children's books and comparable foils.

For the sample of 180 adults, hierarchical regression was used to predict performance on the orthographic processing tasks. In a first step, the phonological processing tasks were used as predictors. In a second step, the Author Recognition Task (ART) was added. If additional variance was accounted for in the second step, then we can conclude that print exposure accounts for variance in orthographic processing skill that is independent of phonological processing abilities or the effects of print exposure on phonological processing abilities. For the orthographic choice task, the phonological processing measures used as predictors in the first step accounted for 13 percent of the variance. When the ART was added as a predictor in the second step, an additional 4 percent of the variance was accounted for. Similar results were found for the homophone choice task, with 11 percent of the variance accounted for by the phonological processing measures, and an additional 5 percent of the variance accounted for by the addition of the ART. Turning to the sample of third- and fourth-grade children, comparable analyses were done using data from 80 of the original 98 children for whom scores on the Title Recognition Test (TRT) were available. For predicting an orthographic composite score (orthographic choice and homophone choice), a phonological composite score (phonological choice and phoneme deletion) accounted for 9 percent of the variance.

When the TRT was added in a second step, an additional 9 percent of variance in the orthographic composite was accounted for. Comparable results were obtained when an IQ measure (Raven's Progressive Matrices) and a paired-associate memory measure were added before the TRT, with 7 percent of the variance uniquely accounted for by the TRT. Thus, both the adult and children data suggest that individual differences in print exposure, quantified by the ART and TRT, uniquely account for variance in orthographic processing skill.

The third important point made by these studies is that not all of the individual differences in orthographic processing skill can be explained by differences in print exposure. The issue here is whether orthographic processing skill should be regarded as an individual difference ability, or merely as a proxy for individual differences in print exposure. The strategy employed by Stanovich et al. (1992) was to predict decoding using (a) phonological processing measures in the first step of a hierarchical multiple regression; (b) print exposure in a second step, and (c) an orthographic processing measure in a third step. Any additional variance accounted for in the third step would be evidence that individual differences in decoding can be accounted for by individual differences in orthographic processing skill that cannot be attributed to mere differences in print exposure or to differences in phonological processing abilities. For the sample of 180 adult readers, the phonological processing measures accounted for 51 percent of the variance in decoding when used as predictors in the first step. Adding two measures of print exposure, the ART and an analogous measure to the TRT but based on magazine titles, resulted in an additional 4 percent of variance accounted for. Finally, adding the orthographic choice task in a third step accounted for yet another 4 percent of the variance in decoding. These results, then, are consistent with viewing orthographic processing skill as an ability that is related to, but not merely a proxy for, print exposure.

Extending Results to a Wider Variety of Reading Situations

With few exceptions, the reading measure used in studies of orthographic processing has been accuracy for words read in isolation. One exception is Stanovich and West (1989), whose measure of reading was a composite speed and accuracy score for words read in isolation. In general, our knowledge of relations between orthographic processing and reading is limited to a very narrow range of reading tasks that are not the kind of reading tasks that children normally encounter in school.

We sought to extend our knowledge about relations between orthographic processing and reading to a wider range of reading tasks in a study of third-grade children (Barker, Torgesen, & Wagner, 1992). Three ideas guided our selection of reading tasks. First, because orthographic processing ability includes having accessible representations for multi-letter units including common words, we predicted that differences in orthographic processing ability would be more pronounced for speed than for accuracy of responses to words presented in isolation. We therefore included a measure of isolated word reading for which latency to respond was the primary dependent variable. Second, because additional processes are involved when children read connected text as opposed to naming words presented in isolation, we included measures of oral and silent reading rate for connected text. We did not have a definite prediction about possible differences in relations between orthographic processing ability and reading for isolated words and for connected text. On the one hand, it is possible that the availability of top-down comprehension processes when reading connected text would lessen the impact of individual differences in orthographic processing ability (and in phonological processing ability, for that matter). In other words, the availability of top-down processing might lessen the impact of factors such as orthographic processing ability that are associated with bottom-up decoding. On the other hand, orthographic processing ability might be more important when reading connected text because the efficient, and relatively automatic means of decoding words and word segments might make it possible to devote more resources or attention to the complex processing operations involved in reading connected text for meaning. The third idea that guided our selection of reading tasks was the idea that because orthographic processing ability can be useful in identifying novel words by relying on analogy to known words (e.g. using the known word CAT to help decode the unknown VAT) (Barron, 1986), we also included a nonword reading task.

Two additional features of this study deserve mention. First, following up on the work just described, we included a measure of print exposure to determine whether a relation between orthographic processing ability and reading existed after controlling for individual differences in print exposure. Second, we included a measure of verbal as well as nonverbal ability. Most previous studies have only included a nonverbal ability task. By including measures of verbal and nonverbal ability, we were able to carry out a more rigorous test of the degree to which relations between orthographic processing ability and reading are independent of general ability.

Our subjects were 87 third-grade children who constituted the entire third-grade class in a rural/suburban elementary school. The children were mostly from lower- to upper-middle class homes. The study was carried out in the second semester of school. We selected third-grade children because orthographic processing ability has developed to a considerable degree by this point (Juel, Griffith, & Gough, 1986), yet word identification skills are still undergoing rapid development.

Our measures of orthographic processing ability were an orthographic choice task and a homophone choice task. The orthographic choice task required children to pick the correct spelling from a pair of words that sounded alike (e.g., BOAT-BOTE). Our measure of performance on this task was median latency for correct trials. The homophone choice task involved reading a sentence and then picking the correct word from a pair of homophones (e.g., "What do you do with a needle and thread? SO-SEW"). Median response time for correct trials was the measure of performance. (In the analyses, all median response time variables were converted to reciprocals of median response times because higher scores presented better performance.)

Our measure of print exposure was a title recognition test modeled after one used by Cunningham and Stanovich (1990). The titles used were drawn from a list of book titles generated by subjects in our samples. There were 25 actual book titles, and 14 foils. Performance was scored in terms of number of correct titles checked minus number of foils checked.

Our measures of phonological processing were Olson et al.'s (1989) phonological choice task, which we described earlier and which also contained the same items used by Cunningham and Stanovich (1990), and a phoneme deletion task. The phoneme deletion task involved asking the children to say a word such as "trick" without the "r" sound (yielding "tick").

Our reading measures included the following. A timed word-recognition measure consisted of median pronunciation latency for correct trials when children were asked to name regular and irregular words drawn from the second- and third-grade readers used in the elementary school where the study was carried out. An untimed word-recognition measure was the Word identification subtest of the Woodcock Reading Mastery Test. For a measure of oral reading of words in context, two passages of 100 words were chosen from the beginning third-grade reader. Performance was measured in words correctly read per second. Two similar passages were selected for a measure of silent reading of words in context. Performance was measured in words read per second. Finally, the Word Attack subtest of the Woodcock Reading Mastery Test served as a measure of accuracy for reading nonwords.

Hierarchical regression analyses were used to address two major questions. First, how much variance in reading is uniquely accounted for by orthographic processing ability, and does this vary across the different kinds of reading tasks that we examined? Second, how much of the variance in reading that is uniquely accounted for by orthographic processing ability is independent of individual differences in print exposure?

Results addressing the question of variance in reading uniquely accounted for by orthographic processing ability and whether this changes across reading tasks are presented in Table 2. For each reading measure, a hierarchical multiple regression was carried out in which age was entered on step one, IQ was entered on step two, the two phonological processing measures were entered on step three, and the two orthographic processing measures were entered on the final step. The variance in reading uniquely accounted for by orthographic processing ability is indicated by the increase in variance accounted for (i.e., R^2 change) on the final step.

These values, which ranged from a low of .05 for accuracy for reading nonwords to a high of .20 for oral reading rate for connected text, indicate two things. First, these results replicate those of Stanovich et al. (1992) and those of others in that orthographic processing ability accounted for variance in reading that was independent of that accounted for by phonological processing abilities or general cognitive ability. Taking the Cunningham and Stanovich (1990) study, for example, they found orthographic processing ability to uniquely account for 10 percent of the variance in Word Identification, whereas, for the present study, the value was a comparable 7 percent.

Table 2

Orthographic Processing as a Unique Predictor of Reading

Dependent variable	Predictors	Beta	R^2	R^2 change
Word Analysis	Age	.02	.00	
	IQ	.05	.03	.03
	PD	.60**		
	PCM	.03	.42	.39**
	OCM	.14		
	HCM	.14	.47	.05*
Word Identification	Age	.02	.00	
	IQ	.03	.04	.04
	PD	.49**		
	PCM	.18	.41	.37**
	OCM	.21*		
	HCM	.12	.48	.07*
Timed Word Identification	Age	.03	.00	
	IQ	.14	.00	.00
	PD	.37**		
	PCM	.09	.22	.22**
	OCM	.21		
	HCM	.14	.32	.10**
Oral Reading Rate	Age	.00	.00	
	IQ	.01	.04	.04
	PD	.19		
	PCM	.15	.25	.21*
	OCM	.54**		
	HCM	.06	.45	.20**
Silent Reading Rate	Age	.06	.01	
	IQ	.06	.04	.04
	PD	.07		
	PCM	.10	.14	.10*
	OCM	.47**		
	HCM	.08	.29	.15**

*$p < .05$. *$p < .01$
Note: IQ = Intelligence; OCM = Orthographic Choice; PD = Phoneme Deletion; HCM = Homophone Choice; PCM = Phonological Choice.

Second, the amount of variance in reading uniquely accounted for by orthographic processing ability is greater for reading connected text than for reading words presented in isolation. These results suggest that fluent access to orthographic representations is especially important when reading connected text. We cannot confirm any particular explanation of this finding using these data, but we can at least make a conjecture about plausible alternative explanations. One explanation is based on differential complexities involved in processing words in isolation compared to connected text. Given the relative complexity of processing connected text for meaning, a premium might be placed on more automatic, less attention-demanding processes (Lesgold & Perfetti, 1981). An alternative explanation is based not on differential complexity but on differential speed. Words in connected text are read more quickly and perhaps not processed as exhaustively as words read in isolation. If, as is usually assumed, phonological processing is not as rapid as orthographic processing, orthographic processing may be more evident when reading connected text. Finally, eye-movement research indicates that information from the parafoveal region (the region spanning about 2 to 4 degrees of visual angle from the point of fixation) is useful in the guidance of eye-movements (Rayner & Pollatsek, 1989). If this information is orthographic in character, it is possible that reading connected text would be facilitated relative to words read in isolation.

Results relevant to answering the second major question of how much of the variance in reading is uniquely accounted for by orthographic processing ability and is independent of individual differences in print exposure are presented in Table 3. These results are from hierarchical multiple regression analyses that differ from those presented in Table 2 in one important way. Our measure of print exposure, a title recognition task, was entered as a predictor before the orthographic processing variables. Thus any increase in reading variance accounted for by the addition of the orthographic processing variables in the final step represents a relation between orthographic processing and reading that is independent of individual differences in print exposure. The results were that although print exposure accounted for reliable proportions of reading variance in the measures that required reading connected text, the attenuation in reading variance accounted for by the orthographic measures was slight. Thus, much of the variance in reading accounted for by individual differences in orthographic processing measures is independent of individual differences in print exposure.

Table 3

Orthographic Processing as a Unique Predictor of Reading After Controlling for Print Exposure

Dependent variable	Predictors	Beta	R^2	R^2 change
Word Analysis	Age	.02	.00	
	IQ	.05	.03	.03
	PD	.60**		
	PCM	.03	.42	.39**
	TRT	.08	.43	.01
	OCM	.11		
	HCM	.15*	.47	.04
Word Identification	Age	.02	.00	
	IQ	.04	.04	.04
	PD	.49**		
	PCM	.18	.41	.37**
	TRT	.05	.42	.01
	OCM	.19**		
	HCM	.12	.48	.05
Timed Word Identification	Age	.02	.00	
	IQ	.08	.00	.01
	PD	.39**		
	PCM	.07	.22	.21**
	TRT	.17	.26	.04*
	OCM	.22		
	HCM	.12	.34	.08*
Oral Reading Rate	Age	.01	.00	
	IQ	.00	.04	.04
	PD	.21*		
	PCM	.12	.25	.21**
	TRT	.21*	.35	.10**
	OCM	.46**		
	HCM	.04	.49	.14**
Silent Reading Rate	Age	.08	.01	
	IQ	.05	.05	.04
	PD	.09		
	PCM	.08	.14	.10*
	TRT	.22*	.24	.10**
	OCM	.39**		
	HCM	.06	.33	.09**

*p < .05. *p < .01
Note: IQ = Intelligence; OCM = Orthographic Choice; PD = Phoneme Deletion; HCM = Homophone Choice; PCM = Phonological Choice.

Our results do not explain the origin of individual differences in orthographic processing ability that appear to be partially independent of print exposure, but we are aware of at least two possibilities. The first possibility is that our results are artifactual. The independence of the relation between orthographic processing ability and reading from print exposure may reflect inadequacies in our measurement of print exposure. This possibility always is a risk when one's phenomenon is represented by residual variance. Alternatively, the possibility we believe to be the most likely is that there exist genuine individual differences in orthographic processing abilities that are not completely accounted for by individual differences in print exposure. Individual differences are the norm in just about every endeavor. It would be remarkable if it turned out to be the case that the facility with which individuals were able to form, store, and manipulate orthographic images was identical across individuals with comparable levels of print exposure.

Alternative Interpretations of the Existing Literature

The consensus view that emerges from the work we have described is that word-level decoding is a composite task, individual differences in which can be attributable to three partially overlapping sources—phonological processing ability, orthographic processing ability, and print exposure—as well as to other sources that have not been the main target of study in the research reviewed (e.g., IQ, SES, type and quality of reading instruction provided). Here we describe one recent critique, and a more general problem that it relates to.

Vellutino, Scanlon, and Tanzman's (1994) critique of orthographic processing research. Vellutino et al. find the evidence for orthographic processing ability as a basic ability that underlies word-level decoding and spelling to be suspect. Their main complaint is that orthographic processing tasks are complex, and that orthographic processing ability per se is not easily distilled form other abilities, including phonological coding ability, word-level decoding ability, and spelling ability. They believe that the tasks most often used to evaluate orthographic coding ability either evaluate word identification or spelling ability, rather than orthographic coding as a basic cognitive ability that is common to both.

For example, consider the orthographic choice task of picking the correct word when presented with CAKE and CAIK. Vellutino et al. argue that children who know the word CAKE will get the item correct, yet this tells us nothing about orthographic coding as a basic cognitive process. Rather, it only distinguishes those who can identify the words from those who cannot. In addition, this task confounds word-specific knowledge with general orthographic knowledge in a way that makes it difficult to determine which is responsible for the correct response. Thus, CAKE may be chosen because its many orthographic neighbors allows a child to choose it by virtue of sensitivity to redundant spelling patterns, rather than from recognition of CAKE as a lexical entry. Vellutino et al. further argue that homophone and orthographic choice tasks require knowledge of word spellings, which makes it possible that they simply are measuring spelling ability rather than a basic process that underlies spelling and reading ability. They consider the homophone choice task (e.g., What falls from clouds, REIN or RAIN?) to be even further removed from orthographic coding ability, because it requires that a child matches word spelling with verbal definitions and requires that the subject hold a descriptive phrase in working memory while making a decision.

Vellutino et al. are correct for the most part. Common orthographic processing tasks are complex indeed, and should not be considered to be pure measures of orthographic processing ability. Of course, the same criticism applies to most any cognitive task, including measures of phonological processing ability, as Vellutino et al. correctly note. The common task of having children read regular nonwords is not a pure measure of the phonological coding ability. Children are able to read nonwords by relying heavily on analogy to pronunciations of known words and spelling patterns with only minimal reliance on phonological coding (e.g., as when CAT and GET are used to arrive at a pronunciation for GAT). Nonwords are not alike, and the more characteristics they share with common words, the more easily they are read (Treiman, Goswami, & Bruck, 1990). Even oral language-based measures of phonological awareness, such as the task of reversing the phonemes in the orally presented word "tab" to get "bat," tasks do not involve any letters, are susceptible to measuring abilities other than phonological awareness, such as orthographic processing ability (Bruck, in press). For a demonstration, pay attention to the strategy that you use to reverse the order of phonemes in the word "mit." Most of us obtain the correct answer, "Tim," by using an orthographic strategy. We visualize the printed word MIT, reverse the order of the letters to form TIM, and then we read the word.

Although we largely agree with Vellutino et al.'s assessment of the situation, we do not find their criticism that common orthographic processing tasks merely measure word-decoding ability or spelling ability to be completely persuasive, because it is not at all clear that word-decoding ability or spelling ability themselves are basic abilities in any real sense of the term. Word-decoding and spelling are both complex tasks, and differences in performance across stimuli and subjects are multiply determined by individual differences in phonological and orthographic coding, and other factors. We completely agree with their recommendation for large scale multivariate studies in which all the major constructs are all represented in a measurement battery. We have found this strategy to be useful in beginning to understand the nature of phonological processing abilities (Wagner, Torgesen, Laughon, Simmons, & Rashotte, 1993).

The problem of competing causal models. An equally troubling problem that Vellutino et al. did not address directly is the problem of competing causal models. The ultimate goal of researchers is a causal model that specifies developmentally-causal relations among orthographic processing, phonological processing, and decoding. Even if we do not seek to explicitly test a given causal model, we rely on causal models implicitly when designing our studies and interpreting their results. For example, an implicit causal model that appears to be shared by a number of researchers in this area is that individual differences in word-level decoding ability are caused by (a) individual differences in phonological processing abilities, (b) individual differences in orthographic processing abilities, (c) print exposure and reading instruction, and (d) other background variables such as IQ, SES, and so on. The problem of competing models is that there typically are multiple causal models that provide an equivalently good fit to the data (McCallum, Wegener, Uchino, & Fabrigar, 1993). Thus, a model in which we simply turn the causal arrows around, in which such things as IQ, SES, print exposure and reading instruction are viewed as being caused by individual differences in word-level decoding, seems highly implausible, yet is likely to provide an equivalently good fit to the data were it tested using path analysis.

The problem of alternative causal models is pernicious in studies in which the variables are measured simultaneously, and less troubling in longitudinal studies. The reason that the problem of alternative causal models is less pernicious in longitudinal studies is that it is at least possible to rule out causal models in which a construct at some time two is viewed as a cause of another construct at a previous time one, in violation of time precedence. The relevance of this issue to the present discussion is that the major correlational studies of relations between orthographic processing, phonological processing, and decoding involve simultaneously collected data.

Longitudinal Correlational Study

In our longitudinal study of causal relations between the development of phonological processing abilities and the acquisition of beginning reading skills from kindergarten through second grade (Wagner, Torgesen, & Rashotte, 1994), we also obtained several measures of orthographic processing and rudimentary knowledge of English orthography. We have reanalyzed these data to examine relations between orthographic processing, phonological processing, and reading; and the longitudinal correlational design provides some protection against the problem of alternative causal models that is not available when variables are measures simultaneously.

Another facet of the design of our study allows us to address some of Vellutino et al.'s (1994) concerns about the existing literature. When testing causal models, it is important that they be specified correctly. Model specification refers to the set of assumptions made by a particular model. Longitudinal correlations studies can be used to test alternative causal models, but misspecified models can yield estimates of causal influences that are erroneous with respect to magnitude and even direction. One common cause of model misspecification is that of omitting known plausible causes. Although one never can be sure that all relevant causes have been included in any causal model, omitting a known plausible cause is reason for concern.

One of the most commonly omitted known plausible causes

is the autoregressive effect of a variable measured at a prior time on the same variable measured at a later time (Gollob & Reichardt, 1987). As we have noted, the best predictor of future behavior often is past behavior. When Vellutino et al.'s (in press) concerns are viewed in terms of the problems of alternative causal models and model misspecification, we can translate them into a testable prediction: If orthographic processing measures merely are proxies for decoding ability, they should not exert a developmental causal effect that is independent of the autoregressive effect of prior decoding ability.

Data from 241 children were included in the analysis. Our measure of decoding was the Word Identification subtest from the Woodcock Reading Mastery Tests. Our orthographic knowledge and processing variables included Clay's (1979) Concepts About Print (CAP) test, letter name knowledge, and a homophone choice task. The homophone choice items are presented in Table 4. Our phonological processing measures included phoneme segmenting and phoneme blending. Finally, the Vocabulary subtest of the Stanford-Binet was used to estimate verbal ability.

Table 4

The Homophone Choice Task

1. You see with your...	I	EYE
2. The smallest number is...	ONE	WON
3. If you don't go out you go...	IN	INN
4. The number after one is...	TO	TWO
5. You use a needle and thread to...	SEW	SO
6. A pretty color is...	BLUE	BLEW
7. What shines in the sky in the day is the...	SUN	SON
8. The number after three is...	FORE	FOUR
9. What makes honey and says buzz is a...	BE	BEE
10. In a garden you pick a...	FLOWER	FLOUR
11. With your eyes you can...	SEE	SEA
12. On your foot you have a big	TOE	TOW
13. If it is not your turn you...	WEIGHT	WAIT
14. If something is not here it is over...	THEIR	THERE
15. You comb your...	HARE	HAIR

The results of main interest are those from hierarchical regression analyses in which the dependent variable was Word Identification in second grade. These analyses involved five steps. For the first step, age served as the sole predictor. In the second step, Word Identification in first grade was added. In the third step, verbal ability was added. In the fourth step, the two phonological processing measures were added. In the final step, the three orthographic processing and knowledge variables were added. The most important result was to determine whether a significant increase in variance accounted for would occur with the last step of adding the orthographic variables, given the fact that the autoregressive effect of first grade Word Identification on second grade Word Identification was already included in the analysis. If the orthographic variables only assessed decoding ability of the sort measured by Word Identification, they should not add to prediction because the better predictor of first-grade Word Identification is already included as a predictor. These results are presented in Table 5.

Table 5

Hierarchical Multiple Regression of Longitudinal Correlational Study

Step	Predictors	R^2	R^2 Change
1.	Age	.00	—
2.	Word ID (1st.)	.58***	.57***
3.	Verbal Ability	.62***	.04***
4.	Segmenting	.67***	.05***
	Blending		
5.	Homophone Choice	.72***	.05***
	Concepts About Print		
	Letter Name Knowledge		

With the exception of age, each step in the hierarchical multiple regression resulted in a significant increase in variance accounted for. As expected, the autoregressive effect of Word

Identification in first grade was the best predictor of Word Identification in second grade. However, phonological processing variables made a contribution to prediction that was independent of that of the autoregressive effect of Word Identification, verbal ability, and age, and the orthographic processing variables made a contribution to prediction that was independent of that made by these same variables and by the phonological processing variables.

CONCLUSIONS

We are convinced of the importance of studying the development of young children's orthographic processing abilities, and of the fact that such study is an important to our understanding of phonological processing as it is of orthographic processing.

A recurrent theme in the work that we have described is that orthography and phonology are related integrally to one another. Once children have acquired some familiarity with English orthography, "pure" measures of orthographic processing or phonological processing are not feasible. Spelling strategies can be employed on many phonological tasks, as evidenced by the fact that older children commonly count four phonemes in three-phoneme words such as GATE that are spelled with four letters (Ehri & Wilce, 1980), and by the fact that an origin of at least some of the residual phonological deficit of adult dyslexics appears to derive from their limited decoding skills and ability to use orthographic strategies on phonological tasks to the same degree as good readers (Bruck, in press). Language tasks are complex, with performance being jointly determined by external factors such as the nature of a child's oral and written language and internal factors such as a child's levels of phonological and orthographic knowledge (Stage & Wagner, 1992).

Historically, researchers in the area of beginning reading have been preoccupied with phonological processing abilities. Relatively recently, researchers have also become preoccupied with orthographic processing abilities. Although phonological processing measures have been employed routinely in recent studies of orthographic processing abilities, their use largely has been a concession to limitations of current measures of orthographic processing ability—a consequence of the fact that orthographic processing abilities have been defined in terms of residual variance in decoding remaining after phonological processing abilities have been held constant. What is now required are approaches that truly integrate orthographic and phonological processing in a comprehensive model.

Acknowledgements

Support for preparation of this chapter and for the research described therein was provided by Grants HD23340 and HD30988 from the National Institute of Child Health and Human Development.

REFERENCES

Adams, M.J. (1990). *Beginning to read: Thinking and learning about print*. Cambridge, MA: MIT Press.

Ball, E., & Blachman, B. (1988). Phonological segmentation training: Effects of reading readiness. *Annals of Dyslexia, 38,* 208-225.

Barker, T.A., Torgesen, J.K., & Wagner, R.K. (1992). The role of orthographic processing skills on five different reading tasks. *Reading Research Quarterly, 27,* 335-345.

Barron, R. W. (1986). Word recognition in early reading: A review of the direct and indirect access hypotheses. *Cognition, 24,* 93-119.

Barron, R.W. (1991). Proto-literacy, literacy and the acquisition of phonological awareness. *Learning and Individual Differences, 3,* 243-255.

Berninger, V.W., & Alsdorf, B. (1988). Are there errors in error analysis? *Journal of Psychoeducational Assessment, 7,* 209-222.

Berninger, V.W., & Lester, K. (1990). *Development of orthographic codes*. Paper presented at the Annual Meeting of the Educational Research Association, Boston.

Bradley, L., & Bryant, P.E. (1978). Difficulties in auditory organization as a possible cause of reading backwardness. *Nature, 271,* 746-747.

Bradley, L., & Bryant, P.E. (1985). *Rhyme and reason in reading and spelling*. Ann Arbor, MI: University of Michigan Press.

Bruck, M. (1990). Word recognition skills of adults with childhood diagnoses of dyslexia. *Developmental Psychology, 26,* 439-454.

Bruck, M. (in press). Persistence of dyslexic's phonological awareness deficits. *Developmental Psychology.*

Bruck, M., & Treiman, R. (1990). Phonological awareness and spelling in normal children and dyslexics: The case of initial consonant clusters. *Journal of Experimental Child Psychology, 50,* 156-178.

Bryant, P.E., Bradley, L., MacLean, M., & Crossland, D. (1989). Nursery rhymes, phonological skills and reading. *Journal of Child Language, 16,* 407-428.

Clay, M.M. (1979). *Reading: The patterning of complex behavior.* Auckland, New Zealand: Heinemann.

Crowder, R.G., & Wagner, R.K. (1991). *The psychology of reading: An introduction.* New York: Oxford University Press.

Cunningham, A.E., & Stanovich, K.E. (1990). Assessing print exposure and orthographic processing skill in children: A quick measure of reading experience. *Journal of Educational Psychology, 82,* 733-740.

Ehri, L.C. (1980). The development of orthographic images. In U. Frith (Ed.), *Cognitive processes in spelling* (pp. 311-338). London: Academic Press.

Ehri, L.C. (1987). Learning to read and spell words. *Journal of Reading Behavior, 19,* 5-31.

Ehri, L.C. (1989). The development of spelling knowledge and its role in reading acquisition and reading disability. *Journal of Learning Disabilities, 22,* 356-365.

Ehri, L.C., & Wilce, L.S. (1980). The influence of orthography on readers' conceptualization of the phonemic structure of words. *Applied Psycholinguistics, 1,* 371-385.

Felton, R.H., & Wood, F.B. (1990). Cognitive deficits in reading disability and attention deficit disorder. In J.K. Torgesen (Ed.), *Cognitive and behavioral characteristics of children with learning disabilities.* Austin, TX: PRO-ED.

Foorman, B.R., & Liberman, D. (1989). Visual and phonological processing of words: A comparison of good and poor readers. *Journal of Learning Disabilities, 22,* 349-355.

Gollob, H.F., & Reichardt, C.S. (1987). Taking account of time lags in causal models. *Child Development, 58,* 80-92.

Goswami, U.C. (1990). Phonological priming and orthographic analogies in reading. *Journal of Experimental Child Psychology, 49,* 323-340.

Jordan, T.R. (1986). Testing the BOSS hypothesis: Evidence for position-insensitive orthographic priming in the lexical decision task. *Memory & Cognition, 14,* 523-532.

Juel, C., Griffith, P., & Gough, P. (1986). Acquisition of literacy: A longitudinal study of children in first and second grade. *Journal of Educational Psychology, 78*, 243-255.

Lesgold, A.M., & Perfetti, C.A. (Eds.) (1981). *Interactive processes in reading*. Hillsdale, NJ: Erlbaum.

Leslie, L., & Thimke, B. (1986). The use of orthographic knowledge in beginning reading. *Journal of Reading Behavior, 18*, 229-241.

Lundberg, I., Frost, J., & Petersen, O. (1988). Effects of an extensive program for stimulating phonological awareness in preschool children. *Reading Research Quarterly, 23*, 263-284.

Manis, F.R., Szeszulski, P., Holt, L., & Graves, K. (1990). Variation in component word recognition and spelling skills among dyslexic children and normal readers. In T. Carr & B.A. Levy (Eds.), *Reading and its development: Component skills approaches*. New York: Academic Press.

McCallum, R.C., Wegener, D.T., Uchino, B.N., & Fabrigar, L.R. (1993). The problem of equivalent models in applications of covariance structure analysis. *Psychological Bulletin, 114*, 185-199.

Olson, R., Forsberg, H., Wise, B., & Rack, J. (1994). Measurement of word recognition, orthographic, and phonological skills. In G.R. Lyon (Ed.), *Frames of reference for the assessment of learning disabilities: New views on measurement issues* (pp.229-277). Baltimore, MD: Brookes.

Olson, R., Wise, B., Conners, F., & Rack, J. (1990). Organization, heritability, and remediation of component word recognition and language skills in disabled readers. In T.H. Carr & B.A. Levy (Eds.), *Reading and its development: Component skills approaches* (pp. 261-322). New York: Academic Press.

Olson, R., Wise, B., Conners, F., Rack. J., & Fulker, D. (1989). Specific deficits in component reading and language skills: Genetic and environmental influences. *Journal of Learning Disabilities, 22*, 339-348.

Perfetti, C.A. (1984). Reading acquisition and beyond: Decoding includes cognition. *American Journal of Education*, 40-57.

Perfetti, C.A., Beck, I., Bell, L., & Hughes, C. (1987). Phonemic knowledge and learning to read are reciprocal: A longitudinal study of first grade children. *Merrill-Palmer Quarterly, 33*, 283-319.

Rack, J.P., Snowling, M.J., & Olson, R.K. (1992). The nonword reading deficit in developmental dyslexia: A review. *Reading Research Quarterly, 27,* 29-53.

Rayner, K., & Pollatsek, A. (1989). *The psychology of reading.* Englewood Cliffs, NJ: Prentice Hall.

Read, C. (1971). Preschool children's knowledge of English orthography. *Harvard Educational Review, 41,* 1-34.

Read, C. (1986). *Children's creative spelling.* London: Routledge & Kegan Paul.

Sattler, J.M. (1988). *Assessment of Children* (3rd ed.). San Diego, CA: J.M. Sattler.

Shankweiler, D., & Liberman, I. (1989). *Phonology and Reading Disability.* IARLD Monograph, No. 6. Ann Arbor, MI: University Press.

Siegel, L.S., & Ryan, E.B. (1988). Reading disability as a language disorder. *Remedial and Special Education, 5(3),* 28-33.

Stage, S.A., & Wagner, R.K. (1992). Development of young children's phonological and orthographic knowledge as revealed by their spellings. *Developmental Psychology, 28,* 287-296.

Stanovich, K.E. (1986). Matthew effects in reading: Some consequences of individual differences in the acquisition of literacy. *Reading Research Quarterly, 21,* 360-407.

Stanovich, K.E. (1988). The right and wrong places to look for the cognitive locus of reading disability. *Annals of Dyslexia, 38,* 154-177.

Stanovich, K.E. (in press). The language code: Issues in word recognition. In S.R. Yussen & M.C. Smith (Eds.), *Reading across the life span.* Springer-Verlag.

Stanovich, K.E., & West, R.F. (1989). Exposure to print and orthographic processing. *Reading Research Quarterly, 24,* 402-433.

Stanovich, K.E., West, R.F., & Cunningham, A.E. (1992). Beyond phonological processes: Print exposure and orthographic processing. In S.A. Brady & D. Shankweiler (Eds.), *Phonological processes in literacy* (pp. 219-235). Hillsdale, NJ: Lawrence Erlbaum Associates.

Szeszulski, P.A., & Manis, F. R. (1990). An examination of familial resemblance among subgroups of dyslexics. *Annals of Dyslexia, 40,* 180-191.

Torgesen, J.K. (1991). Cross-age consistency in phonological processing. In S. Brady & D. Shankweiler (Eds.), *Phonological processes in literacy*. Hillsdale, NJ: Lawrence Erlbaum Associates.

Torgesen, J.K. (in press). Learning disabilities: Historical and conceptual issues. In B.Y.L. Wong (Ed.), *Learning about learning disabilities*. San Diego: Academic Press.

Treiman, R. (1985). Phonemic analysis, spelling, and reading. In T. Carr (Ed.), *New directions for child development: The development of reading skills* (Vol. 27, pp 5-18). San Francisco: Jossey-Bass.

Treiman, R. (1991). Phonological awareness and its roles in learning to read and spell. In D.J. Sawyer & B.J. Fox (Eds.), *Phonological awareness in reading: The evolution of current perspectives* (pp. 159-189). New York: Springer-Verlag.

Treiman, R., Goswami, U., & Bruck, M. (1990). Not all nonwords are alike: Implications for reading development and theory. *Memory & Cognition, 18*, 359-367.

Tunmer, W.E. (1989). The role of language-related factors in reading disability. In D. Shankweiler & I.Y. Liberman (Eds.), *Phonology and reading disability* (pp. 91-131). IARLD Monograph, No. 6. Ann Arbor, MI: University Press.

Tunmer, W.E., & Nesdale, A.R. (1985). Phonemic segmentation skill and beginning reading. *Journal of Educational Psychology, 77*, 417-427.

Vellutino, F.R., Scanlon, D.M., & Tanzman, M.S. (1994). Components of reading ability: Issues and problems in operationalizing word identification, phonological coding, and orthographic coding. In G.R. Lyon (Ed.), *Frames of reference for the assessment of learning disabilities: New views on measurement issues* (pp. 279-332). Baltimore, MD: Brookes.

Wagner, R.K. (1986). Phonological processing abilities and reading: Implications for disabled readers. *Journal of Learning Disabilities, 19*, 623-630.

Wagner, R.K. (1988). Causal relations between the development of phonological processing abilities and the acquisition of reading skills: A meta-analysis. *Merrill-Palmer Quarterly, 34*, 261-279.

Wagner, R.K., Balthazor, M., Hurley, S., Morgan, S. Rashotte, C., Shaner, R., Simmons, K., & Stage, S. (1987). The nature of prereaders' phonological processing abilities. *Cognitive Development, 2*, 355-373.

Wagner, R.K., & Torgesen, J.K. (1987). The nature of phonological processing and its causal role in the acquisition of reading skills. *Psychological Bulletin, 101*, 192-212.

Wagner, R.K., Torgesen, J.K, Laughon, P., Simmons, K., & Rashotte, C.A. (1993). The development of young readers' phonological processing abilities. *Journal of Educational Psychology, 85*, 1-20.

Wagner, R.K., Torgesen, J.K., & Rashotte, C.A. (1994). The development of reading-related phonological processing abilities: New evidence of bi-directional causality from a latent variable longitudinal study. *Development Psychology, 30*, 73-87.

Address Correspondence to:

Richard K. Wagner
Florida State University
Psychology Building R-54
Tallahassee, Florida 32306-1051
U.S.A.

VIRGINIA W. BERNINGER & ROBERT D. ABBOTT

MULTIPLE ORTHOGRAPHIC AND PHONOLOGICAL CODES IN LITERACY ACQUISITION: AN EVOLVING RESEARCH PROGRAM

1. INTRODUCTION

In section 1 we describe how a practical problem—diagnosing and remediating reading disabilities—led to the development of The Multiple Connections Model of orthographic-phonological coding relationships in learning to recognize and spell printed words. In section 2 we review results of a research program based on this model that are relevant to the theoretical issues of whether orthographic and phonological processes are independent, related, or both separate and functionally integrated. In section 3 we compare Dual Route Theory, Connectionism and our model and discuss our transition from assessment to treatment studies for validating the Multiple Connections Model.

1.1 Deriving Theory From Applied Problems

Deese (1992) took the position that "...over the years I have ever more firmly come to the view that a practical problem should be the excuse for erecting an elaborate theory...the prevailing view among psychologists is to the contrary: you start with a theory and then try to bring the world to the theory. The latest efforts in this direction generally go by the name cognitive psychology." A dramatic example of theory being derived from a practical problem is chemical atomic theory, which John Dalton, a meteorologist, conceived while trying to solve practical problems related to absorption of gases by water and of water by the atmosphere (Kuhn, 1970, pp. 132-133). Prevailing theory in chemistry at the time could not solve these problems, whereas atomic theory, derived from practical problems in weather prediction, could.

A relevant example of how theory may not fit real world

V.W. Berninger (ed.), The varieties of orthographic knowledge I: Theoretical and developmental issues, 277-319.

problems was reported by Dale Willows in the acknowledgements for *Visual Processes in Reading and Reading Disabilities* (Willows, Kruk, & Corcos, 1993, p xvii): "...after having spent more than a decade as a basic researcher in the field of reading, I...undertook a clinical internship at the McGill-Montreal Children's Hospital Learning Center. As a result of my experience there, I became convinced that what seemed relatively clear cut in theory was far from it in practice. As someone whose primary research program was focused on the role of linguistic (semantic, syntactic, and phonological) processes in reading, it came as a genuine shock to me to discover a range of phenomena in the reading and writing of the learning disabled that seemed to suggest an involvement of visual processing deficits, in addition to linguistic deficiencies. At the time, the psycholinguistic view was dominant in the field of reading, and reading disabilities were ascribed to linguistic deficits in phonological, morphological, semantic, and syntactic processes, to the exclusion of visual factors."

Likewise, the research reported in this chapter is part of a research program that began as an attempt to solve a practical problem—linking diagnosis of reading disabilities with educational intervention. During her clinical training at Boston's Children's Hospital, the first author was puzzled by the practice of some clinicians, both at the hospital and in the schools, of diagnosing the nature of a reading disability and of prescribing remedial methods on the basis of Verbal IQs and Performance IQ's, a purpose for which IQ tests were never validated. For example, if the Verbal IQ was low, reading disability might be linked to an auditory deficit with the recommendation to avoid phonics, but if the Performance IQ was low, reading disability might be linked to a visual deficit with the recommendation to avoid sight word training. Alternatively, phonics might be recommended if the Verbal IQ was high or sight word training might be recommended if the Performance IQ was high. Sometimes the same logic was applied to other measures of verbal reasoning or visual perception. This approach to assessment and remediation is in keeping with Dual Route Theory (e.g., Coltheart, 1978), which has been influential in basic reading research and assumes separate visual and phonological routes in word recognition.

However, this approach to diagnosis was puzzling for three reasons. First, none of the subtests contributing to a Verbal IQ measures phonemic skills, which a then growing literature and a now sizeable literature showed is a relevant linguistic variable in understanding reading acquisition (see Wagner & Barker, chapter 7). Second, none of the subtests contributing to a Performance IQ measures orthographic skills specific to written language. (See Berninger, 1994 for discussion of why only visual skills specific to orthography and not nonlinguistic visual skills are relevant to clinical assessment of reading.) Third, prior teaching and clinical experience with normally developing and reading disabled children and graduate training in cognitive psychology and psycholinguistics led the first author to conclude that phonics is not a purely auditory method of instruction and sight word training is not a purely visual method. Phonics requires attending to and perceiving component letters in written words and component phonemes in spoken words. Sight word training requires attending to and perceiving a whole written word pattern and retrieving a phonetic or name code for a whole spoken word. That is, each method of reading instruction has both visual (orthographic) and linguistic (phonological) processing requirements. The relevant diagnostic question seemed to be what written language-auditory language connections are functional, allowing a child to benefit from a particular instructional method and which ones need to be remediated so that the child can benefit from the associated instructional method. The relevant theoretical question did not seem to be whether reading was visual or linguistic but rather how visual (orthographic) and linguistic processes are interrelated (Berninger, 1987).

1.2 Alternative Written Language-Auditory Language Connections

To conceptualize alternative ways in which the connections or links might be forged between written and spoken language, linguistic theory about the development of written orthographies in human history was considered. Taylor (1981) described three kinds of writing systems: logographies that map meaning at the whole word level onto a graphic symbol; syllabaries that map syllables in spoken words onto syllables in written words; and alphabets that map phonemes onto letters. Thus, the first working hypothesis was that three kinds of visual-auditory linguistic connections underlie word recognition and that each of these correspond to a different method of teaching word recognition: the whole written word-whole spoken word connection to the look-say method, the letter cluster-oral syllable connection to word families, and the letter-phoneme connection to phonics. In keeping with Dual Route Theory, a whole written word-semantic code connection, underlying sight word recognition in reading, was also included in this schema. However, because phonetic codes automatically activate semantic codes (Tanenhaus, Flanigan, & Seidenberg, 1980), the whole word connections were sometimes grouped together as the whole written word-phonetic/semantic code connection or lexical connection. The original hypothesis has since been modified, based on work by Treiman (1988) on onsets and rimes and by Glushko (1979) and Goswami (1988) on analogies, to include five possible connections (left column) underlying methods of teaching word recognition (right column) (see Berninger, 1994, Table 4.2)

whole word	- name/meaning	look-say/sight words
letter	- phoneme	phonics (single letter-sound)
letter cluster	- phoneme	phonics (blends, digraphs, diphthongs)
letter cluster	- rime	word families (analogies)
letter cluster	- syllable	structural analysis of polysyllabic words

The first step in this research program was to develop measures of the orthographic and phonological codes underlying each of the code connections and associated teaching method. The second step, in which the second author, a statistician specializing in multivariate techniques has been involved, was validating the measures of multiple orthographic and phonological codes, and investigating the relationship of these codes and orthographic-phonological code connections to reading and writing achievement.

1.3 *Operational Measures Of Codes*

Multiple Orthographic Codes. Berninger (1987) used two different tasks to study orthographic processing in nonreaders at the end of kindergarten and the same children at the end of first grade when they were readers. The first task was the Garner attention paradigm (Garner, 1974), which showed that both nonreaders and beginning readers imposed different perceptual structures on shape/terminal letter information and on medial letter information. The second task was memory for orthographic units of varying size, which was based on work by Johnson (1986) and showed that both nonreaders and beginning readers remembered a whole word more accurately and faster than a letter in a word, which they remembered more accurately (and faster) than a letter cluster in a word. Berninger, Yates and Lester (1991) used a different task or different stimuli and replicated this same relative pattern in developing readers in grades 2, 4, and 6 (Study 1) and grades 1, 2, and 3 (Study 2). Johnson (1979) demonstrated that adult readers can encode a word unit without prior encoding of component parts. Johnson (1986) also showed that readers apply component strategies to scan letters in a word after the whole word unit is represented in memory. The finding that nonreaders, beginning readers, and developing readers were able to represent a whole word unit in memory (presented on the stimulus trial) and then make more accurate and faster judgments (on response trials) about that representation at the whole word than at the letter or letter cluster levels suggested that whole word processing might precede component processing of letters both in development and during on-line processing. The best predictor of component reading skill was accuracy (not speed) of coding (second task) and speed (not accuracy) of selective attention to letters (first task). The latter finding is relevant to Bowers et al.'s hypothesis about the relationship between speed of processing orthographic symbols and abstraction of orthographic structure (see chapter 5).

In subsequent work the second task, which required children to first encode a whole written word into short term memory and then to make decisions at the whole word, letter, or letter cluster level, was used instead of the Garner task for two reasons. First, the second task seemed to have better ecological validity for what happens during the act of reading—during fixation pauses written words are first transformed into representations in memory (i.e., coded) and then are translated into linguistic representations (i.e., decoded) based on analysis of orthographic information at the whole word, letter, or letter cluster level. That is, orthographic information is not only attended to and perceived but is also coded and decoded. (See Johnson, 1978 for discussion of the distinction between coding—procedures for translating external stimuli into mental representations—and decoding—accessing the content of a coded representation). Second, the second task yielded measures of orthographic coding at the relevant units of analysis for each of the code connections and teaching methods (see section 1.2).

Multiple Phonological Codes. Initially the focus was on three phonological codes for spoken words—phonetic or name codes for whole words, phonemic codes, and syllable codes. Recently measures of rime codes (Treiman, 1988) have been added. The distinction between phonetic and phonemic levels of analysis was based on Studdert-Kennedy's (1974) review. Prelexical access is phonetic but postlexical access is phonemic (Foss & Blank, 1980). The distinction between phonemic and syllable codes was based on work by Liberman, Shankweiler, Fisher, and Carter (1974) and Rosner (1979). Phoneme and syllable segmentation was measured using a modification of Rosner's (1979) Auditory Analysis Test, which includes syllable and phoneme deletion tasks. The modification (Berninger, Thalberg, DeBruyn, Smith, 1987, Appendix) involved additional items to increase the reliability of the measure.

Phonetic codes cannot be measured independently of semantic codes because of multiple code activation (Tanenhaus et al., 1980). Thus two approaches were used to measure phonetic/semantic codes in the first study (Berninger, 1985, 1986). One was confrontation naming or word finding as measured by the Gardner One-word Expressive Vocabulary Test (Gardner, 1979); both age-corrected standard scores for accuracy, and time scores were obtained. The other was the Vocabulary subtest of the WISC-R (Wechsler, 1974). Both tap phonetic skills—retrieval of name codes to identify a pictured object or concept (Gardner Test) or to explain what a word means (WISC-R Vocabulary)—as well as semantic knowledge of word meaning that is represented pictorially (Gardner Test) or accessed in lexical representations in semantic memory (WISC-R Vocabulary). The WISC-R Vocabulary subtest, which tapped only spoken language, tended to explain more variance in word recognition skills than the Gardner Test, on which many items were visually confusing (see Berninger & Alsdorf, 1989); thus the Gardner Test was dropped in subsequent studies. We did not include a measure of Rapid Automatized Naming (see Wolf et al., chapter 4, and Bowers et al., chapter 5), which taps name codes but also other factors such as visual processing (see Wolf et al., chapter 4). However, the model of orthographic-phonological relationships guiding our research predicts that rapid automatized naming (R.A.N.) is relevant to sight word acquisition, especially to automatization of sight word vocabulary; thus R.A.N. will be used in future work. Converging evidence from a number of studies has shown that rapid automatized naming and phonemic skills contribute independent variance in explaining word recognition (e.g. Bowers et al., chapter 5; Olson et al., chapter 1; Wolf et al., chapter 4; also Blachman, 1984; Bowers & Swanson, 1991; Felton & Brown, 1990). Also, Wolf (1984) has shown that naming speed contributes more to low level word recognition, whereas word finding contributes more to reading comprehension. The Gardner Test is a measure of word finding rather than of rapid automatized naming (R.A.N); although we obtained time scores for sets of items, items varied considerably in familiarity unlike RAN tests which measure speed of naming familiar items (see Bowers et al., chapter 5).

1.4 Validation of Multiple Codes

Three criteria have been used to evaluate the uniqueness of the orthographic codes and the uniqueness of the phonological codes. First, the intercorrelations among the measures of orthographic codes (or phonological codes) were examined. They tend to be low to moderate indicating that the variance in one code cannot be fully explained by variance in the other codes in the same domain, as shown in section 2 for our large-scale cross-sectional study. Second, correlations between each of the codes and criterion measures of component reading and writing skills were examined. The codes are correlated with the criterion reading skills (Berninger, 1984, 1985) and writing skills (Abbott & Berninger, 1993) but differ in their degree of relationship with different component skills especially at different developmental levels (e.g., see Berninger, Yates, & Lester, 1971 for the orthographic codes and Berninger, Proctor, DeBruyn, & Smith, 1988, for phonetic/semantic and phonemic codes). Third, developmental patterns in acquisition of codes were examined. Each of the orthographic codes and each of the phonological codes seems to be on its own developmental trajectory (Berninger, 1987, 1994).

1.5 Operationalizing the Code-Connections

The diagnostic model assumes that connections are forged between orthographic coding and phonological coding procedures of the same unit size (Van Orden, Pennington, & Stone, 1990). Connections are most likely to form if the corresponding orthographic codes and phonological codes are developed to the same level and to a level above a minimum threshold. Thus, measurement of code-connections to date has been indirect—based on inference. If either of the corresponding orthographic or phonological codes is at or below -1 standard deviation, we infer that establishing a code connection is probably problematic. Likewise, if there is a developmental dissociation such that the difference between levels of development of corresponding orthographic and phonological codes is one or more standard deviations, we also infer that establishing a code connection is probably problematic. Thus, we have arbitrarily defined dysfunctional code connections on the basis of (a) one or both of the corresponding codes being at or below -1 standard deviation on grade norms; and (b) a difference of a standard deviation or more between corresponding codes based on grade norms (unreferred sample, Berninger, Chen, & Abbott, 1988; treatment sample, Berninger & Traweek, 1991). In recent analyses with a different unreferred sample we used an alternative approach in which the Mahalanobis statistic (Stevens, 1986) was used to evaluate statistically whether orthographic and phonological codes were developed to reliably different levels; results are reported in section 2.

1.6 Multiple Connections Model

The theoretical model derived from this applied research also assumes that all the multiple orthographic-phonological code connections outlined in section 1.2 are needed for skilled reading. For the rationale based on the cognitive literature and the clinical neuropsychological literature, see Berninger (1994, chapter 4). For the first sample on which this model was tested ($N = 42$), at the end of first grade a composite variable based on whole word orthographic coding and receptive semantic coding (the direct path in Dual Route Theory) and a composite variable based on letter coding and phonemic coding (the indirect path in Dual Route Theory) accounted for significantly more variance in oral reading than either composite alone (Berninger, Chen, & Abbott, 1988). Thus, although the orthographic and phonological codes are separate, as discussed in section 1.4, both code connections play a role in beginning reading and are probably functionally integrated rather than independent paths as predicted by Dual Route Theory. Moreover, the more orthographic-phonological code connections that were functional (using operational criteria in section 1.5), the higher was the reading achievement. In recent analyses with a different unreferred sample (N = 300) we repeated the analysis of the relationship between the number of functional orthographic-phonological code connections (using the new criteria based on the Mahalanobis statistic) and reading, as well as spelling, achievement; results, which replicated the previous finding, are reported in section 2. (In this recent analysis we did not have a measure of receptive semantic coding and thus did not repeat the prior evaluation of the direct and indirect paths.)

1.7 Application Of The Multiple Connections Model To Clinical Practice

For beginning readers (grades 1 to 3 for which we have norms) or for older children who are reading below the third grade level, we follow these procedures in diagnosis. First, we administer the University of Washington Orthographic Coding Test (Berninger et al., 1991, Appendix) to measure whole word coding, letter coding, and letter cluster coding; we also administer the Modified Rosner Test (Berninger et al., 1987) to measure syllable and phoneme coding and the Vocabulary subtest of the WISC-R (Wechsler, 1974) or WISC-III to measure phonetic/semantic coding. Second, we evaluate which orthographic-phonological code connections are probably functional and dysfunctional based on criteria in section 1.5. Third, we evaluate the components of the instructional program (based on teacher interview and classroom observation) to determine whether the necessary instruction and practice are available for each of the code connections in section 1.2. Fourth, based on the second and third step, we identify which code connection(s) is (are) functional and recommend that the associated instructional method (see section 1.2) be used. We also identify the code connection(s) which is(are) dysfunctional and recommend instructional activities to develop the deficient orthographic and/or phonological codes and facilitate connections between them so that the child will benefit from the associated instructional method (see section 1.2). The long-term goal is to get all code connections functional. A balanced program using a variety of instructional methods for word recognition is required to accomplish this goal.

One thing we have learned from application of this theory-based assessment is that we cannot predict a priori whether a child with a problem in word recognition will have a deficit in orthographic coding or phonological coding. This conclusion has held for both unreferred samples, free of referral bias, and referred samples (to treatment studies and to the Clinical Training Laboratory at the University of Washington). For example, in an unreferred sample of 45 children at the end of first grade, 12 were achieving at or below -1 standard deviation on at least one measure of oral or silent reading achievement. Of these 8 (67%) had a disability (at or below -1 standard deviation) in only *one* measurable orthographic or linguistic skill at the end of kindergarten. Of these, half had a disability in an orthographic skill and half had a disability in a linguistic skill. Three of the children with more than one disability had at least one disability in an orthographic skill and one disability in a linguistic skill (Berninger, 1986).

In another unreferred sample of 300 children, we defined disability using three criteria: low functioning (bottom 5% of normal distribution), discrepant from IQ, and low functioning and discrepant from IQ (Berninger, Hart, Abbott, & Karovsky, 1992). Again, disabilities occurred in both orthographic and phonological coding (see Table 1). When patterning of low functioning was analyzed for individual children in the first grade, some had multiple disabilities but most children had a single disability: whole written word coding only ($n = 6$); letter coding only ($n = 4$); letter cluster only ($n = 1$); both whole word and letter ($n = 2$); both letter and letter cluster ($n = 2$); phonemic coding only ($n = 6$); syllable only ($n = 2$); both phonemic and syllable coding ($n = 1$). A few showed disabilities in both orthographic and phonological skills: letter, letter cluster, syllable and phonetic/semantic ($n = 2$); whole written word, phonetic/semantic, phonemic and syllable ($n = 1$); and letter, letter cluster, phonemic, and syllable ($n = 1$) (Berninger & Hart, 1992). (Note that these frequencies do not correspond to those in column LF under grade 1 in Table 1 because some of them are in the column LF+U because they met two criteria.)

The distribution of orthographic and phonological coding skills in referred samples shows a different pattern: Most children have multiple orthographic and phonological coding disabilities but the patterning varies across children as shown in Table 2. In the clinic sample, only three profiles replicated twice: letter cluster + phoneme disability; no disability; and letter cluster + phoneme + syllable disability. In the school sample, only five profiles replicated twice: letter cluster + phonetic/semantic + phonemic + syllabic; phonemic + syllabic; all the codes; all the codes except syllable; and whole word + all the phonological codes.

Taken together, these results show that more than a phonological core variable is contributing to reading disability (also see Wolf et al., chapter 4). They also illustrate the principle of *noncontingent normal variation* (Berninger & Hart, 1992). Not only do coding skills show normal variation along a continuous distribution within a domain but also skill in one code does not necessarily determine skill in another code. Profiles also show normal variation, which is diversity not related to pathology. This normal variation in profiles of coding abilities is probably related to the interaction of genetic constraints and experiences in interacting with print.

Table 1

Incidence of Orthographic and Phonological Coding Disabilities in an Unreferred Sample Based on Three Different Definitions of Disability

	Grade 1 (N=100)			Grade 2 (N=100)			Grade 3 (N-100)		
	LF[a]	U[b]	LF+U[c]	LF[a]	U[b]	LF+U[c]	LF[a]	U[b]	LF+U[c]
Orthographic Coding									
whole word	7	8	5	4	7	3	6	6	2
letter	7	11	7	5	5	2	6	8	3
letter cluster	3	5	2	7	6	2	6	8	2
Phonological Coding									
Phonetic/Semantic	3	4	2	3	6	1	6	8	1
Phonemic	8	9	8	6	6	3	10	7	4
Syllabic	6	6	6	7	5	2	0	4	0

[a]LF = low functioning
[b]U = underachieving relative to IQ
[c]LF+U = combined low functioning and underachieving

Table 2

Incidence of Orthographic and Phonological Coding Disabilities in Two Referred Samples Based on Criteria in Section 1.5

		Orthographic Coding			**Phonological Coding**		
		Whole Word	Letter	Letter Cluster	Phonetic/ Semantic	Phoneme	Syllable
Clinic Sample (n=12)[a]							
M	S1			X		X	
F	S2	X		X			
F	S3					X	
F	S4			X		X	
M	S5						
M	S6						
M	S7				X		
M	S8	X	X				
M	S9	X	X	X		X	X
M	S10					X	
M	S11			X		X	X
M	S12			X		X	X
School Sample (n=20)[b]							
M	S1	X	X	X		X	X
F	S2	X		X	X	X	X
F	S3					X	X
M	S4	X	X			X	X
M	S5			X	X	X	X
M	S6			X		X	X
M	S7				X	X	X
M	S8	X	X				
M	S9	X	X	X		X	
M	S10					X	X
M	S11	X	X		X	X	X
M	S12	X	X	X	X	X	
M	S13	X		X		X	X
M	S14	X	X		X		
M	S15			X	X	X	X
M	S16	X	X	X	X	X	X
F	S17	X	X	X	X	X	
F	S18	X			X	X	X
M	S19	X			X	X	X
F	S20	X	X	X	X	X	X

[a] Mostly children during the summer between first and second grade referred for evaluation of reading problems

[b] Beginning second graders participating in a treatment study for reading disabilities

Another thing we have learned from application of this theory-based assessment to clinical practice is that many children's instructional programs in reading are not well matched to their unique profiles of orthographic and phonological coding abilities. For example, a child for whom only the letter-phoneme connection was functional, indicating that he could benefit from phonics, was in a whole language classroom with no explicit instruction in word attack skills. Another child, for whom only the whole written word-whole spoken word was functional, was in a multisensory phonics program that drilled words in isolation without any practice in reading connected text to develop a sight vocabulary (see Berninger, 1994).

The final thing we are learning is that this theory-based diagnostic system, which takes into account separate orthographic and phonological coding abilities and functional orthographic-phonological relationships, can be used to generate treatment plans that remediate reading disabilities. Berninger and Traweek (1991) described a long term intervention program for reading disabilities in a school setting; the number of functional orthographic-phonological code connections predicted achievement before and after intervention. Berninger, Lester, Sohlberg, and Mateer (1991) reported a short-term and a long-term clinical treatment program for reading disabilities. Berninger, Abbott, Whitaker, and Sylvester (in preparation) discuss results of intensive tutorials in a clinic setting for spelling disabilities and other writing disabilities. We are also preparing detailed case studies of reading disabled children evaluated in our clinic and followed long-term for whom we have provided consultation but other professionals have provided the intervention services.

2.1 Relevance to Theoretical Issues

The Multiple Connections Model was derived from a practical problem, but the empirical results of research designed to validate it have implications for current controversies surrounding orthographic processes in reading and writing.

Whether Orthographic Processing is a Univariate or Multivariate Construct. One reason for the lack of consensus about orthographic processes is that multiple kinds of knowledge are involved and different investigators are focused on different aspects of this multidimensional process (see Introduction to Volume I). To date we have focused on accuracy of orthographic coding (receptive, primary grades; expressive, intermediate grades), speed of orthographic coding (intermediate grades), orthographic-phonological mapping (primary and intermediate grades), and orthographic images (intermediate grades) (see Table 1 in Introduction). The receptive orthographic coding tasks (Berninger et al., 1991), which require a yes/no judgment, are thought to be relevant to procedures used to create orthographic images in memory during the beginning phases of learning to read and write. As can be seen in Table 3a, correlations among whole word, letter, and letter cluster coding are low to moderate, indicating that they are related but not redundant sources of knowledge. The expressive orthographic tasks (Berninger, in press; Berninger, Cartwright, Yates, Swanson, & Abbott, in press), which require processing a briefly presented written word and then reproducing the whole word or a component letter or letter sequence, are thought to be relevant to procedures used to access orthographic images and construct written responses based on them. Speed of encoding written stimuli (measured by the Colorado Perceptual Speed Test, Decker & DeFries, 1981) is thought to be relevant to developing automaticity. Orthographic-phonological mapping is thought to underlie two different mechanisms identified by Carr and Polatsek (1985) in a review of the large literature in experimental psychology on word recognition: word-specific representations (measured by the Word Identification subtest of the WRMT-R, Woodcock, 1987) and rule-governed mechanisms (measured by the Word Attack subtest, WRMT-R, Woodcock, 1987). (Based on recent connectionist models, the latter might be reconceptualized as sub-word rather than rule-governed mechanisms, see section 3). Orthographic images (measured by Olson's homophone/pseudohomophone choice task, Olson, Kliegl, Davidson, & Foltz, 1985; and Stanovich's homophone choice task, Stanovich, West, & Cunningham, 1991) are thought to be the word-specific images represented in memory. As can be seen in Table 3b, correlations among different kinds of orthographic knowledge (speed of coding orthographic symbols, orthographic images, and expressive coding of whole words, letters, and letter clusters) are low to moderate, indicating that they are related but not redundant sources of knowledge.

Development of orthographic images is thought to depend on other kinds of orthographic knowledge—abstraction of orthographic regularity based on permissible and probable letter sequences; procedures for coding units of information in printed words; and code connection procedures for mapping orthographic information onto corresponding units of phonological information represented in memory or for mapping phonological information onto corresponding units of orthographic information. Orthographic-phonological mapping can occur in either direction, beginning with orthography or beginning with phonology (see Barron, chapter 6). We have used structural equation modeling to investigate executive functions in managing print to sound mappings versus sound to print mappings (Berninger, 1994).

Thus, like Olson et al. (chapter 1) we concur with Ehri's (1992) interactive view between orthography and phonology. Where the Multiple Connections Model differs from other interactive models is in specification of multiple codes and multiple phonological codes and the goal of determining which connections between corresponding codes are functional for *individual* children. Correlations reported in Table 3a show that at best 44% of the variance in one orthographic code is explained by variance in another orthographic code. A similar pattern occurred for the orthographic skills in the intermediate grade sample (Table 3b). Likewise, correlations show that the multiple phonological coding procedures are related but not redundant in primary grade (Table 4a) and intermediate grade (Table 4b) samples. At best 27% of the variance in one phonological code is explained by variance in another phonological code. From these *interindividual* differences in the levels to which the various orthographic and phonological codes are developed it follows that *intraindividual* differences may occur in which connections between corresponding codes are functional. Another feature of the Multiple Connections Model is its inclusion of both phonetic name codes and phonemic codes, both of which contribute independent variance to word recognition (see Olson et al., chapter 1, Bowers et al., chapter 5, Wolf et al., chapter 4). Presumably rapid automatized naming taps phonetic codes as well as other processes (see Wolf et al., chapter 4).

Table 3a

Intercorrelations among Orthographic Measures. Primary Grade Sample

	V1	V2	V3
Grade 1 (*N*=100)			
V1 whole word			
V2 letter	.65		
V3 letter cluster	.62	.19	
Grade 2 (*N*=100)			
V1			
V2	.48		
V3	.45	.66	
Grade 3 (*N*=100)			
V1			
V2	.39		
V3	.28	.50	

Table 3b

Intercorrelations among Orthographic Measures. Intermediate Grade Sample

	V1	V2	V3	V4
Grade 4 (*N*=100)				
V1 Colorado Perceptual Speed				
V2 Homophone Choice	.52			
V3 Homophone/Pseudohomophone Choice	.62	.64		
V4 Expressive Orthographic Coding	.52	.44	.55	
Grade 5 (*N*=100)				
V1				
V2	.25			
V3	.60	.56		
V4	.25	.21	.53	
Grade 6 (*N*=100)				
V1				
V2	.35			
V3	.48	.67		
V4	.35	.14	.36	

Table 4a

Intercorrelations among Phonological Measures. Primary Grade Sample

	V1	V2	V3
Grade 1 (*N*=100)			
V1 Phonetic/Semantic			
V2 Phonemic	.33		
V3 Syllabic	.27	.33	
Grade 2 (*N*=100)			
V1			
V2	.52		
V3	.38	.38	
Grade 3 (*N*=100)			
V1			
V2	.37		
V3	.16	.26	

Table 4b

Intercorrelations among Phonological Measures. Intermediate Grade Sample

	V1	V2	V3
Grade 4 (*N*=100)			
V1 Phonetic/Semantic			
V2 Phonemic	.41		
V3 Rime	.34	.45	
Grade 5 (*N*=100)			
V1			
V2	.33		
V3	.36	.26	
Grade 6 (*N*=100)			
V1			
V2	.24		
V3	.35	.44	

In summary, based on others' work and our own, we conclude that orthographic processing is a multivariate construct. Based on our own work we conclude that one source of orthographic knowledge—orthographic coding involves multiple coding procedures.

Whether Orthographic Skills Are the Same or Separate from Reading and Writing Skills. In response to issues raised by Vellutino et al. (1994) (also see Wagner & Barker, chapter 7), we summarized the correlations between orthographic measures and component reading and writing skills in our primary grade sample (Table 5a) and our intermediate grade sample (Table 5b). Although most of the correlations are statistically significant, they are low to moderate at best. In particular the criticism that the homophone/pseudohomophone choice task or homophone choice task merely measures spelling (correlations range from .38 to .58) or word recognition skill (correlations range from .40 to .58) does not seem to be warranted.

Whether Orthographic and Phonological Skills Are Unique Contributors. Multiple regression analyses replicated findings of other research groups (see Olson et al., chapter 1; Wagner & Barker, chapter 7), who used other measures of orthographic and phonological skills, showing that orthographic and phonological skills add unique variance to explaining word recognition. Our results show that *multiple orthographic* and *multiple phonological* skills contribute unique increments of variance in reading real words, reading pronounceable nonwords, and spelling dictated words in both the primary grade (Table 6a) and intermediate grade samples (Table 6b). In the primary grade sample all three orthographic coding and all three phonological coding skills (same as in Tables 3a and 4a) contributed unique increments of variance to reading real words; and all these codes except letter coding contributed unique increments of variance to reading nonwords. All these codes, except whole word coding, *and* the interaction between letter cluster and syllable contributed unique increments of variance to spelling dictated words. In the intermediate grade sample (Berninger et al., in press) three orthographic measures (homophone choice, homophone/pseudohomophone choice, and expressive orthographic coding) and three phonological skills (phoneme localization and phoneme articulation,

Table 5a

Correlations Between Orthographic Coding and Reading and Writing Skills. Primary Grades ($N = 300$)[a]

	Whole Word Coding	Letter Coding	Letter Cluster Coding
Reading Real Words	.41	.47	.47
Reading Pronounceable Nonwords	.39	.45	.49
Handwriting Fluency	.52	.51	.60
Spelling Dictated Words	.24	.33	.37
Compositional Fluency–Narrative	.48	.48	.54
Compositional Fluency–Expository	.40	.41	.46

[a] All correlations are statistically significant

Table 5b

Correlations Between Orthographic Skills and Reading and Writing Skills. Intermediate Grades ($N = 300$)[a]

	Colorado Perceptual Speed (Timed)	Homophone Choice	Homophone/ Pseudo-homophone	Expressive Orthographic Coding (untimed)
Reading Real Words	.40	.46	.58	.48
Reading Pronounceable Nonwords	.33	.40	.54	.55
Handwriting Fluency	.36	.16	.33	.30
Spelling Dictated Words	.36	.46	.58	.47
Spontaneous Spelling–Narrative	.26	.45	.53	.34
Spontaneous Spelling–Expository	.30	.38	.44	.41
Compositional Fluency–Narrative	.28	.11	.18	.07
Compositional Fluency–Expository	.25	.14	.21	.09
Compositional Quality–Narrative	.34	.27	.32	.24
Compositional Quality–Expository	.34	.28	.38	.29

[a]All correlations are statistically significant except for those that are underlined.

Table 6a

Contribution of Orthogrpahic and Phonological Codes to Reading and Spelling Single Words.
Primary Grade Sample ($N = 300$)

Dependent Measure	Independent Measure	Standardized Coefficient	t	p	R^2	F (9, 290)	p
Reading Real Words					.48	29.90	.001
	Whole Word	.13	2.37	.018*			
	Letter	.18	3.10	.002*			
	Letter Cluster	.18	3.32	.001*			
	Phonetic/Semantic	.22	4.41	.001*			
	Syllable	.10	2.15	.033*			
	Phoneme	.21	4.01	.001*			
	Whole Word x Phonetic/Semantic	-.03	-.72	.473			
	Letter x Phoneme	.02	.38	.702			
	Letter Cluster x Syllable	.03	.69	.491			
Reading Pronounceable Nonwords					.50	31.95	.001
	Whole Word	.12	2.30	.022*			
	Letter	.09	1.53	.128			
	Letter Cluster	.22	4.10	.001*			
	Phonetic/Semantic	.14	3.01	.003*			
	Syllable	.17	3.73	.001*			
	Phoneme	.29	5.75	.001*			
	Whole Word x Phonetic/Semantic	-.02	-.47	.636			
	Letter x Phoneme	.07	1.47	.143			
	Letter Cluster x Syllable	.10	2.18	.030*			
Spelling Dictated Words					.42	23.41	.001
	Whole Word	.08	1.51	.131			
	Letter	.15	2.42	.016*			
	Letter Cluster	.24	4.06	.001*			
	Phonetic/Semantic	.16	3.18	.002*			
	Syllable	.17	3.46	.001*			
	Phoneme	.14	2.60	.010*			
	Whole Word x Phonetic/Semantic	-.04	-.77	.444			
	Letter x Phoneme	-.02	-.34	.738			
	Letter Cluster x Syllable	.11	2.16	.031*			

* Adds significant increment of variance at $p < .05$ or better

Table 6b

Contribution of Orthogrpahic and Phonological Codes to Reading and Spelling Single Words. Intermediate Grade Sample ($N = 300$)

Dependent Measure	Independent Measure	Standardized Coefficient	t	p	R^2	F (9, 290)	p
Reading Real Words					.55	51.31	.001
	Homophone Choice	.12	2.33	.020*			
	Homophone/Pseudohomophone Choice	.27	4.75	.001*			
	Expressive Orthographic Coding	.14	3.03	.003*			
	Phoneme Localization	.10	2.29	.023*			
	Phoneme Articulation	.12	2.46	.015*			
	Syllable/Rime/Phoneme Deletion	.12	2.51	.013*			
	Verbal IQ	.25`	5.50	.001*			
Reading Pronounceable Nonwords					.50	41.54	.001
	Homophone Choice	.10	1.91	.057			
	Homophone/Pseudohomophone Choice	.22	3.67	.001*			
	Expressive Orthographic Coding	.28	5.56	.001*			
	Phoneme Localization	.15	3.35	.001*			
	Phoneme Articulation	.17	3.11	.002*			
	Syllable/Rime/Phoneme Deletion	.13	2.46	.015*			
	Verbal IQ	.00`	-.03	.973			
Spelling Dictated Real Words				.44	33.07	.001	
	Homophone Choice	.13	2.32	.021*			
	Homophone/Pseudohomophone Choice	.32	5.18	.001*			
	Expressive Orthographic Coding	.17	3.24	.001*			
	Phonetic Memory	.06	1.32	.187			
	Syllable/Rime/Phoneme Deletion	.06	1.03	.302			
	Phoneme Articulation	.11	1.96	.051*			
	Verbal IQ	.11`	2.14	.033*			

*Adds significant increment of variance at $p < .05$ or better

Vellutino & Scanlon, 1987; and syllable, rime, phoneme deletion of nonwords, Berninger, in press) contributed unique increments of variance to reading real words. All these codes except homophone choice, which requires choosing the homophone to answer a question and thus semantic as well as orthographic address, contributed unique increments of variance to reading pronounceable nonwords. All three orthographic skills and one phonological skill (phoneme articulation) contributed unique increments to spelling dictated words. The results for reading nonwords are theoretically important because they show that in the primary and intermediate grades *both orthographic and phonological codes contribute to nonword reading, which cannot be considered a pure phonological task.*

Whether Orthographic-Phonological Codes Have Functional Connections. Just because orthographic and phonological codes contribute unique variance demonstrating their separate existence in the functional reading or writing system, it does not mean that they are not functionally related. To demonstrate the importance of achieving functional connections between corresponding orthographic and phonological codes (whole written words and phonetic/ semantic codes; letter and phoneme codes; and letter cluster and syllable codes), we used the following criteria to determine which orthographic-phonological code connections were functional or dysfunctional for *individual* children in an unreferred primary grade sample ($N = 300$). A code connection was deemed dysfunctional if (a) the corresponding codes were developed to reliably different levels based on the Mahalanobis statistic (Stevens, 1986) at the .05 level, one tail test; and (b) at least one of the codes fell in the lowest 5% of the normal distribution. These dual criteria, which were more stringent than those used in previous studies (see section 1.5), offered the advantage of reducing the chance of identifying a connection as functional when it is really dysfunctional but the disadvantage of having to exclude 58 cases (19.3% of the sample) as indeterminant because they met one but not both criteria. If a connection did not meet criteria for dysfunctionality or was not indeterminant, it was considered functional.

The results are summarized in Table 7. All three orthographic-phonological code connections were functional for almost 70% of the sample. Only two orthographic-phonological code connections were functional for about 10% of the sample. Only one orthographic-phonological code connection was functional for about 2% of the sample. No functional orthographic-phonological code connections were identified for 0.3% of the sample.

The groups with all code connections read real words 0.90 standard deviations better, read nonwords 0.86 standard deviations better, and spelled 0.67 standard deviations better, on the average, than the group with only two code connections functional. The group with two code connections spelled 0.50 standard deviations better, on the average, than the group with only one code connection; the difference in their reading achievement was minimal but in the predicted direction. The group with one connection read real words over 1 standard deviation better and nonwords 0.80 standard deviations better and spelled 0.50 standard deviations better than the one child with zero connections, who read and spelled poorly—over 1 1/2 standard deviations or 2 standard deviations below the mean, respectively. Consistently, mean reading and spelling achievement dropped as the number of functional code connections decreased. Thus, failure of orthographic and phonological codes to develop beyond minimal thresholds and failure of corresponding codes to develop to comparable levels can interfere with forming of code connections and consequently with reading and spelling achievement.

Analysis of spelling errors in our corpus of dictated spelling tests and compositions also supported the interactive view of orthographic and phonological processes. Initially we analyzed the most frequent errors for a constant set of 15 words on the WRAT-R (Jastak & Wilkinson, 1984) in grades 1, 2, and 3 (see Table 8). We coded whether the errors were in the onset or the rime and whether they reflected primarily phonological problems (e.g., deletion, substitution, or addition of sound representations), primarily orthographic problems (e.g., letter reversal or transposition of letters), or phonological-to-orthographic mapping errors—what Barron, chapter 6, calls the sound-to-print connection (e.g., incorrect representation of a vowel sound, substituting a plausible alternative representation of a particular sound, failure to apply a final e rule for marking a vowel long, failure to double a letter, etc.). As can be seen in

Table 7

Mean Reading and Spelling Achievement for Individuals with Different Numbers of Functional Code Connections

	Reading Real Words		**Reading Nonwords**		**Spelling**	
	M	**SD**	**M**	**SD**	**M**	**SD**
3 Connections Functional (*N* = 209)[a]	109.5	16.6	106.7	13.9	99.5	17.5
2 Connections Functional (*N* = 31)[b]	96.0	12.1	93.8	12.7	89.3	14.1
1 Connection Functional (*N* = 6)[b]	95.3	17.9	90.5	6.1	81.0	17.9
0 Connections Functional (*N* = 1)[b]	76.0	—	78.0	—	73.0	—

[a] Excluding 58 cases meeting one criterion but not both criteria for dysfunctional code connections (see text)

[b] Meet both criteria for a dysfunctional code connection (see text)

Table 8, onsets of syllables both in monosyllabic and polysyllabic words were almost always spelled correctly. Most errors occurred in rime units. Phonological errors, as defined in our coding scheme, occurred occasionally, and orthographic errors, as defined in our coding scheme, occurred rarely. Most errors reflected problems in phonological-orthographic mapping—in misrepresenting vowel sounds or in substituting a plausible alternative that can only be ruled out with word-specific knowledge (e.g., whach, macke, saye, lite, nacher). Inspection of the spelling errors made by individual children in their narrative and expository compositions revealed the same pattern—most errors occurred in the rime of syllables and involved errors in phonological-orthographic mapping rather than pure orthographic or pure phonological problems.

Much has been written about the invented spellings during the protoliteracy period (see Barron, chapter 6), which reflect emerging knowledge of letter-sound relationships. Likewise, most spelling errors of developing spellers reflect emerging knowledge of letter-sound relationships. Few words are completely misspelled—often the error involves only one or two letter-sound representations. Some errors actually reflect plausible alternatives for representing sounds in the orthography.

The spelling errors of a boy referred to our clinic for severe writing disabilities illustrate these points (see Table 9). The teacher had written on his spelling test: "If you would spend half as much effort studying your spelling, as you do in fabricating excuses and blaming others for your poor grades, you would learn better. It's high time that you take responsibility for your own learning. It takes a teacher of strong character not to give up on someone who has to be pushed and corrected every inch of the way. When 20 out of 26 kids earn 18 or more points out of 20, that shows that your grades are not my fault. They are your fault and it's time you realize the truth and act upon it. I don't understand why your parents listen to your excuses." A teacher more knowledgeable about the processes underlying spelling acquisition would have noted that most of the spellings were close to the mark. The boy may have added a sound to some words such as "scrambuling" or deleted a sound for some words like "studing," because he has trouble analyzing the representation of the spoken word. Only one reversal (orthographic error) occurred (ba<u>d</u>es). Most of his errors reflected inadequate

Table 8

Most frequent spelling errors for a set of 15 words on the Wide Range Achievement Test-Revised (*N* = 100 at each grade level in this unreferred sample)

Word	Grade 1	Frequency	Grade 2	Frequency	Grade 3	Frequency
make	mak	13	mack	3	mack	4
	mack	10	mak	1		
	macke	5	mac	1		
	mace	2	mike	1		
	maak	1				
say	sa	15	sae	3	saye	1
	sae	4	sa	2	sa	1
	saye	4	saa	2		
	saay	5	sai	1		
	saa	1	siy	1		
cut	kat	10	kut	1	cet	1
	kut	7	ket	1		
	cat	7	cat	1		
	cot	2	ckut	1		
	cate	2	kute	1		
light	lit	25	lite	12	lite	4
	lite	20	lit	2	litte	1
	litt	3	ligh	2		
	liht	1	litht	1		
	lihte	1	liate	1		
order	ordr	18	oder	9	oder	13
	odr	10	ordr	6	orter	2
	rdr	3	odr	4	ordr	2
	ordre	3	ortr	3	ordre	1
	orbr	3	odor	2		
watch	woch	16	wach	14	wach	20
	wach	13	woch	6	woch	5
	woh	4	wath		wotch	2
	woc	2	whach	4	wache	1
	wot	2	wacht	2	wacth	1
nature	nacher	12	nacher	13	nacher	17
	nachr	9	nachr	8	natcher	11
	nachre	2	natcher	4	nather	4
	nacr	2	nather	4	natcer	3
	naecher	1	naher	2	nater	2

Word	Grade 1	Frequency	Grade 2	Frequency	Grade 3	Frequency
explain	explan	5	explan	8	explane	19
	explane	3	explanle	7	explan	11
	icksplan	3	exsplane	7	exsplane	7
	iksplan	2	icsplan	5	exsplan	4
	xplan	2	exsplan	3	iscplan	3
edge	eg	8	ege	16	ege	15
	ege	7	eg	9	eage	7
	ej	6	age	4	edg	4
	eje	2	edg	2	egde	3
	egg	2	egde	1	eg	2
kitchen	kichin	7	kichin	11	kichen	22
	kichen	5	kichen	6	kitchin	3
	cichin	4	cichin	4	cichin	3
	cichn	2	kittchen	3	kichin	3
	cichen	2	kichn	1	kechen	2
surprise	spris	7	supris	8	suprise	14
	suprise	3	sprise	7	surprize	8
	saprise	3	suprise	6	sprise	3
	srpris	2	spris	4	suprize	3
	serpris	2	srpis	3	srprise	2
success	secses	2	sexses	8	sucsess	9
	sexses	1	secses	6	sixses	7
	sekses	1	sicses	4	sucses	6
	sicses	1	sixses	3	sexses	6
	sucses	1	sickses	2	sicses	4
reasonable	reasnable	1	resenable	3	resenable	8
	resenbl	1	resnable	2	resonable	6
	resenebl	1	resenuble	2	resinable	4
	resinable	1	resinable	2	resanable	3
	resinabl	1	resnabal	1	resnable	3
imaginary	amadg	1	imagenary	3	imaganary	5
	amagein	1	amaganary	2	imagenary	5
	amangenery	1	inmagenary	2	amaganary	4
	emaginary	1	imajenary	1	amagenary	3
	emaginary	1	imaganare	1	amaginary	3
character	carecter	1	charecter	4	caricter	5
	careckter	1	caricter	2	cariter	3
	caricker	1	cerecter	2	caracter	2
	caricter	1	carector	2	carector	2
	carrickter	1	chareter	2	carictor	2

learning of phonological-orthographic correspondences. For example "pul" is an alternative way of representing the same sound as "ple"; and "sc" in scemming is an alternative way of spelling the same sound as represented by "sk." The distinction between short e and short i is not always made in the spoken form of "habets." He did not know or failed to apply rules for doubling letters (e.g., "drumer") or marking long vowels (e.g., hatful). He is caught in a circular loop. Because of underdeveloped knowledge of phonological-orthographic correspondences, his orthographic images are probably partial rather than complete representations (see Ehri, 1992); thus, he cannot rely on word-specific representations when unsure about how to translate sound into print. His dilemma cannot be solved by relying on a pure orthographic or pure phonological strategy. It can only be solved by helping him continue to build knowledge of the interrelationships between orthography and phonology.

Table 9

Spelling Test for Boy Referred for Clinical Assessment

His written spelling	Dictated word
bumping	
crumpul	crumple
scrambuling	scrambling
splis	supplies
liking	
drumer	drummer
studing	studying
bloking	blocking
studed	studied
habets	habits
contres	countries
scemming	skimming
ugliest	
shadeiest	shadiest
slopper	sloppier
tidest	tidiest
bades	babies
ponies	
wavest	waviest
hatful	hateful

Whether Similar Conclusions Are Drawn for the Acquired as for the Developmental Dyslexias. McCarthy and Warrington (1990) reviewed the clinical neuropsychology literature and subtyped acquired dyslexias into two broad categories: visual word-form dyslexias and central dyslexias. The visual word-form dyslexias were further subtyped into spelling dyslexia, neglect dyslexia, and attentional dyslexia. In spelling dyslexia the patient can only recognize words if he or she first spells them letter by letter in left to right sequence. In neglect dyslexia the patient misreads the initial or terminal parts of words. In attentional dyslexia the patient can read single words in isolation but has difficulty reading words embedded in connected text. We argue that these acquired visual form dyslexias have parallels in developmental reading disorders related to deficits in orthographic coding of printed words in isolation or context. The central dyslexias were further subtyped into reading by sound dyslexia or reading by sight dyslexia. In reading by sound dyslexia the patient has difficulty translating spelling into sound. In reading by sight vocabulary the patient has difficulty translating spelling into meaning. We argue that the reading by sound dyslexia results from deficits in orthographic-phonological code connections at the whole word or subword levels, and that reading by sight dyslexia results from deficits in orthographic-semantic code connections at the whole word level. Thus, research on the acquired dyslexias and research on developmental dyslexias have yielded similar conclusions: orthographic coding and orthographic-phonological code connections are separable components in the reading system. Any aspect of the orthographic coding of the visual form of the word or of the process of translating that visual form into sound or meaning may dissociate in the developing reader or break down in the skilled reader. Yet, in normal reading both components—orthographic coding and orthographic-phonological connections—function in an integrated manner. This conclusion of both separable *and* integrated orthographic and phonological processes is consistent with the genetic findings of Olson et al. (chapter 1, this volume). They showed that orthographic and phonological deficits have a shared genetic etiology (correlated variance) and also different genetic pathways (independent variance).

3.1 *Implications For Theories Of Word Recognition*

Dual Route Theory. According to Dual Route Theory (e.g.,

Coltheart, 1978), independent and noninteractive lexical and nonlexical routes exist for reading. The lexical route, which is direct and based on word-specific representations, is used to read irregular words which have exceptions to grapheme-phoneme correspondence. The nonlexical route, which is indirect and based on representations of rules, is used to read regular words (for further discussion, see Barron, 1986; Carr & Polatsek, 1985; Chase & Tallal, 1991; and Humphreys & Evett, 1985).

Soon after its appearance in the literature a number of criticisms were leveled against Dual Route Theory. Marcel (1980) argued that the crucial issue was not regularity of words in terms of grapheme-phoneme correspondence but whether the graphemes had competing pronunciations. Shallice and Warrington (1980) argued that the phonological route does not just operate on graphemes but also on syllables and short words. Shallice, Warrington, and McCarthy (1983) argued that the phonological route can also operate on sub-syllabic units such as consonant clusters and morphemes. Morton and Patterson (1980) proposed three different procedures for obtaining a phonological code from a visual input: (a) grapheme-phoneme correspondence rules; (b) direct route from visual input to phonological output; and (c) indirect route from the input visual system to semantic system to output phonological system. Likewise, Baron (1979) pointed out that word-specific associations can be formed between a whole printed word and its sound or its meaning whether or not the word is regular or irregular in grapheme-phoneme correspondence. Shallice et al. (1983) found that degree of irregularity affected pronunciation of written words: mildly irregular words with a single exception to grapheme-phoneme correspondence are read better than highly irregular words with several exceptions to grapheme-phoneme correspondences. Glushko (1979) and Seidenberg, Waters, Sanders, and Lagner (1984) showed that regularity does not have to reflect grapheme-phoneme correspondence; it can be defined on the basis of analogies to known words, which involve comparison of common sub-syllable patterns across words. Humphreys and Evett (1985) reviewed evidence showing that brain damage does not selectively eliminate either the lexical or nonlexical route. Taken together, these arguments and findings cast doubt on the claim that oral reading depends on two separate mechanisms—one for purely regular words in terms of grapheme-phoneme correspondence and one for purely irregular words in terms of grapheme-phoneme correspondence.

Another claim of Dual Route theorists (e.g., Doctor & Coltheart, 1980) which has been criticized is that beginning readers use the indirect, nonlexical route, which is phonological, while skilled readers use the direct, lexical route, which is visual. Barron (1986) reviewed evidence that both routes may be used by beginning readers. Van Orden (1987) showed that skilled readers also use an indirect, phonological route. Also, recent research reviewed by Jackson et al. (chapter 2) shows the importance of phonological processing in adult skilled reading in all languages. Berninger (1985, 1986, 1994) reported evidence that both visual (orthographic) and phonological processes are involved in beginning reading. The use of the term route is also problematic because it assumes that the lexicon is a place is the brain where words go—an assumption not consistent with current evidence in neuroscience. An alternative view is a computational model that assumes lexical level procedures that coordinate multiple kinds of codes (see Berninger, 1989).

Despite the mounting criticisms (for review, see Chase & Tallal, 1991; Van Orden et al., 1991), Dual Route Theory still has its advocates (e.g., Posner, Peterson, Fox, & Raichle, 1988). One possible reason for its survival is the phenomenological experiences of reading researchers, who as adult skilled readers perceive that they go directly from print to meaning in silent reading and remember sounding out words when they learned to read. The psychological reality of orthographic-phonological connections underlying word recognition may be more obvious when one adopts the developmental perspective of the child learning to read (Berninger, 1994).

Connectionism. Although Dual Route Theory has survived despite much criticism, an alternative, competing theory has also flourished: connectionism which is a computational model that treats orthographic and phonological processes as interactive in a parallel, distributed system rather than as insular and independent in a serial processing system (see Chase & Tallal, 1991). For example, Seidenberg and McClelland (1989) used computer simulation to evaluate a distributed, developmental model of word recognition based on a single computational procedure that is applied to all words, whether or not they are regular, and nonwords. In this model words do not activate entries in a lexicon. Rather knowledge of words is encoded in terms of the weights or connections between the orthographic input and "hidden" units between the input and output units and between the hidden and phonological output units in a distributed memory network. Learning occurs as those weights are modified through experience in reading words. When the number of hidden units was reduced, learning still occurred but performance was impaired for exception words. This model has been criticized because it does not adequately account for experimental results with human subjects, particularly for nonwords (Besner, Twilley, McCann, & Seergobin, 1990).

In another version of a connectionist model, not based on computer simulation, is the *Covariant Learning Hypothesis* (Van Orden et al., 1990), which proposes subsymbols, which are rule-like but not rule-governed, as an alternative to the symbolic indirect route in Dual Route Theory, which is rule-governed. Subsymbols are microfeatures that emerge momentarily and behave as a single, functional entity when activated in univariant patterns in a dynamic system. Orthographic and phonological subsymbols, which are connected to each other by modifiable weights, can function at any unit size—whole word, single letter, or letter groups—but the combination of subsymbols represented in an orthographic-phonological mapping must be at the appropriate unit-size of correspondence, which can vary from time to time. Learning occurs as the weights between the subsymbols are adjusted through *whole word crosstalk* or *subword crosstalk,* which can occur independently of one another. Consistent cross-talk across a set of words allows connection weights to grow faster than when there is inconsistent cross-talk. The resulting matrix of connection weights reflects patterns of orthographic-phonological covariance or regularity of the language, which is continuous rather than categorical as in Dual Route Theory. Thus, one learning algorithm can account for both word-specific and rule-governed learning, as in Seidenberg and McClelland's (1989) model. However, cross-talk follows a predictable developmental pattern. Initially, associations are formed on a stimulus specific basis at the word level, but after sufficient experience with specific input-output pairs, the correlational structure begins to appear rule-like at the subword level. That is, instead of dual routes, covariance structures emerge at two levels—whole word and subword.

The Covariant Learning Hypothesis explains how word recognition can be learned inductively from experience with words without explicit instruction in orthographic-phonological covariances. In the case of humans learning to read, however, not all children abstract these covariances inductively. Many children benefit from deductive learning in which teachers explicitly draw their attention to these covariances; educators call this metacognitive awareness of these covariances "rules." Thus, although the computational network may not use rules, it does *not* follow that explicit instruction about these covariances in the form of "rules" plays no role in learning to read (see Foorman, Francis, Novy, & Liberman, 1991). Thus, if Carr and Polatsek's (1985) distinction between word-specific and rule-governed learning is modified to a distinction between word-specific and subword orthographic-phonological covariances, their conclusions seem consistent with the Covariant Learning Hypothesis. There is one computational network from which two levels of orthographic-phonological mappings emerge—whole word and subword—and these mappings can be abstracted inductively, as in the case of computer simulations and early, natural readers, or learned deductively through explicit "rules" that bring to metacognitive awareness orthographic-phonological covariances.

Connectionist models have two limitations for explaining how children learn to read. First, connectionist architectures require far more learning trials than does human learning; for example, 50,000 trials may be required to reach 95% accuracy in oral reading of text. Hybrid models that combine symbolic learning with connectionist input-output pairings hold promise for handling learning from instruction in fewer learning trials. (See Schneider & Graham, 1992, for discussion of these issues.) Second, current connectionist models cannot explain individual differences in how children learn to read. Although developmental dyslexia is being modeled, dyslexia is not a homogeneous disorder. Not only do children with reading disabilities show heterogeneity but also normally developing readers show normal variation in the reading acquisition process (Berninger, 1994).

Multiple Connections Model. Like connectionist models, this model assumes that connections among neural networks are fundamental to brain organization. However, the purpose of the model is not to make explicit, testable predictions about computational processes. Rather, the purpose of the model is theory-based diagnosis and remediation of reading or spelling disabilities. When children have problems in word recognition, clinicians and teachers cannot directly alter the hidden units that compute orthographic-phonological covariances; but they can assess whether children may have problems in coding orthographic or phonological information at a particular unit size and they can design instructional activities to facilitate forming connections between corresponding orthographic and phonological codes of a certain unit size and abstracting their covariances. That is, the model was explicitly designed to measure and deal with individual differences in the reading acquisition process (see Berninger, Chen, & Abbott, 1988) and to link assessment and educational intervention (see Berninger & Traweek, 1991).

If we were to investigate computational issues within the context of the Multiple Connections Model, we would focus on the timing mechanism for the coding operations and for the coordination of code-connections (see Berninger, 1989). A growing body of evidence shows that dyslexics have temporal deficits in the transient visual system (Lovegrove, 1993, Lovegrove & Williams, 1993), the auditory processing system (Tallal, 1980), motor coordination (Wolff, Cohen, & Drake, 1984), and naming speed (Bowers & Swanson, 1991; Wolf & Goodglass, 1986; also Bowers et al., chapter 5, and Wolf et al., chapter 4).

Currently we are making a transition from investigating the Multiple Connections Model within an assessment framework to a treatment framework (Berninger & Abbott, 1994). Bronfenbrenner (1979) argued that to show that one really understands a process one must be able to demonstrate that one can change that process in predictable ways. Our treatment studies in progress are therefore comparing growth curves when treatment focuses on a discrete orthographic-phonological connection compared to multiple orthographic-phonological connections. Results of a recent study (Hart, Berninger, & Abbott, in preparation) are consistent with the hypothesis that training multiple code connections results in faster learning over time than does training in one code connection (letter-phoneme) coupled with prior and concurrent training in phonological and orthographic awareness. Results of another study (Traweek, Cartwright, & Berninger, 1994) showed that instructional program affects which code connections form; both whole word and subword code connections tended to be functional in an integrated reading-writing program whereas only subword connections tended to be functional in a direct phonics instructional program.

4.1 Conclusions

The Multiple Connections Model grew out of an attempt to solve a practical problem—assessing individual differences in orthographic and phonological skills to prevent and remediate reading disabilities. Theory was derived from an integration of information in diverse literatures, including linguistics, cognitive psychology, neuropsychology, and education, and clinical observation. Theory also guided the basic research conducted to validate the theoretical model. Thus the relationship between theory and practice was bidirectional, with practice informing theory and theory informing practice. As researchers continue to investigate the role of orthographic processes in literacy we hope that links between basic research and applied practice will be strengthened.

Acknowledgements

Preparation of this chapter and much of the research described was supported by grant No. 25858-04 from the National Institute of Child Health and Human Development. The authors thank Ana Cartwright for her assistance in analyzing the spelling errors on the dictated spelling tests and compositions.

REFERENCES

Abbott, R., & Berninger, V. (1993). Structural equation modeling of relationships among developmental skills and writing skills in primary and intermediate grade students. *Journal of Educational Psychology, 85(3)*, 478-508.

Baron, J. (1979). Orthographic and word-specific mechanisms in children's reading of words. *Child Development, 50*, 60-72.

Barron, R. (1986). Word recognition in early reading: A review of the direct and indirect access hypotheses. *Cognition, 24*, 93-119.

Barron, R. (1994). The sound-to-spelling connection: Orthographic-activation in auditory word recognition and its implications for the acquisition of phonological awareness and literary skills. In V. Berninger (Ed.), *The varieties of orthographic knowledge I: Theoretical and developmental issues* (pp. 219-242). Dordrecht, The Netherlands: Kluwer Academic Publishers.

Berninger, V. (1985). Preliminary findings of year-long longitudinal study of normal variation in learning to read. *Perceptual and Motor Skills, 60*, 665-666.

Berninger, V. (1986). Normal variation in reading acquisition. *Perceptual and Motor Skills, 62*, 691-716.

Berninger, V. (1987). Global, component, and serial processing of printed words in beginning reading. *Journal of Experimental Child Psychology, 43*, 387-418.

Berninger, V. (1989). Orchestration of multiple codes in developing readers: An alternative model of lexical access. *International Journal of Neuroscience, 48*, 85-104.

Berninger, V. (1994). *Reading and writing acquisition. A developmental neuropsychological perspective.* Dubuque, Iowa: Brown & Benchmark.

Berninger, V. (in press). Codes, connections, context, and constructive processes: Integrating the Vygotskian and Lurian perspectives. In E. Assink (Ed.), *Literacy acquisition and social context*. Hertfordshire, United Kingdom: Harvester Wheatsheaf.

Berninger, V., & Abbott, R. (1994). Redefining learning disabilities: Moving beyond IQ-achievement discrepancies to failure to respond to validated treatment protocols. In G.R. Lyon (Ed.), *Frames of references for the assessment of learning disabilities: New views on measurement issues* (pp. 163-183). Baltimore, MD: Paul H. Brookes.

Berninger, V., Abbott, R., Whitaker, D., & Sylvester, L. (in preparation). Integrating explicit instruction in low-level skills and process instruction in high-level skills in treatment protocols for writing disabled children. To appear in *Learning Disabilities Quarterly*.

Berninger, V., & Alsdorf, B. (1989). Are there errors in error analysis? *Journal of Psychoeducational Assessment, 7*, 209-222.

Berninger, V., Cartwright, A., Yates, C., Swanson, H.L., & Abbott, R. (in press). Developmental skills related to writing and reading acquisition in the intermediate grades: Shared and unique functional systems. *Reading and Writing: An Interdisciplinary Journal.*

Berninger, V., Chen, A., & Abbott, R. (1988). A test of the multiple connections model of reading acquisition. *International Journal of Neuroscience, 42,* 283-295.

Berninger, V., & Hart, T. (1992). A developmental neuropsychological perspective for reading and writing acquisition. *Educational Psychologist, 27,* 415-434.

Berninger, V., Hart, T., Abbott, R., & Karovsky, P. (1992). Defining reading and writing disabilities with and without IQ: A flexible developmental perspective. *Learning Disability Quarterly, 15,* 103-118.

Berninger, V., Lester, K., Sohlberg, M., & Mateer, C. (1991). Intervention based on the multiple connections model for developmental dyslexia and acquired deep dyslexia. *Archives of Clinical Neuropsychology, 6,* 375-391.

Berninger, V., Proctor, A., DeBruyn, I., & Smith, R. (1988). Relationship between levels of oral and written language in beginning readers. *Journal of School Psychology, 26,* 341-357.

Berninger, V., Thalberg, S., DeBruyn, I., & Smith, R. (1987). Preventing reading disabilities by assessing and remediating phonemic skills. *School Psychology Review, 16,* 554-565.

Berninger, V., & Traweek, D. (1991). Effects of two-phase intervention on three orthographic-phonological code connections. *Learning and Individual Differences, 3,* 323-338.

Berninger, V., Yates, C., & Lester, K. (1991). Multiple orthographic codes in reading and writing acquisition. *Reading and Writing: An Interdisciplinary Journal, 3,* 115-149.

Besner, D., Twilley, L., McCann, R., & Seergobin, K. (1990). On the association between connectionism and data: Are a few words necessary? *Psychological Review, 97,* 432-446.

Blachman, B.A. (1984). Relationship of rapid naming ability and language analysis skills to kindergarten and first-grade reading achievement. *Journal of Educational Psychology, 76,* 610-622.

Bowers, P., Golden, J., Kennedy, A., & Young, A. (1994). Limits upon orthographic knowledge due to processes indexed by naming speed. In V. Berninger (Ed.), *The varieties of orthographic knowledge I: Theoretical and developmental issues* (pp. 173-218). Dordrecht, The Netherlands: Kluwer Academic Publishers.

Bowers, P., & Swanson, L. (1991). Naming speed deficits in reading disability: Multiple measures of a singular process. *Journal of Experimental Child Psychology, 51,* 195-219.

Bronfenbrenner, U. (1979). *The ecology of human development.* Cambridge, MA: Harvard University Press.

Carr, T., & Pollatsek, A. (1985). Recognizing printed words: A look at current models. In *Reading research: Advances in theory and practice,* Vol. 5 (pp. 1-82). New York: Academic Press.

Chase, C., & Tallal, P. (1991). Cognitive models of developmental reading disorders. In J. Obrzut & G. Hynd (Eds.), *Neuropsychological Foundations of Learning Disabilities* (pp. 199-240). New York: Academic Press.

Coltheart, M. (1978). Lexical access in simple reading tasks. In G. Underwood (Ed.), *Strategies of information processing* (pp. 151-216). London: Academic Press.

Decker, S., & DeFries, J. (1981). Cognitive ability profiles in families of reading-disabled children. *Developmental Medicine and Child Neurology, 23,* 217-227.

Deese, J. (1992). Foreword. In S. Templeton & D. Bear (Eds.), *Development of orthographic knowledge and the foundations of literacy* (p. ix). Hillsdale, NJ: Lawrence Erlbaum Associates.

Doctor, E.A., & Coltheart, M. (1980). Children's use of phonological encoding when reading for meaning. *Memory & Cognition, 8,* 195-209.

Ehri, L.C. (1992). Reconceptualizing the development of sight word reading and its relationship to recoding. In P.B. Gough, L.C. Ehri, & R. Treiman (Eds.), *Reading acquisition* (pp. 107-143). Hillsdale, NJ: Lawrence Erlbaum Associates.

Felton, R., & Brown, I. (1990). Phonological processes as predictors of specific reading skills in children at risk for reading failure. *Reading and Writing. An Interdisciplinary Journal, 2,* 39-59.

Foorman, B., Francis, D., Novy, D., & Liberman, D. (1991). How letter-sound instruction mediates progress in first-grade reading and spelling. *Journal of Educational Psychology, 83,* 456-469.

Foss, D., & Blank, M. (1980). Identifying the speech codes. *Cognitive Psychology, 12,* 1-31.

Gardner, M. (1979). *Expressive one-word picture vocabulary test.* Novato, CA: Academic Therapy Publications.

Garner, W.R. (1974). *The processing of information and structure.* Potomac, MD: Erlbaum.

Glushko, R. (1979). The organization and activation of orthographic knowledge in reading aloud. *Journal of Experimental Psychology: Human Perception and Performance, 5,* 674-691.

Goswami, U. (1988). Orthographic analogies and reading development. *Quarterly Journal of Experimental Psychology, 40A,* 239-268.

Hart, T., Berninger, V., & Abbott, R. (in preparation). Comparison of combined phonemic and phonics training with combined sight word, phonics, and word family training on reading and spelling growth.

Humphreys, G., & Evett, L. (1985). Are there independent lexical and nonlexical routes in word processing? An evaluation of the dual-route theory of reading. *The Behavioral and Brain Sciences, 8,* 689-740.

Jackson, N., Lu, W-H., & Ju, D. (1994). Reading Chinese and reading English: Similarities, differences, and second language learning. In V. Berninger (Ed.), *The varieties of orthographic knowledge I: Theoretical and developmental issues* (pp. 73-109). Dordrecht, The Netherlands: Kluwer Academic Publishers.

Jastak, S., & Wilkinson, G. (1984). *Wide Range Achievement Test-Revised.* Wilmington, DE: Jastak Associates.

Johnson, N. (1978). Coding processes in memory. In W.K. Estes (Ed.), *Handbook of learning and cognitive processes* (Vol. 6, pp. 87-129). Hillsdale, NJ: Erlbaum.

Johnson, N. (1979). The role of letters in word identification: A test of the pattern-unit model. *Memory & Cognition, 7,* 496-504.

Johnson, N. (1986). On looking at letters within words: Do we "see" them in memory? *Journal of Memory and Language, 25,* 558-570.

Kuhn, T. (1970). *The structure of scientific revolutions.* Chicago: The University of Chicago Press.

Liberman, I., Shankweiler, D., Fischer, F., & Carter, B. (1974). Explicit syllable and phoneme segmentation in the young child. *Journal of Experimental Child Psychology, 18,* 201-212.

Lovegrove, W. (1993). Weakness in the transient visual system: A causal factor in dyslexia? In P. Tallal, A. Galaburda, R. Llinas, & C. von Euler (Eds.), *Temporal information processing in the nervous system: Special reference to dyslexia and dysphasia* (pp. 57-69). New York: New York Academy of Sciences.

Lovegrove, W., & Williams, M. (1993). *Visual processes in reading and reading disabilities*. Hillsdale: NJ: Lawrence Erlbaum.

Marcel, T. (1980). Surface dyslexia and beginning reading: A revised hypothesis of the pronunciation of print and its impairments. In M. Coltheart, K. Patterson, & J. Marshall (Eds.), *Deep dyslexia* (pp. 227-258). London: Routledge & Kegan Paul.

McCarthy, R., & Warrington, E. (1990). *Cognitive neuropsychology. A clinical introduction*. New York: Academic Press.

Morton, J., & Patterson, K. (1980). A new attempt at an interpretation, or, an attempt at a new interpretation. In M. Coltheart, K. Patterson, & J. Marshall (Eds.), *Deep dyslexia*, (pp. 91-118). London: Routledge & Kegan Paul.

Olson, R., Forsberg, H., & Wise, B. (1994). Genes, environment, and the development of orthographic skills. In V. Berninger (Ed.), *The varieties of orthographic knowledge I: Theoretical and developmental issues* (pp. 27-71). Dordrecht, The Netherlands: Kluwer Academic Publishers.

Olson, R.K., Kliegl, R., Davidson, B., & Foltz, G. (1985). Individual and development differences in reading disability. In G.E. MacKinnon & T.G. Waller (Eds.), *Reading research: Advances in theory and practice* (Vol. 4, pp. 1-64). New York: Academic Press.

Posner, M., Peterson, S., Fox, P., & Reichle, M. (1988). Localization of cognitive operations in the human brain. *Science, 240*, 1627-1631.

Rosner, J. (1979). *Helping children overcome learning disabilities*, 2nd ed. New York: Walker.

Schneider, W., & Graham, D. (1992). Introduction to connectionist modeling in education. *Educational Psychologist, 27*, 513-530.

Seidenberg, M., & McClelland, J. (1989). A distributed, developmental model of word recognition and naming. *Psychological Review, 96*, 523-568.

Seidenberg, M., Waters, G., Sanders, W., & Lagner, P. (1984). Pre- and postlexical foci of contextual effects on word recognition. *Memory & Cognition, 12,* 315-328.

Shallice, T., & Warrington, E. (1980). Single and multiple component central dyslexic syndromes. In M. Coltheart, K. Patterson, & J. Marshall (Eds.), *Deep dyslexia* (pp. 119-145). London: Routledge & Kegan Paul.

Shallice, T., Warrington, E., & McCarthy, R. (1983). Reading without semantics. *Quarterly Journal of Experimental Psychology, 35A,* 111-138.

Stanovich, K.E., West, R.F., & Cunningham, A.E. (1991). Beyond phonological processes: Print-exposure and orthographic processing. In S. Brady & D. Shankweiler (Eds.), *Phonological processes in literacy,* pp. 219-235. Hillsdale, NJ: Erlbaum.

Stevens, J. (1986). *Applied multivariate statistics for the sciences.* Hillsdale, NJ: Erlbaum.

Studdert-Kennedy, M. (1974). The perception of speech. In T. Sebeok (Ed.), *Current trends in linguistics* (Vol. 12, pp. 2349-2385). The Hague: Mouton.

Tallal, P. (1980). Auditory temporal perception phonics and reading disabilities in children. *Brain and Language, 9,* 182-198.

Tanenhaus, M., Flanigan, H., & Seidenberg, M. (1980). Orthographic and phonological activation in auditory and visual word recognition. *Memory & Cognition, 8,* 513-520.

Taylor, I. (1981). Writing systems and reading. In *Reading research: Advances in theory and practice* (Vol. 2, pp. 1-51). New York: Academic Press.

Traweek, D., Cartwright, A., & Berninger, V. (1994). *Relationships between learner characteristics and instructional programs in learning to read and write: Implications for assessment and intervention.* Submitted.

Treiman, R. (1988). The internal structure of the syllable. In G. Carlson & M. Tanenhaus (Eds.), *Linguistic structure in language processing* (pp. 27-52). Dordrecht, Holland: Kluwer.

Van Orden, G. (1987). A ROWS is a ROSE: Spelling, sound, and reading. *Memory & Cognition, 15,* 181-198.

Van Orden, G., Pennington, B., & Stone, G. (1990). Word identification in reading and the promise of subsymbolic psycholinguistics. *Psychological Review, 97,* 1-35.

Vellutino, F., & Scanlon, D.C. (1987). Phonological coding, phonological awareness, and reading ability: Evidence from a longitudinal and experimental study. *Merrill-Palmer Quarterly, 33,* 321-363.

Vellutino, F., Scanlon, D., & Tanzman. M. (1994). Components of reading ability: Issues and problems in operationalizing word identification, phonological coding, and orthographic coding. In G.R. Lyon (Ed.), *Frames of reference for the assessment of learning disabilities: New views on measurement issues* (pp. 279-332). Baltimore, MD: Paul Brookes Publishing.

Wagner, R., & Barker, T. (1994). The development of orthographic processing ability. In V. Berninger (Ed.), *The varieties of orthographic knowledge I: Theoretical and developmental issues* (pp. 243-276). Dordrecht, The Netherlands: Kluwer Academic Publishers.

Wechsler, D. (1974). *Wechsler Intelligence Scale-Revised.* New York: Psychological Corporation.

Willows, D., Kruk, R., & Corcos, E. (1993). *Visual processes in reading and reading disabilities.* Hillsdale, NJ: Lawrence Erlbaum.

Wolf, M. (1984). Naming, reading, and the dyslexias: A longitudinal overview. *Annals of Dyslexia, 34,* 87-115.

Wolf, M., & Goodglass, H. (1986). Dyslexia, dysnomia, and lexical retrieval: A longitudinal investigation. *Brain and Language, 28,* 154-168.

Wolf, M., Pfeil, C., Lotz, R., & Biddle, K. (1994). Towards a more universal understanding of the developmental dyslexias: The contribution of orthographic factors. In V. Berninger (Ed.), *The varieties of orthographic knowledge I: Theoretical and developmental issues* (pp. 137-171). Dordrecht, The Netherlands: Kluwer Academic Publishers.

Wolff, P.H., Cohen, C., & Drake, C. (1984). Impaired motor timing control in specific reading retardation. *Neuropsychologia, 22,* 587-600.

Woodcock, R. (1987). *Woodcock Reading Mastery Test-Revised.* Circle Pines, MN: American Guidance Service.

Address correspondence to:

Virginia W. Berninger
University of Washington
Miller Hall DQ-12
Seattle, WA 98195
U.S.A.

BARBARA R. FOORMAN

PHONOLOGICAL AND ORTHOGRAPHIC PROCESSING: SEPARATE BUT EQUAL?

INTRODUCTION

The title of this volume is *The varieties of orthographic knowledge I: Theoretical and developmental issues*. The authors have met this charge so well that the reader may be overwhelmed by the varieties of orthographic knowledge and despairing of any hope for consensus. Yet there are at least three points of consensus among the authors. First, in studying reading, phonological processing skill has been over-emphasized at the expense of orthographic processing skill. Second, orthographic processing can be operationalized and assessed separately from phonological processing. Third, although orthographic and phonological processing can be dissociated statistically, they are conceptually intertwined.

In spite of these areas of consensus, questions of construct validity remain. If an orthography is defined as a system for writing a language, then orthographic skill is how good a person is at producing (i.e., encoding) and comprehending (i.e., decoding or, more appropriately, deciphering) written characters or scripts. Only in extreme cases is it plausible to think of one's skill in writing characters as separable from one's skill in pronouncing characters. One such case is the congenitally deaf person who manages to become a fluent reader. Another case is the reader of Japanese characters (*kanji*) who knows the meaning of a character but does not know the Japanese or Chinese pronunciation. Yet in most speaker/hearers of a language, deciphering script is a matter of associating written units with sound, perhaps only to aid in remembering the gist. Thus, when reading Dostoevski, I assign private sound values to the hopelessly long and unpronounceable Russian names. I know I'm wrong in these sound values, but I need a place marker in the verbal narrative I create in order to retell the story later, perhaps only to myself. In contrast, when my third grade daughter reads an unfamiliar

V.W. Berninger (ed.), The varieties of orthographic knowledge I: Theretical and developmental issues, 321-357.

word, she "sounds it out" as a way to index its meaning. For her, "sounding out" or phonological encoding (unfortunately referred to as phonological decoding in the literature) is primarily a strategy to *gain* meaning. For me, phonological encoding is primarily a strategy to *maintain* meaning. In both cases, orthography has activated phonology, in the one case, prelexically, and, in the other case, postlexically. Believers in the dual routes of (1) phonological decoding—an indirect route governed by grapheme-phoneme correspondences—and (2) direct "visual" access of orthography see these two routes as distinct, both in terms of their conceptual mechanisms and their functional brain architectures. This tradition of separate routes has spawned different tests for assessing phonological processing and for assessing orthographic processing. Justification for this tradition of separate but equal is provided by: a) statistical analyses revealing unique contributions to variation in word recognition for each type of processing; b) unique patterns of reading deficits in the acquired dyslexias and, perhaps, in the developmental dyslexias; and 3) variable emphases in the orthographies of the world on each route.

In the remarks to follow I will discuss how the authors of this volume address these issues. I will first review the research on reading and spelling German, Dutch, and Chinese presented in this volume to assess universal claims of separate processing routes. Then I will summarize how the constructs of phonological and orthographic processing are typically operationalized and comment on the individual differences in orthographic and phonological processing that the authors in this volume have presented. Finally, I will return to the assumption of dual routes that underlies so much of the research in this area but which is increasingly seen as problematic by the authors in this volume. I will speak in favor of a connectionist architecture and of the promise of connectionist models for capturing the mechanism by which orthographic patterns are recognized as words.

PROCESSING ORTHOGRAPHIES OTHER THAN ENGLISH

This book has been written in English—or, more appropriately, in Latin script. Latin script is just one of the 29 writing systems of the world currently used in major newspapers (Nakanishi, 1980). However, Latin script is used by the majority of countries of the world, countries influenced by Christianity:

Countries in North and South America and the majority of countries in Africa, Europe, and Oceania. Arabic script is used by Moslem countries: countries of northern Africa, the Middle East, Afghanistan, and Malaysia. Cyrillic script is used by countries influenced by the Greek Orthodox religion: Russia and Balkin countries. In addition to Japanese, Korean, and Southeast Asian scripts, there are 15 official scripts recognized in India. Finally—or shall I say, firstly—there are Chinese characters. Approximately one in five people in the world is Chinese. Therefore, to relegate mention of Chinese characters to last seems short-sighted.

Ten years ago I hosted a conference, later a book, entitled *Acquisition of reading skills: Cultural constraints and cognitive universals* (Foorman & Siegel, 1986). I was particularly interested in the universality of Bradley and Bryant's (1983, 1985) claim of phonological awareness—specifically rhyme and alliteration skills—as the causal factor in learning to read. As a student and researcher of the Japanese language (Foorman & Kinoshita, 1983), I was struck by the fact that ubiquitious homophony made meter, not rhyme, the primary poetic device in the Japanese language. And yet literacy rates in Japan are among the highest in the world. I was also struck by the rhyming skills of members of nonliterate cultures and members of literate cultures with marginal literacy skills (e.g., Roazzi, Dowker, & Bryant, 1993; Labov, 1972; Morais, 1988). In short, the role of phonology in learning to read had to be contextualized within characteristics of the writing system and of the spoken language, as well as within the opportunity to, and value of, becoming literate. Consequently, contributions to my conference and book by Hatano (1986) on the Japanese orthographies (Chinese characters and hiragana and katakana syllabaries) and by Lee, Stigler, and Stevenson (1986) on Chinese characters were particularly helpful.

In the current volume, the contributions of Jackson, Lu, and Lu on Chinese, Wolf, Pfeil, Lotz, and Biddle on German, and Assink and Kattenberg on Dutch highlight trade-offs between orthography and phonology. In German the relation between sounds in the spoken language and alphabetic letters is close to one-to-one, although not nearly as close as in Finnish, Hungarian, Serbo-Croatian, Spanish, and Italian. These are referred to as "shallow" orthographies because the sound-symbol correspondence is so close, in contrast to the opaque correspondence of a "deep" orthography like English.

According to Wolf et al. (chapter 4), German children are relatively good at decoding and phonemic segmentaion compared to English readers. In fact, the hallmark of dyslexia in English (Rack, Snowling, & Olson, 1992)—poor nonword decoding—is not a good indicator in German. Wolf et al. (chapter 4) found no difference in nonword reading between severely impaired German readers and average readers. Instead, the differences lay in speed of lexical access as measured by rapid naming tasks. Thus, by studying readers of a more "shallow" orthography such as German, where poor reading is not a consequence of inability to decode, Wolf et al. (chapter 4) cast doubt on implicit universal claims about phonological core deficits of dyslexia. They also argue for a deficit in the precise, rapid access and retrieval of visually presented linguistic information.

Jackson et al.'s (chapter 2) chapter goes a long way toward straightening out misconceptions regarding the Chinese orthography. The major misconception is that Chinese characters are pictorial logographs, devoid of phonological attributes. Pictorial logographs are word-like pictures. In contrast, Chinese characters are morphosyllabic, that is, meaningful syllables. The spoken language consists of about 400 syllables, with pitch contour playing a major role in determining meaning. The characters consist of strokes written in a fixed order and organized into semantic radicals and phonetic radicals. It is possible to construct pseudo-characters because of the customary positions of the semantic-phonetic compound. Interestingly, Sacks (1989) reports that born deaf Chinese are better at copying pseudo-characters than hearing Chinese, presumably because the hearing Chinese are distracted by phonological processing and deaf Chinese are more adept at depicting graphic forms. In a similar vein, Jackson et al. (chapter 2) point out that reading Chinese characters is primarily a left hemisphere function because dyslexia is likely to include parietal-occipital cortex lesions.

In studies of adult readers of Chinese, Jackson et al. (chapter 2) found that character recognition is determined by frequency of usage (which is inversely associated with the number of strokes) and by degree to which pronunciation is predicted from the phonetic radical. Jackson et al. (chapter 2) point out that priming and backward masking studies indicate that phonological information is available relatively early in the identification of characters. Also, the "tongue-twister" effect showing that phonological representations are automatically activated and used in reading English text is also apparent when native speakers of Mandarin read stories written in Chinese (Zhang & Perfetti, 1993). Additionally, in alphabetic orthographies the meaning and role of *word* is central. Researchers speak of the "word superiority effect" in eye movement studies (see Rayner & Pollatsek, 1989, for a review), and text comprehension is affected by word-level predictors. However, in Chinese, once there is more than a single character presented, the role and meaning of *word* is less clear cut. Readers of Chinese seem to pause at physical or syntactic boundaries rather than at word-level boundaries.

By way of summary, let me requote Jackson et al.'s (chapter 2) quote of Perfetti, Zhang, and Berent's (1992) listing of principles guiding recent research.

> (1) 'across writing systems, encounters with most printed words...automatically lead to phonological activation, beginning with phoneme constituents of the word and including the word's pronunciation;' (2) 'writing systems constrain the extent to which this activation includes sublexical phonology, but not whether activation occurs;'and (3) 'activated phonology serves memory and comprehension, with phonological rehearsal but not activation itself under reader control.' (p. 231)

What we have learned from Chinese is that phonology is activated even in the case of reading a nonalphabetic orthography. What we have learned from German is that in a highly regular orthography where phonological demands are relatively controlled, non-phonological sources of reading disruption can become more apparent. Thus, it is *not* the case that Chinese characters are read via a direct, visual route. Nor is it adequate to ascribe German reading to an indirect, grapheme-phoneme route. A single route of interconnecting orthographic and phonological codes appears to be a more accurate description of the reading process in the world's orthographies. Or, to shift the focus from the orthography to the reader, Jackson et al. (chapter 2) point out that "universal properties of the human mind are more important than specific properties of different orthographies in determining how written language is processed."

Finally, we turn to Assink and Kattenberg's (chapter 3) chapter on Dutch. Dutch, like English, is a deep orthography in terms of the complexity of sound-symbol correspondences. In fact, it is deeper than English in the sense that spelling preserves syntax as well as morphology. So, in English we often preserve the morphological structure of words when we spell (e.g., *courage-courageous*). In Dutch, grammatical functions absent in the spoken language are preserved as well (e.g., *wig wachten/wachtten* for *we wait/waited*). Consequently, the Dutch spelling system is difficult for novices to learn. Assink and Kattenberg (chapter 3) distinguish knowledge of word images from knowledge of spelling. The former refers to implicit knowledge of orthographic structure that enables one to detect and reject system-illegal orthographic options, regardless of context (e.g., *bcat* for *boat* is system illegal, whereas *boap* is not). In contrast, spelling knowledge requires explicit command of orthographic rules. I shall return to a discussion of the role of explicit, or conscious, rule learning in orthographic processing in the final section on connectionism. But first let us consider how the constructs of phonological and orthographic processing are operationalized in studies of reading English.

MEASURING PHONOLOGICAL AND ORTHOGRAPHIC PROCESSING

Phonological Processing

Phonological processing belongs to a well mapped domain, thanks to the more than two decades of pioneering research from the Haskins Laboratory (see Brady & Shankweiler, 1990, for a review). The causal links between phonological processing skill and learning to read and spell are well established (see Adams, 1990; Goswami & Bryant, 1990; Wagner & Torgesen, 1987; and Vellutino, 1991). This link is generally assumed to be bi-directional, that is, that phonological skill promotes success in reading and spelling and, in turn, success in reading and spelling promotes phonological skill (Foorman & Francis, 1994; Stanovich, 1986; Wagner, Torgesen, & Rashotte, 1994). However, Bryant and his colleagues have a strong argument that it is the preliterate skill in rhyming gained through nursery rhymes that promotes learning to read and spell (MacLean, Bryant, & Bradley, 1987).

The construct of phonological processing is typically operationalized in terms of phonological awareness measures of rhyming, synthesis, and analysis tests, as well as in terms of phonological memory, phonological decoding, and rapid naming tests. The memory tasks address phonological coding in short-term memory by asking the subject to repeat nonwords or strings of digits of varying length. Note that here the emphasis is on short-term rather than working memory. Wagner and Barker (chapter 7, p. 1) say that "*phonological coding in working memory* refers to the ability to use phonological information or codes to represent speech-based information for short-term storage." Because these tasks demand only brief storage, it is more appropriate to refer to them as short-term memory tasks and to reserve the name working memory for tasks that assess the efficiency with which the products of operations are stored for subsequent use. An example of a working memory measure is Case's (1985) counting span test where subjects are asked to count outloud a set of objects and to recall the number of objects in each set after it is removed. Then the number of sets of objects they are asked to count increases until the point is reached where they can no longer keep track of all the totals. The point I want to emphasize is that working memory tasks tap executive functions that demand much more than the brief memory for speech-based information entailed by the construct of phonological processing.

Phonological decoding measures are nonword reading tests. Nonwords are pronounceable letter strings used to guarantee an emphasis on phonological rather than orthographic processing. Olson, Forsberg, and Wise (chapter 1) use both oral and silent nonword reading tests. In the oral version, nonwords are presented one at a time on a computer and response latencies are measured with a voice key. In the silent version, three nonwords are presented on the computer screen (e.g., *coam-baim-goam; dysical-fotograph-barmacy*). The subjects push one of three buttons as quickly as possible to indicate which nonwords sounds like a real word if read aloud.

Rapid Automatized Naming (R.A.N.) tests consist of a simultaneous presentation of stimuli that are to be named sequentially as quickly as possible. Wolf, Bally, and Morris (1986) added an object task to the original Denckla and Rudel (1974, 1976) tests for color, letters, and numbers. These *serial naming* tests stand in contrast to *discrete naming* tests where stimuli are presented in isolation and naming latencies are measured. Both serial and discrete naming tests differentiate good from poor or dyslexic readers and contribute variance to word recognition beyond that accounted for by other phonological processing measures. However, according to

Wolf et al. (chapter 4, p. 5), "the deficit appears differentially more powerful in serial vs. discrete (or isolated) presentation." Wolf et al. (chapter 4) and Bowers, Golden, Kennedy, and Young (chapter 5) regard dyslexia as a deficit in the precise, rapid access and retrieval of visually presented linguistic information. Thus, in addition to deficits in phonological processing, Wolf et al. (chapter 4) and Bowers et al. (chapter 5) argue that dyslexia is also caused by core deficits in naming speed. They refer to this as the "double-deficit hypothesis."

Rhyming, analysis, and synthesis tests are often referred to as phonological awareness tasks. These tasks typically include the following:

1. Rhyme production
2. Detection of rhyme and alliteration, where the odd word in a series of words is to be identified (e.g., "slam,""jam,""ram,""gun;""best,""sand,"" bake,""bear").
3. Blending of syllables and phonemes (e.g., "cow-boy" to "cowboy;""c-at" to "cat;""c-a-t" to "cat").
4. Segmenting words into syllables and phonemes ("cowboy" to "cow-boy;""cat" to "c-a-t").
5. Segmentation plus transposition of syllables or phonemes (e.g., reversing "bat" to "tab" either verbally or by manipulating colored blocks or Pig Latin instructions to delete the initial sound of a word such as "hope" and add /ay/ to yield "ope-hay").

Factor analytic studies of these measures tend to support a single phonological processing measure consisting of tasks involving blending, segmenting, and transpositions, with rhyme tasks loading on a separate factor (Stanovich, Cunningham, & Cramer, 1984; Yopp, 1988). Typically, kindergarteners can do only rhyme tasks, first and second graders also can do the blending and analysis tasks, and third graders and above can do the transposition tasks in addition to the other tasks. This décalage appears to be due to cognitive and reading development. In other words, between the ages of 5 and 7 there is a developmental shift toward increasing reflectivity on the child's part and an instructional shift toward more formal reading activities on the teacher's part. A transposition task like Pig Latin requires memory of the instructions, memory of the target word—often in the form of an "orthographic image"—and mental space for the operations of deleting the initial sound and adding /ay/ to the end of the word.

In contrast to a transposition task, a segmentation task like that developed by Bruce (1964) or Rosner and Simon (1971) is less demanding of cognitive and reading development than one might think. A sample item of Rosner and Simon's (1971) *Test of Auditory Analysis Skills (TAAS)* is "Say *carpet*, now say it again without *car*" (*pet*). Other items are the following, with the sound to be deleted noted parenthetically: *bel(t)* and *ti(me); (l)end* and *(s)mile; cr(e)ate* and *cont(in)ent*. Rosner and Simon found that 5 and 6 year olds were better at deleting final sounds than initial sounds (see also Content, Kolinsky, Morais, & Bertelson, 1986), and that deletion of medial sounds was difficult even for 10 and 11 year olds, a finding confirmed by Bruce (1964).

My colleagues and I (Foorman, Jenkins, & Francis, 1993) empirically tested the relation between reading and spelling knowledge, on the one hand, and phonological processing on the other, by examining on a word by word, child by child basis first and second graders' ability to segment, read, and spell 50 words. A multivariate analysis of variance was conducted on difference scores among segmentation, reading, and spelling. Generally, differences favored segmentation and were maximized when final sounds were deleted and minimized when medial sounds were deleted. In other words, children could delete final sounds of words they could neither read nor spell. However, deletion of medial sounds appeared contingent on being able to read and spell the word. In addition, graphical analyses showed a greater probability of correct reading and spelling given correct segmentation than incorrect segmentation. In sum, segmentation of beginning and ending sounds appeared to be a prerequisite to learning to read and spell.

It is informative that when these first and second graders made errors in deleting the initial or second consonant in a blend, they tended to produce the rime of the word. For example, when asked to say "crib" without the /k/, they tended to say "ib." When asked to say "swing" without the /w/, they tended to say "ing." These kinds of errors lend support to Goswami and Bryant's (1990) claim that beginning readers do as well as they do on a segmentation test because they adopt a strategy of dropping either the initial or ending sounds. These units correspond to Treiman's (1985) intrasyllabic divisions of onset and rime, and are for Goswami (1993) the phonological basis for analogizing to new orthographic forms.

In another study of 80 first graders (Foorman, Francis, Novy, & Liberman, 1991) individual growth curve analysis indicated that segmentation scores obtained in October predicted overall performance in reading and spelling on a list of 60 words. Growth in segmentation predicted overall performance in spelling but only predicted end-of-year differences in reading words with regular compared to exceptional spelling patterns. Finally, better reading of regular words in October was associated with faster growth in spelling, and better spelling of regular words in October was predictive of May word reading. Thus, it appears that the ability to segment sounds in the speech stream is predictive of improvement in spelling words to dictation, which, in turn, enables more accurate identification of printed words. The link between segmentation and spelling is logical and has been empirically supported by other research (e.g., Lundberg, Frost, & Petersen, 1988). When children are asked to spell words they cannot read, they must segment the sounds in the word and associate each sound with a letter. As spellings progress through phases of inventedness to conventional, the orthographic representation becomes complete. Hence, it is not surprising that knowledge of a word's spelling facilitates its accurate identification. On the other hand, accurate identification of a printed word may be based on partial orthographic representation and good guessing. Consequently, accuracy of word identification usually exceeds that of spelling.

Another factor affecting these links among phonological processing, spelling, and reading is the method of reading instruction. In our first grade study described above (Foorman et al., 1991), 40 of the children were in three classrooms receiving approximately 45 minutes a day of explicit letter-sound (LS) instruction, and 40 were in classrooms receiving approximately 15 minutes a day of explicit letter-sound instruction. Thus, we called the groups the More-LS and Less-LS classrooms. The More-LS teachers referred to their approach to instruction as phonics. The Less-LS teachers referred to their approach as whole language and justified the 15 minutes of daily LS instruction during spelling as preparation for decoding items on the standardized test given at the end of the year. (In the meantime, the school district has eliminated standardized tests at the end of grade 1 and has integrated spelling into language arts in the form of writing activities.)

Classrooms were comparable in the beginning of the school year on grade equivalencies on a standardized reading test and on raw scores on the *Peabody Picture Vocabulary Test-Revised* (Dunn & Dunn, 1981). They were also similar in diversity of ethnic make-up and socio-economic status. Using a repeated measures approach, we examined classroom differences in segmentation, word reading, and spelling scores in October, February, and May. There were no classroom differences in segmentation. However, classrooms with more letter-sound instruction improved at a faster rate in correct spellings and readings of words with regular and exceptional spelling patterns. The error patterns of both groups' reading and spelling progressed from nonphonetic to phonetic to correct responses. On the reading task the More-LS group progressed through this pattern at a faster rate for both types of words. However, on the spelling task the instructional groups did not differ in the rate of reduction of nonphonetic errors. The Less-LS group progressed to a predominance of phonetic spellings at the end of the year, whereas the More-LS group moved on to a greater proportion of correct spellings. Interestingly, it was in the correct spelling of exception words that the More-LS classrooms's *rate* of progress was significant. Remember that students in the Less-LS classrooms received LS instruction during spelling where for 15 minutes each day they segmented into syllables or onset-rimes the word the teacher presented on a transparency. When the projector was turned off, they wrote the word from memory, and when it was turned on again, they corrected any misspelling. In contrast, spelling instruction in the More-LS classrooms was the more traditional, visually oriented approach of writing and rewriting. This emphasis on writing accurate visual-orthographic representations of words is certainly a plausible explanation for the More-LS classes' impressive gains on spelling words with exceptional spelling patterns (e.g., *comb*) relative to the Less-LS classes.

The lack of group differences in segmentation seems surprising, especially in light of other research supporting the conclusion that children taught by phonics are better at segmenting sounds than children taught by a whole word method (Alegria, Pignot, & Morais, 1982; Baron & Treiman, 1980; Perfetti, Beck, Bell, & Hughes, 1987). However, it is possible that the phonological emphasis of the spelling instruction in the Less-LS classes was sufficient to prevent *group* differences in segmentation. But lack of group differences does not mean there were not individual differences in how LS instruction mediated the links among segmentation and progress in reading and spelling. Using exploratory data techniques, we were able to detect some of these individual differences (Foorman & Francis, 1994). Specifically, we plotted October segmentation scores against estimated growth in segmentation for all children. We selected 4 first graders—2 from each LS group—who were similarly low on the segmentaion test at the beginning of the year. Two of the 4 children had high segmentation growth across the year and 2 had low growth, with one child in each LS group, respectively. As might be expected, the two children with high segmentation growth moved faster through the sequence of nonphonetic error to phonetic error to correct response in reading and spelling compared to the two segmenters with low growth. Additionally, the two More-LS children moved through this sequence faster than the other two children. But, importantly, the low growth segmenter who received More-LS instruction appeared to move through the sequence at a comparable or even slightly faster rate than the high growth segmenter who received Less-LS instruction. Thus, letter-sound instruction appears to ameliorate the rate at which segmentation skill changes during first grade, especially for children with poor development of phonological skills.

The benefits of explicit letter-sound instruction for learning to read, spell, and segment words is echoed by Wolf et al. (chapter 4) in their study of German children in grades 2 and 4, some of whom received explicit letter-sound (LS) instruction and some of whom engaged in "creative writing experiences... through which the child was expected to infer decoding principles" (p. 156). Both groups of children received a rapid automatized naming (R.A.N.) test of objects and a parallel form of words (rapid automatized words; R.A.W.). Good readers were able to automatize their word reading so that by grade 4 the discrepancy between R.A.N. and R.A.W. latencies favored R.A.W. In contrast, poor readers' latencies for word reading (R.A.W.) never dropped below those for object naming (R.A.N.). In addition to these anticipated findings, Wolf et al.

found a difference in discrepancy scores in grade 2 depending on which method of reading instruction the children received. Those receiving the traditional emphasis on structured, phonic rules in the German orthography were significantly faster in word reading relative to object naming compared to the group that was expected to infer decoding principles. However, by grade 4 there were no differences between the instructional groups. But this lack of differences in grade 4 may not reveal differences in comprehension processes fostered by early acceleration in automaticity. In addition, it is important to look at reading level by reading method interactions. In particular, among poor readers in grade 4, one would expect explicit letter-sound instruction to speed automaticity relative to instructional activities where decoding principles had to be inferred.

In summary, phonological processing has been operationalized with measures of phonological memory, rapid naming, rhyme, analysis, and synthesis. To the extent that the input is auditory and the subject does not know how to spell the word to be manipulated, cognitive processing of these measures can be described as phonological. In these cases, the ability to hold speech-based information in memory long enough to recognize and manipulate beginning and ending sounds in words is clearly a prerequisite to successful literacy development. However, as soon as the auditory input evokes a visual-orthographic image in the subject, the processing can no longer be described as purely phonological. To reiterate the conclusion of other researchers (e.g., Juel, Griffith, & Gough, 1986; Tunmer & Nesdale, 1985), efficient phonological processing is a necessary but not sufficient condition for skilled word recognition. Let us turn to one of the other key ingredients in word recognition—orthographic processing.

Orthographic Processing

Typical measures of orthographic processing are:

1. Word-pseudohomophone choice where the subject presses a button as quickly as possible to indicate which member of a pair is the correct orthographic pattern (e.g., *rain rane; sammon salmon*) (Olson, Kliegl, Davidson, & Foltz, 1985).
2. Nonlexical choice where the subject selects the nonword most like an English word (e.g., *filv filk;*

moke moje; vism visn; powl lowp) (Siegel, Geva, & Share, 1993).

3. Orthographic verification where the subject listens to a word ("street") and then confirms if the subsequent word on the screen *(street or streat)* is correct (Manis, Szeszulski, Holt, & Graves, 1990).
4. Homophone choice where the subject responds to a sentence such as "Which is a fruit?"by pressing a button to indicate which member of a pair *(pair pear)* is a fruit (Olson et al., chapter 1; Barker, Torgesen & Wagner, 1992; Stanovich & West, 1989).
5. Homophone verification where the subject listens to a sentence and decides which member of a pair is correct *(week weak)*. The *Peabody Individual Achievement Test* (PIAT; Dunn & Markwardt, 1970) for spelling is similar but has four orthographically and often phonologically similar choices printed on a card (e.g., "cloudy": *clowdy cloady cloudey cloudy).*
6. Detection of letter clusters in words (e.g., brief presentation of *clock,* followed by *cl* or *c o)* (Berninger, Yates, & Lester, 1991).
7. Exception word spelling (e.g., *comb)*

All of these measures demand some degree of phonological processing. However, it is the orthographic processing that determines the accuracy of the response. An exception is the PIAT, where the lack of homophony among the four choices invites additional phonological processing.

As mentioned in the previous section, phonological processing can be thought of as distinct from orthographic processing if the stimulus is auditory and the subject has no knowledge of the word's spelling. However, it is controversial whether orthographic processing can be dissociated from phonological processing. Those that argue for the dissociation emphasize the visual processing demanded by deciphering print. Thus, for example, Carr and Posner (in press) define orthography as "the visual organization of the writing system." According to this view, orthographic processing relies on a visual code based on the redundancy of letter sequences and their positions within words (Corcos & Willows, 1993). Tasks used to assess the quality of this visual code typically ask the subject to look at a pair of stimuli and indicate the one that looks most like a word. Sample items from Leslie and Shannon's (1981) study of preschoolers, kindergarteners, first and second graders include: *GSP G8P*; *WOC RSD*; and *grisp tsacl*. Leslie and Shannon found that accuracy was directly related to reading ability, a finding they argue supports word recognition as a process of extracting visual features. However, an alternate interpretation is that phonological processing, not orthographic processing, mediates accuracy. At least in the cases of *WOC-RSD* and *grisp-tsacl*, pronounceability would seem to play a major role in the decision process. Tasks such as these prompt Vellutino, Scanlon, and Tanzman (1994) to argue that orthographic processing tasks are merely word recognition and spelling tasks. But Wagner and Barker (chapter 7) show that orthographic processing tasks are not merely proxies for decoding and spelling by the fact that they exert a developmental causal effect that is independent of the autoregressive effect of prior decoding ability.

Those who argue for the visual nature of orthographic processing do have one key point. Orthography is a visual stimulus. If there is distortion in the initial sensory input, then subsequent processing will be jeopardized. Such reasoning has led to the recent hypothesis of a deficit in the transient visual system as a cause of dyslexia (Lovegrove, Garcia, & Nicholson, 1990) and to the development of visual processing tasks sensitive to impairments in parallel processing of word-like symbol arrays. For example, Wimmer (1993) presented digits in word-like arrays so briefly that sequential processing was not possible. After presentation and a mask, the child was asked to name one of the digits at a specified position. Wimmer found that performance on this task was not related to naming speed in German-speaking dyslexic children at grades 2, 3, and 4. However, performance on the visual processing tasks was not very different between dyslexics and age-matched controls at grades 2 and 3. There were larger differences at grade 4 but the dyslexics' performance was still better than that of grade 2 controls, "thus leaving open the possibility that the low performance on the visual-processing tasks reflects a consequence, and not a cause, of impaired reading speed" (p. 27).

Bowers et al. (chapter 5) agree with Stanovich (1988) that the group of dyslexics with problems with the "automatic and nonintentional induction of orthographic patterns" (p. 601) is likely to be very small. Although admitting that "a more 'hard-wired' process of orthographic pattern learning is possible" (p. 321), Stanovich (1992) endorses exploring a more "strategic interpretation of the underlying processing problem" (p. 321). He points to the work of Vellutino and Scanlon (1984) and Frith (1985) as suggesting that the deficit in forming orthographic representations may be due to overly global processing with insufficient attention to individual letters or groupings of letters. Insufficient attention to individual letters would seem to lead to incomplete or inaccurate orthographic representations. Thus, as Olson et al. (chapter 1) point out, on tasks demanding precise representations, such as choosing the correct orthographic pattern between *sammon-salmon*, dyslexics do worse than younger normal readers. However, on nonword choice tasks (e.g., *filv filk*), dyslexics are comparable or even superior to younger normals. Olson et al. reason that because this latter task does not require a response to a word, the task may be tapping a more general level of orthographic processing, a level at which dyslexics function within a normal range. Perfetti (1992) argues that imprecise orthographic representations are due to poor underlying phonological representations, an argument based on an integrative view of phonological and orthographic processing. But Olson et al. counter that the near-normal performance of dyslexics when nonword targets and foils are presented simultaneously supports a more separatist view of orthographic and phonological processing.

Orthographic processing as a distinct construct, dissociable from phonological processing, has received recent support from studies of brain imaging. Carr and Posner (in press) point out that studies utilizing Positron Emission Tomography (PET) with adult readers of English support two anatomically localized structures. One structure, that they call the Prestriate Visual Word Form System (Prestriate VWFS), is an orthographic encoding mechanism that resides in the left-medial prestriate visual cortex. The Prestriate VWFS serves as a primary gateway for connecting the visual system with the second structure, the language system. Carr and Posner (in press) argue for two pathways that transmit orthographic codes from the Prestriate VWFS to the linguistic system.

> One is an inferior pathway toward temporal cortex that treats written words as visual objects. The other is a more superior pathway toward temporoparietal cortex that gives orthographic codes access to phonological analysis. The two pathways appear to differ in biological preparedness, with substantially greater heritability of individual differences in the temporoparietal phonological analysis pathway than in the temporal object recognition pathway. (p. 35)

Olson et al.'s (chapter 1) recent behavior-genetic analyses with a larger sample of twins than the previous analyses (Olson, Wise, Conners, Rack, & Fulker, 1989) no longer support deficits in phonological coding as more heritable than deficits in orthographic coding. Instead, univariate results suggest little difference in levels of heritability for group deficits in the two types of coding. Furthermore, bivariate results suggest that the covariance between the deficits is due to the same genetic mechanisms. Consequently, Olson et al. (chapter 1) abandon the dual-route view defended in their previous research and, instead, adopt Ehri's (1989, 1992) integrative view of the development of orthographic and phonological skills. I will return to a discussion of Ehri's integrative view and dual-route theory in the final section on connectionist models.

Olson et al. (chapter 1) report that in spite of covariance between phonological and orthographic coding deficits and significant correlations between the orthographic and phonological factors, the two types of codes do account for significant independent variance in word recognition. The key variable that loaded differentially high on the phonological factor was, not surprisingly, phonological awareness. On the orthographic factor it was print exposure that loaded differentially high. Print exposure is usually assessed by giving the subject a list of age-appropriate book or magazine titles or names of authors mixed in with foils (Stanovich & West, 1989; Cunningham & Stanovich, 1991). The idea is that the more titles or authors the subject correctly identifies, minus foils, the more reading the subject has probably done. With children, the idea is to eliminate names of books used in the curriculum so as to assess print exposure outside of school (Cunningham & Stanovich, 1991). However, the more common technique is to present students with a list of popular book titles without attempting to eliminate titles from the school curriculum. Using this popularity approach, Olson et al. (chapter 1), Wagner and Barker (chapter 7), and Stanovich, West, and

Cunningham (1992) found that individual differences in print exposure uniquely account for variance in orthographic processing skill.

Print exposure is not merely a proxy for orthographic processing because the latter accounts for additional variance in multiple regression analyses where decoding is predicted by entering phonological processing first, then print exposure, and, finally, orthographic processing. But Olson et al. (chapter 1) also report a very high loading of title recognition on the orthographic factor. They explain this and similar findings by reasoning that exposure to print helps the development of orthographic codes, which, in turn, enhances word recognition. Even more concretely, the ability to choose the correct orthographic pattern from the pair *rain-rane* is dependent upon previous exposure to *rain* in print. Yet, Olson et al. (chapter 1) present us with a puzzle. Deficits in print exposure appear to have no significant level of heritability but appear to have significant shared-environment effects. Thus, the high loading of print exposure on the orthographic factor would lead one to expect significant shared-environment effects for orthographic coding. But this expectation is not supported. On a final note, Olson et al. wonder, given the strength of the overall correlation between phonological and orthographic processing measures, whether the unique contribution of print exposure to orthographic coding deficits might not be considered relatively weak after all.

There are obvious difficulties in trying to assess print exposure with beginning readers. First of all, because they are beginners, their exposure to print comes primarily from their parents reading to them. Parental readings tend to focus on content rather than on characteristics of print or the title (Yaden, Smolkin, & Conlin, 1989). Moreover, with the advent of literature-based instruction, it is difficult to find popular titles that the children have not been exposed to in the curriculum. One of my students worked hard to find such titles only to discover a virtual floor effect in the data (Glazier, 1993). In fact, out of a list of 20 actual titles and 13 foils, the 71 second graders recognized an average of only 4 titles. These scores were sufficient to yield significant correlations with spelling and word recognition measures ($r = .32$ and $.77$, $p < .01$ and $.001$, respectively) and to contribute unique variation in spelling and word recognition beyond that accounted for by phonological awareness. But further analysis revealed the list of 4 titles to be virtually the same for all students. Because the probability of the same 4 titles showing up in children's homes is extremely low, one concludes that the children were exposed to these titles somewhere in a school activity, such as in trips to the library. Thus, print exposure and instructional exposure become one and the same. The most useful measure of print exposure would be a record of the frequency with which a beginning reader has been exposed to particular printed words, both in and out of school. That record of exposures would serve as a measure of opportunity to practice orthographic and phonological processing skills. The cumulative vocabulary lists of basal readers provide a start to such a record, but with the demise of basal readers and the advent of literature-based instruction, the task of accumulating such a record is daunting indeed.

The final factor to consider in a discussion of orthographic processing is letter name knowledge. A decade of research on emergent literacy (see Adams, 1990, and Sulzby & Teale, 1991, for reviews) points out that children in a literate culture come to school with thousands of hours of exposure to the letter names and sounds of the characters in their orthography (or orthographies). Some homes will afford much more exposure than others, depending upon such things as availability and access to print materials and educational television.

Why is letter name knowledge important? One often cited reason is that knowledge of letter names in kindergarten or the beginning of first grade is the best predictor of success in beginning reading (e.g., Bond & Dykstra, 1967; Stevenson, Parker, Wilkinson, Hegion, & Fish, 1976). However, it should be pointed out that early ability to name letters is not predictive of success in second or third grade reading (Stevenson et al., 1976). The question is: What is it about knowing letter names that seems to facilitate learning to read? First, correct letter naming assumes correct recognition, which, in turn, involves discriminating the distinctive features of letters. In cases where the number of distinguishing features is minimal (e.g., the 180º rotation between *b* and *d*), recognition can become quite effortful for the young child. Second, letter names provide a first strategy for decoding that will be successful for almost all consonants in English. In the case of vowels, the names provide at least one source of identity. Third, Barron (chapter 6) believes that prereaders' letter-name and letter-sound associations signal an important shift in language development toward the "activation of orthographic information during the process of auditory word recognition" (p. 2). Drawing upon Ehri's idea that letters come to symbolize sound during the development of reading and spelling (see Ehri, 1994, for a review), Barron wants to emphasize just how early on in literacy development such orthographic information is activated. In fact, he has coined the term *proto-literacy* to capture that phase when the prereader is able to activate letter-name and letter-sound associations to aid in such auditory tasks as phonological awareness.

In summary, orthographic processing has been operationalized with tasks requiring verification or choice of conventional spellings or legal spelling patterns, exposure to print, and knowledge of letter names and sounds. In fact, there appears to be a developmental hierarchy in these tasks such that letter-name knowledge and exposure to print help in the development of the orthographic code needed to identify words in the verification and choice tasks. Orthographic processing does appear to dissociate from phonological processing in brain imaging studies of skilled readers and in multiple regression analyses where orthographic processing accounts for unique variation in word recognition beyond that accounted for by phonological processing and print exposure. Recent research emphasizes the visual processing inherent in orthographic codes and hypotheses a deficit in the transient visual system as a cause of dyslexia. Problems of "hard-wiring" in the visual systems or, for that matter in the auditory system, probably account for a very small percentage of the causes of dyslexia. A more realistic possibility is the overly global strategy for forming orthographic representations that Frith (1985) and Vellutino and Scanlon (1984) ascribe to dyslexics.

IN SEARCH OF AN ADEQUATE PSYCHOLOGICAL MODEL OF READING

The authors of this volume and I too are searching for an adequate psychological model of the reading process. Bowers et al. (chapter 5) appear to be committed to a dual-route view. Olson et al. (chapter 1) abandon the separatist, dual-route view (Olson, Kliegl, Davidson, & Foltz, 1985) in favor of an integrative view of the development of phonological and orthographic processes (Ehri, 1989, 1992). Assink and Kattenberg (chapter 3) find that Karmiloff-Smith's (1985; 1987) model fits their data better than Ehri and Wilce's (1979; 1983) model of "unitization" in word identification. Berninger and Abbott (chapter 8) embrace the connectionist framework of Van Orden, Pennington, and Stone (1990). And I (Foorman, 1994) have shifted from the dual-route perspective evident in the Foorman and Liberman (1989) definition of orthographic skills given in Wagner and Barker's (chapter 7) Table 1 to the connectionist—specifically, parallel distributed processing (PDP) view of Seidenberg and McClelland (1989). In this section I will distinguish connectionist models from interactive models that do and do not entail dual routes. I will argue that Ehri's (1992, 1994) integrative view of the development of phonological and orthographic processing in fact fits well with the PDP view of reading development (Seidenberg & McClelland, 1989).

Interactive Models of Reading

Interactive models of reading integrate bottom-up processing of sublexical units with top-down contextual knowledge. A frequently cited interactive model focusing on the parallel rather than serial nature of levels of processing letters is that of McClelland and Rumelhart (1981). More comprehensive models are offered by Just and Carpenter (1980), Rayner and Pollatsek (1989), and Perfetti (1991). Both the Just and Carpenter and Rayner and Pollatsek models emphasize the bottom-up process of eye fixations interacting with the top-down information drawn from long-term memory into short-term (or working) memory. Perfetti (1991) named his model Restrictive-Interactive to emphasize the constraints his parallel, interactive model places on interactions.

> Its interactions are restricted to occur only within the specific data structures of lexical formation (i.e., letters, phonemes, and words). It allows no influences from outside lexical data structures, no importation of knowledge, expectancies, and beliefs. Skilled word recognition is context free. (p. 34)

A key feature of Perfetti's model is the distinction between the functional and autonomous lexicons. The functional lexicon consists of all the words that can be accessed through reading but have not yet reached an autonomous state. Once words have been "moved over" into the autonomous lexicon they become part of abstract spelling knowledge that allows for "automatic" recognition of spelling patterns.

All of these interactive models belong to the symbol manipulation paradigm of information processing in that words are identified through access to a mental lexicon. This access is said to occur through one of two routes: an "indirect" route that converts letters to sounds and a "direct,"lexical route that entails a dictionary lookup procedure (see Coltheart, Curtis, Atkins, & Haller,1993, for a review).

Connectionist Models of Reading

Connectionist models of reading emphasize (1) a single, rather than dual, mechanism for processing words, and (2) distributed representations and weighted connections between units rather than symbolic rules for mapping letters and sounds (see Foorman, 1994, for a review). In short, there is no mental dictionary, no lookup procedure, no lexical route. Instead, there are *computed* orthographic, phonological, and semantic codes. These codes are computed each time a word is recognized, not retrieved from memory. Hence, connectionism is rooted in the principle of *distributed* representations of knowledge. Learning is a matter of adjusting the weights between connections. Learning to recognize words involves encoding the frequency and consistency of correspondences between orthography and phonology. A key concept to understanding individual differences in reading is the architectural constraint of *computational capacity* (Seidenberg, 1993). According to this notion, performance of connectionist nets may be limited by factors such as the number of units and patterns of interconnectivity among them. A central implication of connectionism for the teaching of reading is that letter-sound correspondences are important—not as rules to be memorized, but rather as characteristics of spelling patterns to be recognized through training.

Seidenberg and McClelland's (1989) model has been criticized for its poor performance on nonwords, inability to simulate acquired and developmental dyslexia (Coltheart et al., 1993, for a review), and its inability to capture the role of structured phonological representations in the development of word reading (Rack, Hulme, Snowling, & Wightman, 1994). However, poor performance on nonwords has virtually been eliminated through the notion of componential attractors. A componential attractor is a stable activity pattern. In the case of a quasiregular task such as word reading, "networks generalize because the attractors it develops for regular words are *componential*—they have substructure that reflects common sublexical correspondences between orthography and phonology" (Plaut & McClelland, 1993, p. 824). In this attractor network, "componential attractors for regular words coexist with much less componential attractors for exception words,"thereby "challenging 'dual-route' assumptions that multiple, independent mechanisms are required for quasiregular tasks" (Plaut & McClelland, 1993, p. 824).

In addition, simulations have been "damaged" to successfully imitate behaviors of acquired and developmental dyslexia. In one simulation the number of hidden units was reduced, with a consequential reduction in computational capacity (Seidenberg & McClelland, 1989). In another simulation, orthographic units were degraded to simulate a deficit in visual processing (Seidenberg, 1992). Both simulations produced similar behavioral profiles, what Seidenberg (1993, p. 303) refers to as "a modal pattern of impairment among English-reading dyslexics:"

> They are typically impaired in reading single words, especially irregularly pronounced words such as *have* and *some* and pseudowords such as *mave* and *lome*. Compared with normal readers, they are relatively less impaired in reading regular, rule-governed words such as *like* or *must*. (p. 303)

Thus, the "damage" simulations help us understand that (1) similar dyslexic behaviors can emanate from different underlying causes, and (2) exception words as well as nonwords are impaired in the modal pattern. Dual-route theory predicts the pattern of impairments referred to as *surface dyslexia* and *phonological dyslexia*. In the former, exception word reading is impaired, while regular and nonword reading is preserved. In *phonological dyslexia*, reading of nonwords is impaired, while word reading is preserved. Because the modal pattern of impairments in exception word and nonword reading simulated by connectionist models cuts across the patterns predicted by the dual-route model, the explanatory and predictive validity of dual-route theory is seriously questioned and the single mechanism explanation of connectionism is supported. Thus, the separatist view of orthographic processing is challenged by the successful simulations of dyslexia by the connectionist architecture (Stanovich, 1993).

Finally, a criticism of connectionism that is more difficult to counter is its inability to capture the role of structured phonological representations in the development of word reading (Rack et al., 1994). Most children come to beginning reading instruction with five or six years of oral language development in syntax, phonology, and semantics. Many children will also have thousands of hours of orthographic experiences as well. As summarized above, research supports a certain degree of phonological and orthographic (i.e., letter-name) knowledge as a prerequisite to reading success. Yet, the Seidenberg and McClelland (1989) model begins its simulation of word reading development with a corpus of 2897 monosyllabic words and no accounting for these prerequisite phonological abilities. Consequently, quite a lot of training is needed to produce accurate word reading. There is, however, at least one connectionist network that does take phonological development into account. Its name is NETalk and it was developed by Sejnowski and Rosenberg (1987) to demonstrate how a parallel, distributed network rather than a set of pronunciation rules can learn to convert English text to speech. Significantly, the network was trained on phonetic transcriptions from informal, continuous speech of a child.

Ehri's Integrative View

Ehri (1992, 1994) refers to her alternative theory of sight word learning as amalgamation theory. Central to amalgamation theory is skill in phonological recoding. According to Ehri (1994):

> ...when mature alphabetic readers practice reading specific words by phonologically recoding the words, they form access routes for those words into memory. Readers build these access routes by using their knowledge of grapheme-phoneme correspondences to amalgamate letters in spellings to phonemes in pronunciations of the words. The letters are processed as visual symbols for the phonemes and the sequence of letters is retained in memory as an alphabetic, phonological representation of the word. (p. 25)

Ehri goes on to explain that once this word-specific access route is established in memory, phonological rules drop out and the spelling alone activates the connections that produce correct pronunciations that lead to meaning.

Ehri's view of the shift from an alphabetic phase of reading to skilled reading is similar to Perfetti's (1992) explanation of the shift from a functional to an autonomous lexicon. However, prior to alphabetic reading, Ehri (1992, 1994) describes a phase of *phonetic cue reading* based on forming access routes out of partial letter-sound correspondences. Typically, it is the initial and/or final letters that become linked to phonetic units in pronunciation. Ehri (1994) explains:

> To illustrate, the first few times a phonetic cue reader sees and hears *milk*, she recognizes how the initial and final letters correspond to /m/ and /k/ in pronunciation. This creates an access route into lexical memory that enables her to retrieve the pronunciation when she sees the spelling again. (p. 10)

In over a decade and a half of careful experimental study of phonetic cue reading, Ehri has demonstrated the "unitization" of letter-sound knowledge that precedes alphabetic reading. Ehri (1994) is critical of connectionist models for not explaining the development of amalgamations:

> By eliminating the lexicon, by focusing upon separate orthographic, phonological, and semantic codes, and by obscuring how the *integration* or *unitization process* among these codes works in learning to process words, connectionist theorists have not captured the key constructs and mechanisms necessary to account for acquisition. (p. 39)

In spite of Ehri's (1994) criticism of connectionism and her allegiance to information processing concepts of mental lexicon and rules for relating graphemes to phonemes, researchers such as Rack et al. (1994) regard her description of phonetic cue reading as consistent with connectionist theory. Connectionist learning entails direct mappings from orthography to phonology. During the acquisition phase—Ehri's phonetic cue reading phase—the mappings will undoubtedly be based on partial information about words' pronunciations from cues available in the printed words' letter-sounds or letter names. Rather than being converted to a rule-governed process, this direct mapping mechanism of connectionist theory develops into what Van Orden et al. (1990) call "covariant learning."

> A mapping process that is acquired through covariant learning must exhibit a predictable pattern of development. Initially, input codes and output codes are associated on a stimulus-specific basis. Thus, early in development, performance will appear to be governed by stimulus-specific knowledge. Eventually, however, rule-like performance emerges as performance is affected by the subtle, distributional structure across input-output pairs. Finally, with sufficient experience of specific input-output pairs, performance will converge toward an asymptote. (p. 514)

Thus, covariant learning hypothesizes Piagetian stagelike transitions in behavior, but from a subsymbolic perspective. There are researchers who complain that connectionism accounts for behavioral mastery but not for the transition from implicit representations to explicit ones (e.g., Holyoak, 1991; Karmiloff-Smith, 1987; Schneider, 1987). These researchers argue for a hybrid model—"symbolic connectionism"—where parallel, distributed processing is combined with sequential, symbol manipulation. As I have written elsewhere (Foorman, 1994), connectionism does not have to borrow from information processing in order to explain how implicit representations become explicit or conscious. The process by which information is re-represented to ourselves or to others is but one of many plausible, coherent "drafts" of reality (Dennett, 1991). To the extent a response requires public display in verbal form, sequential symbol manipulation may indeed be an adequate description. However, in my opinion, such description fits only the tip of an iceberg most persuasively characterized by learning where the effects of consistency and frequency emanate from a common process, the adjustment of weights according to experience. Rather than the explicit-implicit dichotomy, it may prove more useful to think of awareness or consciousness as a continuum. At opposite ends of the continuum are *automatic* behaviors and *attended* behaviors (Carr, 1992). With respect to word reading, position on the continuum will be determined by familiarity and consistency of the words being read. In such a view, the integration of phonological and orthographic processing becomes the "stable attractor" of reading development.

CONCLUSION

The title of this chapter poses a challenging question, "Phonological and Orthographic Processing: Separate but

Equal?" The authors of this volume all agree to the conceptual intertwining of these constructs, yet point to their dissociation statistically, especially in studies of dyslexics performing orthographic tasks demanding more general visual processing and in brain-imaging studies of skilled reading. Thus, are we to conclude that phonological and orthographic processing are separate?

I will boldly answer my question with: No! I find the evidence to be in favor of *integration* of phonological and orthographic processing. First, from an evolutionary perspective, it makes sense that orthographic processing "piggybacks" on the language system evolved in humans. However, there will be a period in development when the piggybacking will seem disjointed, indeed even separate. Thus, Ehri (1992, 1994) wants to highlight the separate strands of knowledge that become amalgamated during phonetic cue reading, whereas Barron (chapter 6) wants to stress the integration of orthographic knowledge and phonological awareness during the period of proto-literacy. Both are right, for how can one understand an integrated product without some attention to the units in the process and their "unitization." Hence, tasks that dissociate conceptually in terms of their phonological and orthographic demands can be designed to be distinct. The fact that these tasks dissociate statistically is not, therefore, surprising, but the degree of the dissociation over time with different populations of readers is of theoretical and practical interest.

But I advise that we not become carried away with unraveling the integrated whole. The bigger picture of the reading process favors integration. Remember Olson et al.'s (chapter 1) new data supportive of *comparable* levels of heritability and *common* genetic mechanisms for phonological and orthographic processing. Remember the universal involvement of *both* phonology and orthography across Chinese, Dutch, English, and German. Remember that Seidenberg's (1992, 1993) various "damage" simulations produced the *common* modal pattern of dyslexia, a finding supportive of the *single* mechanism of connectionism and not of the *dual* mechanism of dual-route theory. But the story of integration has only begun. And, in the meantime, research emanating from the belief of "separate but equal" will enrich our scientific endeavors into phonological and orthographic processing.

Acknowledgements

Preparation of this chapter was supported by grants HD30995 and HD28172 from the National Institutes of Child Health and Human Development. Collaborators on these grants are David Francis and Jack Fletcher.

REFERENCES

Adams, M.J. (1990). *Beginning to read.* Cambridge, MA: MIT Press.

Alegria, J., Pignot, E., & Morais, J. (1982). Phonetic analysis of speech and memory codes in beginning readers. *Memory and Cognition*, 10, 451-456.

Assink, E., & Kattenberg, G. (1994). Higher-order linguistic influences on development of orthographic knowledge: Illustrations from spelling problems in Dutch and assessment tools. In V.W. Berninger (Ed.), *The varieties of orthographic knowledge I: Theoretical and developmental issues* (pp. 111-136). Dordrecht, The Netherlands: Kluwer Academic Press.

Barker, T.A., Torgesen, J.K., & Wagner, R.K. (1992). The role of orthographic processing skills on five different reading tasks. *Reading Research Quarterly*, 27, 335-345.

Baron, J., & Treiman, R. (1980). Some problems in the study of differences in cognitive processes. *Memory and Cognition*, 8, 313-321.

Barron, R. (1994). The sound-to-spelling connection: Orthographic activation in auditory word recognition and its implications for the acquisition of phonological awareness and literacy skills. In V.W. Berninger (Ed.), *The varieties of orthographic knowledge I: Theoretical and developmental issues* (pp. 219-242). Dordrecht, The Netherlands: Kluwer Academic Press.

Berninger, V., & Abbott, R. (1994). Multiple orthographic and phonological codes in literacy acquisition: An evolving research program. In V.W. Berninger (Ed.), *The varieties of orthographic knowledge I: Theoretical and developmental issues* (pp. 277-317). Dordrecht, The Netherlands: Kluwer Academic Press.

Berninger, V., Yates, C., & Lester, K. (1991). Multiple orthographic codes in reading and writing acquisition. *Reading and Writing: An Interdisciplinary Journal*, 3, 115-149.

Bond, G.L., & Dykstra, R. (1967). The cooperative research program in first-grade reading instruction. *Reading Research Quarterly*, 2, 5-142..

Bowers, P., Golden, J., Kennedy, A., & Young, A. (1994). Limits upon orthographic knowledge due to processes indexed by naming speed. In V.W. Berninger (Ed.), *The varieties of orthographic knowledge I: Theoretical and developmental issues* (pp. 173-218). Dordrecht, The Netherlands: Kluwer Academic Press.

Bradley, L., & Bryant, P.E. (1983). Categorizing sounds and learning to read—a causal connection. *Nature*, 301, 419-421.

Bradley, L., & Bryant, P.E. (1985). *Rhyme and reason in reading and spelling*. I.A.R.L.D. Monographs No. 1, Ann Arbor: University of Michigan Press.

Brady, S.A., & Shankweiler, D.P. (1990). *Phonological processes in literacy*. Hillsdale, NJ: Erlbaum.

Bruce, L.J. (1964). The analysis of word sounds. *British Journal of Educational Psychology*, 34, 158-170.

Carr, T.H. (1992). Automaticity and cognitive anatomy: Is word recognition "automatic"? *American Journal of Psychology*, 105, 201-237.

Carr, T.H., & Posner, M.I. (in press). The impact of learning to read on the functional anatomy of language processing. In B. de Gelder & J. Morais (Eds.), *Language and literacy: Comparative approaches*. Cambridge, MA: MIT Press.

Case, R. (1985). *Intellectual development: Birth to adulthood*. New York, NY: Academic Press.

Coltheart M., Curtis, B., Atkins, P., & Haller, M. (1993). Models of reading aloud: Dual-route and parallel-distributed-processing approaches. *Psychological Review*, 100, 589-608.

Content, A., Kolinsky, R., Morais, J., & Bertelson, P. (1986). Phonetic segmentation in pre-readers: Effect of corrective information. *Journal of Experimental Child Psychology*, 42, 49-72.

Corcos, E., & Willows, D. (1993). The processing of orthographic information. In D.M. Willows, R.S. Kruk, & E. Corcos (Eds.), *Visual processes in reading and reading disabilities* (pp. 163-190). Hillsdale, NJ: Erlbaum.

Cunningham, A.E., & Stanovich, K.E. (1991). Tracking the unique effects of print exposure in children: Associations with vocabulary, general knowledge, and spelling. *Journal of Educational Psychology*, 83, 264-274.

Denckla, M., & Rudel, R.G. (1974). Rapid "automatized" naming of pictured objects, colors, letters and numbers by normal children. *Cortex*, 10, 186-202.

Denckla, M., & Rudel, R.G. (1976). Rapid "automaticed" naming (R.A.N.): Dyslexia differentiated from other learning disabilities. *Neuropsychologia*, 14, 471-479.

Dennett, D. (1991). *Consciousness explained.* Boston, MA: Little, Brown & Co.

Dunn, L.M., & Dunn, L. (1981). *Peabody Picture Vocabulary Test.* Circle Pines, MD: American Guidance Service.

Dunn, L.M., & Markwardt, F.C. (1970). *Examiner's manual: Peabody Individual Achievement Test.* Circle Pines, MD: American Guidance Service.

Ehri, L.C. (1989). Movement into word reading and spelling: How spelling contributes to reading. In J. Mason (Ed.), *Reading and writing connections* (pp. 65-81). Boston, MA: Allyn Bacon.

Ehri, L.C. (1992). Reconceptualizing the development of sight word reading and its relationship to recoding. In P.B. Gough, L.C. Ehri, & R. Treiman (Eds.), *Reading acquisition* (pp. 107-143). Hillsdale, NJ: Erlbaum.

Ehri, L.C. (1994). Development of the ability to read words: Update. In R. Ruddell, M. Ruddell, & H. Singer (Eds.), *Theoretical models and processes of reading* (pp. 323-353). Newark, DE: IRA.

Ehri, L.C., & Wilce, L.S. (1979). The mnemonic value of orthography among beginning readers. *Journal of Educational Psychology*, 71, 26-40.

Ehri, L.C., & Wilce, L.S. (1983). Development of word identification speed in skilled and less skilled beginning readers. *Journal of Educational Psychology*, 75, 3-18.

Foorman, B.R. (1994). The relevance of a connectionist model of reading for "The Great Debate." *Educational Psychology Review*, 6, 25-47.

Foorman, B.R., & Francis, D.J. (1994). Exploring connections among reading, spelling, and phonemic segmentation during first grade. *Reading and Writing: An Interdisciplinary Journal*, 6, 1-26.

Foorman, B.R., & Francis, D.J., Novy, D., & Liberman, D. (1991). How letter-sound instruction mediates progress in first-grade reading and spelling. *Journal of Educational Psychology*, 83, 456-469.

Foorman, B.R., Jenkins, L., & Francis, D.J. (1993). Links among segmenting, spelling, and reading words in first and second grades. *Reading and Writing: An Interdisciplinary Journal*, 5, 1-16.

Foorman, B.R., & Kinoshita, Y. (1983). Linguistic effects on children's encoding and decoding performance in Japan, the United States, and England. *Child Development*, 54, 69-77.

Foorman, B.R., & Liberman, D. (1989). Visual and phonological processing of words: A comparison of good and poor readers. *Journal of Learning Disabilities*, 22, 349-355.

Foorman, B.R., & Siegel, A.W. (Eds.) (1986). *Acquisition of reading skills: Cultural constraints and cognitive universals.* Hillsdale, NJ: Erlbaum.

Frith, U. (1985). Beneath the surface of developmental dyslexia. In K.E. Patterson, J.C. Marshall, & M. Coltheart (Eds.), *Surface dyslexia* (pp. 301-390). Hillsdale, NJ: Erlbaum.

Glazier, C.R. (1993). *Orthographic and Phonological Spelling Patterns in Second Grade Children.* Unpublished Master's Thesis, University of Houston, Houston, TX

Goswami, U. (1993). Toward an interactive analogy model of reading development: Decoding vowel graphemes in beginning reading. *Journal of Experimental Child Psychology*, 56, 443-475.

Goswami, U., & Bryant, P.E. (1990). *Phonological skills and learning to read.* Hillsdale, NJ: Erlbaum.

Hatano, G. (1986). How do Japanese children learn to read?: Orthographic and eco-cultural variables. In B.R. Foorman & A.W. Siegel (Eds.), *Acquisition of reading skills: Cultural constraints and cognitive universals* (pp. 81-114). Hillsdale, NJ: Erlbaum.

Holyoak, K.J. (1991). Symbolic connectionism: Toward third-generation theories of expertise. In K.A. Ericsson & J. Smith (Eds.), *Toward a general theory of expertise* (pp. 301-335). Cambridge, UK: Cambridge University Press.

Jackson, N., Lu, W-H, & Ju, D. (1994). Reading Chinese and reading English: Similarities, differences, and second-language learning. In V. W. Berninger (Ed.), *The varieties of orthographic knowledge I: Theoretical and developmental issues* (pp. 73-109). Dordrecht, The Netherlands: Kluwer Academic Publishers.

Juel, C., Griffith, P.L, & Gough, P.B. (1986). Acquisition of literacy: A longitudinal study of children in first and second grades. *Journal of Educational Psychology*, 78, 243-255.

Just, M.A., & Carpenter, P.A. (1980). A theory of reading: From eye fixations to comprehension. *Psychological Review*, 87, 329-354.

Karmiloff-Smith, A. (1985). Language and cognitive processes from a developmental perspective. *Language and Cognitive Processes*, 1, 61-85.

Karmiloff-Smith, A. (1987). Function and process in comparing language and cognition. In M. Hickmann (Ed.), *Social and functional approaches to language and thought*. New York, NY: Academic Press.

Labov, W. (1972). *Language in the inter-city: Studies in the Black English vernacular*. Philadelphia, PA: University of Pennsylvania Press.

Lee, S., Stigler, J.W., & Stevenson, H. (1986). Beginning reading in Chinese and English. In B.R. Foorman & A.W. Siegel (Eds.), *Acquisition of reading skills: Cultural constraints and cognitive universals* (p. 123-150).

Leslie, L., & Shannon, A.J. (1981). Recognition of orthographic structure during beginning reading. *Journal of Reading Behavior*, 13, 313-324.

Lovegrove, W., Garcia, R.P., & Nicholson, S.B. (1990). Experimental evidence for a transient system deficit in specific reading disability. *Journal of the American Optometric Association*, 61, 137-146.

Lundberg, I., Frost, J., & Petersen, O. (1988). Effects of an extensive program for stimulating phonological awareness in preschool children. *Reading Research Quarterly*, 23, 263-284.

MacLean, M., Bryant, P., & Bradley, L. (1987). Rhymes, nursery rhymes, and reading in early childhood. *Merrill-Palmer Quarterly*, 33, 255-281.

Manis, F.R., Szeszulski, P.A., Holt, L.K., & Graves, K. (1990). Variation in component word recognition and spelling skills among dyslexic children and normal readers. In T. Carr & B.A. Levy (Eds.), *Reading and its development: Component skills approaches* (pp. 207-259). New York, NY: Academic Press.

McClelland, J.L., & Rumelhart, D.E. (1981). An interactive activation model of context effects in letter perception: Part 1, An account of basic findings. *Psychological Review*, 88, 375-407.

Morais, J. (1988, November). *Constraints on the development of phonemic awareness.* Paper presented in the Symposium on Phonological Processing in Literacy to honor the research of Isabelle Y. Liberman, 39th Annual Conference of the Orton Society, Tampa, FL.

Nakanishi, A. (1980). *Writing systems of the world.* Rutland, VT: Charles E. Tuttle Co.

Olson, R., Forsberg, H., & Wise, B. (1994). Genes, environment, and the development of orthographic skills. In V. W. Berninger (Ed.), *The varieties of orthographic knowledge I: Theoretical and developmental issues* (pp. 27-71). Dordrecht, The Netherlands: Kluwer Academic Publishers.

Olson, R.K., Kliegl, R., Davidson, B.J., & Foltz, G. (1985). Individual and developmental differences in reading disability. In G.E. MacKinnon & T.G. Waller (Eds.), *Reading research: Advances in theory and practice, Vol 4* (pp. 1-64). New York, NY: Academic Press.

Olson, R.K., Wise, B., Conners, F., Rack, J., & Fulker, D. (1989). Specific deficits in component reading and language skills: Genetic and environmental influences. *Journal of Learning Disabilities*, 22, 339-348.

Plaut, D.C., & McClelland, J.L. (1993). Generalization with componential attractors: Word and nonword reading in an attractor network. In *Proceedings of the 15th annual conference of the Cognitive Science Society*. Hillsdale, NJ: Erlbaum.

Perfetti, C.A. (1991). Representations and awareness in the acquisition of reading competence. In L. Rieben & C.A. Perfetti (Eds.), *Learning to read: Basic research and its implications* (pp. 33-46). Hillsdale, NJ: Erlbaum.

Perfetti, C.A. (1992). The representation problem in reading acquisition. In P.R. Gough, L.C. Ehri, & R. Treiman (Eds.), *Reading acquisition* (pp. 145-174). Hillsdale, NJ: Erlbaum.

Perfetti, C.A., Beck, I., Bell, L., & Hughes, C. (1987). Phonemic knowledge and learning to read are reciprocal: A longitudinal study of first grade children. *Merrill-Palmer Quarterly*, 33, 283-319.

Perfetti, C.A., Zhang, S., & Berent, I. (1992). Reading in English and Chinese: Evidence for a "universal" phonological principle. In R. Frost & L. Katz (Eds.), *Orthography, phonology, morphology, and meaning* (pp. 227-248). Amsterdam: North-Holland.

Rack, J., Hulme, C., Snowling, M., & Wightman, J. (1994). The role of phonology in young children learning to read words: The direct-mapping hypothesis. *Journal of Experimental Child Psychology*, 57, 42-71.

Rack, J., Snowling, M., & Olson, R.K. (1992). The nonword reading deficit in developmental dyslexia: A review. *Reading Research Quarterly*, 27, 28-53.

Rayner, K., & Pollatsek, A. (1989). *The psychology of reading*. Englewood Cliffs, NJ: Prentice-Hall.

Roazzi, A., Dowker, A., & Bryant, P.E. (1993). Phonological abilities of Brazilian street poets. *Applied Psycholinguistics*, 14, 535-551.

Rosner, J., & Simon, D. (1971). The Auditory Analysis Test: An initial report. *Journal of Learning Disabilities*, 4, 384-392.

Sacks, O. (1989). *Seeing voices*. Berkeley, CA: University of California, Berkeley, Press.

Schneider, W. (1987). Connectionism: Is it a paradigm shift for psychology? *Behavior Research Methods, Instruments and Computers*, 19, 73-83.

Seidenberg, M. (1992). Dyslexia in a computational model of word recognition in reading. In P.B. Gough, L.C. Ehri, & R. Treiman (Eds.), *Reading acquisition* (pp. 243-274). Hillsdale, NH: Erlbaum.

Seidenberg, M. (1993). A connectionist modeling approach to word recognition and dyslexia. *Psychological Science*, 4, 299-304.

Seidenberg, M., & McClelland, J.L. (1989). A distributed, developmental model of word recognition and naming. *Psychological Review*, 96, 523-568.

Sejnowski, T.J., & Rosenberg, C.R. (1987). Parallel networds that learn to pronounce English test. *Complex Systems*, 1, 145-168.

Siegel, L.S., Geva, E., & Share, D. (1993). The development of orthographic skills in normal and disabled readers. Unpublished manuscript.

Stanovich, K.E. (1986). Matthew effects in reading: Some consequences of individual differences in the acquisition of literacy. *Reading Research Quarterly*, 21, 360-407.

Stanovich, K.E. (1988). The dyslexic and the garden-variety poor reader: The phonological-core variable-difference model. *Journal of Learning Disabilities*, 21, 590-604.

Stanovich, K.E. (1992). Speculations on the causes and consequences of individual differences in early reading acquisition. In P.B. Gough, L.C. Ehri, & R. Treiman (Eds.), *Reading acquisition* (pp. 307-342). Hillsdale, NJ: Erlbaum.

Stanovich, K.E. (1993). The construct validity of discrepancy definitions of reading disability. In G.R. Lyon, D.B. Gray, J.F. Kavanagh, & N.A. Krasnegor (Eds.), *Better understanding of learning disabilities* (pp. 273-308). Baltimore, MD: Brookes.

Stanovich, K.E., Cunningham, A.E., & Cramer, B. (1984). Assessing phonological awareness in kindergarten children: Issues of task comparability. *Journal of Experimental Child Psychology*, 38, 175-190.

Stanovich, K.E., & West, R.F. (1989). Exposure to print and orthographic processing. *Reading Research Quarterly*, 24, 402-433.

Stanovich, K.E., West, R.F., & Cunningham, A.E. (1992). Beyond phonological processes: Print exposure and orthographic processing. In S.A. Brady & D. Shankweiler (Eds.), *Phonological processes in literacy* (pp. 219-235). Hillsdale, NJ: Erlbaum.

Stevenson, H.W., Parker, T., Wilkinson, A., Hegion, A., & Fish, E. (1976). Longitudinal study of individual differences in cognitive development and scholastic achievement. *Journal of Educational Psychology*, 68, 377-400.

Sulzby, E., & Teale, W. (1991). Emergent literacy. In R. Barr, M.L. Kamil, P. Mosenthal, & P.D. Pearson (Eds.), *Handbook of reading research, Vol. II* (pp. 727-758). New York, NY: Longman.

Treiman, R. (1985). Onsets and rimes as units of spoken syllables: Evidence from children. *Journal of Experimental Child Psychology*, 39, 161-181.

Tunmer, W.E., & Nesdale, A.R. (1985). Phonemic segmentation skill and beginning reading. *Journal of Educational Psychology*, 77, 417-427.

Van Orden, G.C., Pennington, B.F., & Stone, G.O. (1990). Word identificaion in reading and the promise of subsymbolic psycholinguistics. *Psychological Review*, 97, 488-522.

Vellutino, F.R. (1991). Introduction to three studies on reading acquisition: Convergent findings on theoretical foundations of code-oriented versus whole-language approaches to reading instruction. *Journal of Educational Psychology*, 83, 437-443.

Vellutino, F.R., & Scanlon, D.M. (1984). Converging perspectives in the study of the reading process: Reactions to the papers presented by Morrison, Siegel and Ryan, and Stanovich. *Remedial and Special Education*, 5, 39-44.

Vellutino, F.R., Scanlon, D.M., & Tanzman, M.S. (1994). Components of reading ability: Issues and problems in operationalizing word identification, phonological coding, and orthographic coding. In G.R. Lyon (Ed.), *Frames of reference for the assessment of learning disabilities: New views on measurement issues* (pp. 279-332). Baltimore, MD: Brookes.

Wagner, R., & Barker, T. (1994). The development of orthographic processing ability. In V. W. Berninger (Ed.), *The varieties of orthographic knowledge I: Theoretical and developmental issues* (pp. 243-275). Dordrecht, The Netherlands: Kluwer Academic Publishers.

Wagner, R.K., & Torgesen, J.K. (1987). The nature of phonological processing and its causal role in the acquisition of reading skills. *Psychological Bulletin*, 101, 192-212.

Wagner, R.K., Torgesen, J.K., & Rashotte, C.A. (1994). The development of reading-related phonological processing abilities: New evidence of bi-directional causality from a latent variable longitudinal study. *Developmental Psychology*, 30, 73-87.

Wimmer, H. (1993). Characteristics of developmental dyslexia in a regular writing system. *Applied Psycholinguistics*, 14, 1-34.

Wolf, M., Pfeil, C., Lotz, R., & Biddle, K. (1994). Towards a more universal understanding of the developmental dyslexias: The contribution of orthographic factors. In V. W. Berninger (Ed.), *The varieties of orthographic knowledge I: Theoretical and developmental issues* (pp. 131-171). Dordrecht, The Netherlands: Klwer Academic Publishers.

Wolf, M., Bally, H., & Morris, R. (1986). Automaticity, retrieval processes and reading: A longitudinal study in average and impaired readers. *Child Development*, 57, 988-1005.

Yaden, D.B., Smolkin, L.B., & Conlin, A. (1989). Preschoolers' questions about pictures, print convention, and story text during reading aloud at home. *Reading Research Quarterly*, 24, 188-214.

Yopp, H.K. (1988). The validity and reliability of phonemic awareness tests. *Reading Research Quarterly*, 23, 159-177.

Zhang, S., & Perfetti, C.A. (1993). The tongue-twister effect in reading Chinese. *Journal of Experimental Psychology: Learning, Memory, and Cognition*, 19, 1082-1093.

Address correspondence to:

Barbara R. Foorman
Educational Psychology
University of Houston
Houston, TX 77204-5874
U.S.A.

ESTHER GEVA & DALE WILLOWS

ORTHOGRAPHIC KNOWLEDGE IS ORTHOGRAPHIC KNOWLEDGE IS ORTHOGRAPHIC KNOWLEDGE

Why are we studying orthographic knowledge? Over the last 15 years, a majority of investigations of reading have been concerned with word recognition processes. In particular, they have focused on the role of cognitive and phonological processes in reading acquisition and reading disabilities. These studies have led most researchers and theoreticians to the conclusion that "automatic" word recognition is the primary factor underlying reading fluency and reading comprehension, that word recognition proficiency is based on the development of phonological processing abilities, and that the variance unaccounted for is relatively minimal (Cunningham & Stanovich, 1990; Stanovich & West, 1989; Stanovich, West & Cunningham, 1992). It would seem, then, that research on orthographic processing can contribute in only a minor way to our understanding of reading acquisition and disability.

On the other hand, perhaps orthographic processing and phonological processing share a great deal of common variance. If one examines the types of tasks ostensibly measuring each, the overlap is readily apparent. Although phonological processes have been the subject of an enormous amount of research, and terms such as phonemic awareness and phonological coding have become commonplace in the literature, the definition of these terms has not always been consistent or explicit. To some extent their meaning is best inferred from the measures that are used to test them. The vast majority of measures of phonological processes are not unrelated to knowledge of letters and spelling, sometimes quite explicitly (e.g., pseudoword reading) but at other times more implicitly (e.g., try to perform the Rosner task of saying "black" leaving off the /b/, without thinking about how the word is spelled). The work of Seidenberg and Tannenhaus (1979) who

V.W. Berninger (ed.), The varieties of orthographic knowledge I: Theoretical and developmental issues, 359-380.

found automatic orthographic activation in rhyme judgment tasks (e.g., do dune-tune rhyme? do stuff-tough rhyme?) suggested that it is difficult to separate orthographic and phonological processes. So did the more recent work of Bruck, (1992) involving a phoneme counting task (e.g., how many phonemes in "tisk" and "leem"). Bruck reports that normals were more likely than reading disabled (RD) children to activate the spelling of the words in performing the task and count the number of letters. These are examples par excellence of the interconnectedness, and perhaps the bi-directional activation between phonology and orthography (Barron, chapter 6, this volume): In fact, the term phonological "coding" is referring to the connection between the processing of phonology and the orthographic code that represents the phonology. Thus, as Wagner and Barker (chapter 7, this volume) have suggested, the line between phonological and orthographic processes is not an unambiguous one:

> Our view is that it is premature to close in on any one conceptualization or task [of orthographic processing]. We are particularly doubtful about the feasibility of constructing "pure" measures of orthographic processing ability, just as we doubt whether measures such as decoding nonwords provide as pure a measure of phonological coding as most of us once thought they did (Treiman, Goswami, & Bruck, 1990). Perhaps, the best we can do is to construct tasks that differ in the degree to which they elicit or, at least, encourage orthographic or phonological coding, (p. 248).

The backbone of this chapter is a critical examination of the task types used to measure orthographic knowledge and what it is they purport to measure. To provide a comprehensive discussion of theoretical and methodological issues arising out of the rich and multidimensional information printed on these pages would be redundant, since some of the authors have already done so in their respective chapters. To repeat what was already said would also be tedious. Instead, we chose to assemble our comments around three themes. The first is a global view account of what develops in orthographic knowledge. The second revolves around general conceptual issues and conceptual issues in cross-linguistic research and in second language learning. In particular, we raise some questions about the extent to which specific findings regarding orthographic knowledge in various age and ability groups apply across different orthographies and across various second language (L_2) contexts. The third cluster revolves around some persistent methodological issues in research concerned with orthographic processing. More specifically, we discuss linguistic, metalinguistic, cognitive and visual processing factors which may be confounded with measures purporting to assess orthographic processing. We end the chapter with a brief discussion of visual components in orthographic processing which may distinguish it from phonological knowledge.

ORTHOGRAPHIC PROCESSING—WHAT DEVELOPS?

Unarguably, the studies described in this volume have demonstrated that (a) with development the nature and components of orthographic knowledge change, and (b) that individual and developmental differences in word recognition and in word spelling accuracy can be somewhat better understood by considering the contributions of orthographic knowledge over and above the contributions of phonological processing.

As is evident from the comprehensive introduction provided by Berninger to Volume I, as well as the integrative discussion in the respective chapters by Barron and by Wagner and Barker, orthographic knowledge is not a unidimensional construct which can be measured by a simple continuous measure and on which one could anticipate to find individual and developmental differences. Rather, it seems that different measures address different aspects of this complex construct, whose very nature changes with development and exposure to the written forms of one's own language and possibly through exposure to other writing systems. Orthographic knowledge is like a moving target: What it means varies as a function of task, orthographic characteristics, reading ability, research design and sample characteristics.

To illustrate, it seems that prior to, or perhaps simultaneously with, the emergence of "proto-literacy" à-la Barron (chapter 6, this volume) and Ehri (1993), it is possible to detect global, visually and spatially based orthographic knowledge. This type of global orthographic knowledge is displayed by non-reading Taiwanese children attending kindergarten, who can distinguish between appropriately oriented right-side-up Chinese characters and upside-down

Chinese characters, even though they may still have trouble in distinguishing appropriate orientation from mirror-image characters (Lu & Jackson, 1993). It is evidenced, likewise, by the type of orthographic knowledge displayed by non-reading pre-school children growing up in an English environment, who, when presented with texts in different languages, can assert that the Chinese text is not English even though they may not be able yet to tell Russian and English apart (Geva, 1994).

The type of orthographic knowledge described above is gradually augmented with the ability to notice sublexical clusters (Berninger & Abbott, chapter 8; Bowers, Golden, Kennedy & Young, chapter 5, this volume). It is also augmented by the learner's growing competence in distinguishing legal from illegal sub-lexical clusters (Assink & Kattenberg, chapter 3, this volume; Siegel, Share & Geva, 1994; Geva & Share, in preparation). Being able to select the appropriate homophone while spelling (e.g., pair - pear) (Assink & Kattenberg, chapter 3, this volume; Olson, Forsberg & Wise, chapter 1, this volume; Stanovich, West & Cunningham, 1992; Wagner & Barker, chapter 7, this volume), constitutes yet another building block.

Another milestone in the development of orthographic knowledge, involving the ability to integrate orthographic and syntactic information, is evidenced when the middle-school student or the L_2 learner becomes cognizant of the fact that /ðer/ can be written in a number of ways (i.e., "their," "there," or "they're") (Assink & Kattenberg, chapter 3, this volume). This milestone does not reflect only more analyzed orthographic knowledge. Instead, it involves resource-demanding processes and development along a number of dimensions. Assink and Kattenberg (chapter 3, this volume) have shown that children's ability to integrate syntactic information with spelling accuracy increases gradually with age, and that higher order oral language processes contribute to what we call "orthographic knowledge." This point, which has been overlooked by some researchers who study orthographic knowledge, is relevant to English, but it may be even more relevant to growth in orthographic knowledge in highly inflected languages such as French, Dutch and Hebrew. Moreover, to be able to carry out successfully a task requiring the coordination of linguistic information from a number of sources does not reflect growth along a single dimension. Instead, it means that the learners have at their disposal the benefits of encapsulated fast naming speed (Bowers & Wolf, 1993; Bowers et al, chapter 5; Wolf, Pfeil, Lotz & Biddle, chapter 4, this volume) and the metalinguistic knowledge needed to focus on clusterable sublexical units (Berninger & Abbott, chapter 8; Bowers, et al, chapter 5, this volume). It also includes efficient recognition and search strategies of legal and illegal orthographic clusters (Assink & Kattenberg, chapter 3; Jackson, Lu & Ju, chapter 2; Wolf et al, chapter 4, this volume). Moreover, accurate performance means that the learner has the metacognitive strategies and the working memory capacity needed to simultaneously analyze and consider functional linguistic properties such as parts of speech, gender and tense, and form properties such as identical phonology (Bialystok & Ryan, 1985).

UNRESOLVED CONCEPTUAL ISSUES

Two unstated assumptions are common to a large number of studies in which orthographic knowledge is measured with forced-choice, multiple-choice and yes-no tasks: (a) subjects are familiar with the meaning of the target lexical items in a homophone choice task, or with the meaning of the real word in pseudohomophone tasks; (b) subjects are aware of the identical phonology associated with the written form of each of the items. These assumptions are implied by the fact that researchers tend to include in these tasks only high frequency lexical items.

The assumption that subjects are familiar with the target items may be only partially valid, however, when subjects are novices, learning to read in their first language (L_1) or second language (L_2). Questions concerning the second assumption are not trivial either. It may be true that one of the building blocks of a higher degree of orthographic knowledge entails the ability to distinguish among homophones in reading and spelling tasks. However, the English writing system does not consist only of homophones. More importantly, this knowledge may be related to other underlying cognitive and metalinguistic skills. To be able to perform homophone or pseudohomophone choice tasks the readers need to be aware of the fact that words that sound the same may nevertheless be spelled differently and mean different things. Once this awareness is in place they then need to be able to recall or recognize with minimum effort alternative legal spelling candidates, and develop a strategy to deal with potential ambiguities.

It is not rare to observe young readers and L_2 learners who overgeneralize a particular spelling rule they have just acquired. For example, the "silent e" strategy may be highly salient as learners become cognizant of spelling rules and begin to apply them systematically. During this transitory stage they may not be aware yet that "oa" is an acceptable orthographic alternative to the /ou/ diphthong. As a result, they may opt systematically for word spellings conforming to the "silent e" rule in English. This may lead them to prefer "rane" over "rain" and "sope" over "soap." In other words, their repertoire of alternative spellings for identical phonemes may not be fully developed yet, and they may rely on a subset of orthographic features, made salient by instruction. The size and range of this repertoire may depend on print exposure and instruction (Cunningham & Stanovich, 1990; Stanovich & West, 1989). Yet, it may also depend on basic cognitive and metalinguistic prerequisite skills such as verbal memory and the ability to analyze separately form (i.e., spelling), sound, and meaning, and to integrate information from all these sources. In other words, what may be taken by researchers as evidence for development along a single continuum from less developed to more developed orthographic knowledge, may be intricately entangled with underlying developmental, metacognitive, and metalinguistic factors.

Gradually the young readers will also increase their repertoire of homographs, identically written words whose pronunciation is determined on the basis of meaning and of syntactic constraints (e.g., bow /bou/-bow /bau/). To illustrate, consider the type of orthographic knowledge implicated in determining that even though "invalid" (with stress on the first syllable) and "invalid" (with stress on the second syllable) sound different, their spelling is identical. This knowledge would require an awareness of the two meanings of this word, coupled with the ability to coordinate pronunciation with orthographic, semantic and syntactic information. Interestingly, so far, this component of orthographic knowledge has not received much attention among researchers, perhaps because of the persistent influence of bottom-up processing models, coupled possibly with theoretical biases favoring the phonology-to-orthography route.

The difficulty in separating orthographic knowledge from other forms of linguistic knowledge is as apparent when we consider the interplay between orthographic and morphemic knowledge. Imagine that while reading a text in a magazine catering to the health-conscious, you encounter a word you have never seen or heard before, say "nutraceuticals." Good readers can make an educated guess about how to pronounce this new word, and manage to infer its meaning. With the help of an ill-defined process one is able to separate this new word into the three morphemes "nutra" and "ceutical(s)," each of which consists of distinct meaning carrying clusters. At a more detailed level the expert reader knows that in English "ceu" is a legitimate and pronounceable cluster, and that sometimes, though quite rarely, English words may end with the /ä/ sound as in "(nut)ra." Does the ability to parse this word into morphemes belong exclusively to the domain of morphemic knowledge, or does it interact with orthographic knowledge? Is it possible that aptitude in noticing morphemes in compound words is an extension of the reader's growing ability to notice sublexical clusters, as noted by Berninger and Abbott (chapter 8, this volume)?

Researchers have been ingenious in inventing tasks to measure orthographic knowledge. At the same time, subjects rarely actually have to spell. Selecting a spelling option from a given array, deciding whether a given spelling is accurate, or reading an irregular word may be demanding to the novice. Yet, none seem to capture the task demands of an authentic spelling task where the writer needs to coordinate and monitor phonological, orthographic, syntactic and semantic information in producing complex texts.

Cross-linguistic comparisons. The chapters by Assink and Kattenberg (chapter 3, this volume), Wolf et al (chapter 4, this volume) and Jackson et al. (chapter 2, this volume) highlight the importance of examining carefully in different writing systems what is meant by orthographic knowledge, and the contribution of underlying cognitive and linguistic factors to its development in different orthographic systems. It is clear that theoretical claims regarding the universal role of orthographic and phonological processing in reading and spelling, based on learning to read and spell in English and other Roman-based alphabets, need to be examined carefully.

The "Orthographic Depth Hypothesis" (Frost, Katz & Bentin, 1987; Katz & Frost, 1992; Turvey, Feldman & Lukatela, 1984) has been proposed as one way of addressing potential differences in basic reading processes in different orthographies. According to this hypothesis there are differences between alphabetic orthographies in terms of how systematically spelling and pronunciations can be mapped onto each other. A shallow orthography allows a simple one-to-one correspondence between letters and sounds. A more complex, or "deep" orthography, while still abiding by the alphabetic principle, employs a more elaborate set of relationships between letters and sounds. One hypothesis, therefore, is that individuals will learn to read and spell accurately faster when a shallow orthography is involved.

Orthographic depth is typically used to describe a factor relevant to the process of decoding. The fact that it influences spelling, as well, is generally tacitly assumed. However, Venezky (1970) cautioned us long ago, that the translation of phonemes to graphemes and graphemes to phonemes may require different rules. Some recent research evidence suggests that indeed, this tacit assumption is not necessarily applicable. For example, in Hebrew some sounds are associated with more than one graphemic candidate, but no grapheme has more than one corresponding phoneme. Geva, Wade-Woolley and Shany (1993) found that the less complex (voweled) Hebrew orthography facilitated the decoding accuracy of grade 1 and 2 children for whom Hebrew was L_2. However, it failed to maintain that facilitation in spelling. Depressed second language effects were apparent in spelling but not in decoding, which actually favored the L_2 subjects. In other words, the level of orthographic depth does not necessarily remain the same for decoding and encoding, and it is possible for the same language to be relatively shallow for readers but deeper for spellers.

In much of the research discussed in this volume there is a close affinity between the conceptualization of orthographic knowledge and spelling. Some of the researchers (e.g., Assink & Kattenberg, chapter 3) tend to treat as interchangeable the relationships between orthographic knowledge and spelling. Yet, the results reported by Geva et al. (1993) suggest that in some languages there may be a "depth differential" between the processing demands of decoding and spelling tasks. It is likewise possible that in some languages the type of orthographic knowledge encapsulated in recognition tasks may not be isomorphic with the knowledge required by "real" spelling tasks.

Another issue that needs to be explored across orthographies involves the nature of the phoneme-grapheme correspondences yielding homophones and pseudohomophones in different alphabetic and non-alphabetic writing systems. For example, while exact statistics are not available, it seems that in English homophones (and pseudohomophones) are a result of vowel identity manipulation or the presence of certain silent consonants in word initial or word final positions. The vowels whose manipulation results in homophones can appear in word initial, word medial, as well as word final positions (e.g., or/oar; flour/flower; blue/blew). Relatedly, Stage and Wagner (1992) report that English vowels tend to occur more frequently in the medial position, while consonants tend to occur more often in word initial and word final positions. They found that by controlling for phoneme position the average proportion of correctly spelled vowels in words was comparable to that of consonants. The consonants "k" and "g" are silent when they are followed by "n" and "w" is silent when followed by "r," resulting in homophones such as" knead-need" and "wrack-rack." The silent "n" in final position, preceded by "m" yields homophones such as damn-dam.

It seems though that in different orthographies homophones may be based on different linguistic elements. For example, in modern spoken Hebrew one can find consonant pairs that lost their unique historical phonemic representations, and are associated with identical phonemes (Berman, 1978). Thus, the phoneme /x/ can be represented by two distinct graphemes: /xeth/ח and /xaf/כ , and the phoneme /s/ is associated with the grapheme /samex/ס and /sin/שׂ. Relatedly, Hebrew homophones and pseudohomophones are the result of consonant-based phoneme ambiguity. The ambiguous consonants can occur in word initial, word medial and word final positions, for example, /al/אל (don't) and /al/על (on); /sum/שׂם ([he] put) and /sum/סם (drug); /ax/אך (but) and /ax/אח (brother).[1] As may be expected, spelling errors in Hebrew often involve phonologically interchangeable consonant pairs. They do not involve vowel ambiguity, since in Hebrew the pronunciation of vowels (when they are present) is unambiguous (Berman, 1978). What we do not know yet is whether such differences in orthographic structure yield differences in the strategies used to process homophones in different orthographies, and whether differences in writing systems result in orthography-specific processing requirements and in different distributions of error types. At the same time, it is reasonable that there may be cross-orthography processing commonalties as well.

Another issue that needs to be addressed in cross-orthography research concerns the question of "what develops?" To illustrate, a child for whom English is the L_1 or an individual acquiring literacy skills in English as L_2 may not recognize or spell "pain" automatically. Yet, he or she may nevertheless derive the correct response in a pseudohomophone or homophone choice task by being strategic. They may have learned to focus and examine the vowels in similarly sounding words such as "pain" and "pane," even when they are unable yet to recognize the words "on sight." This approach may reflect a productive strategy based on the salience of vowels as "trouble makers" in English spelling. Poor readers and reading disabled readers may be slower in developing this strategic knowledge as well as in recalling the specific competing spelling candidates.

Languages may differ also in the relative complexity and processing demands presented by the need to consider higher level syntactic information in making decisions about word meanings, spellings and ultimately, text comprehension. For example, alphabetic languages such as Dutch, French and Hebrew are highly inflected. Assink and Kattenberg (chapter 3, this volume) help to draw our attention to the influence of the development of syntactic and semantic skills on orthographic knowledge. Furthermore, Jackson et al (chapter 2, this volume) remind us that :

> ...word level predictors that are major contributors to reading times for English text are less important sources of variance in the time allocated to processing Chinese text. Instead, readers of Chinese tend to pause at physical or syntactic boundaries, perhaps to integrate what they have read so far. (p. 86)

Such findings should caution researchers to be more mindful in assuming that findings from English-based studies are directly relevant to orthographic knowledge in other languages. We still do not agree as to the nature of orthographic knowledge, the precise role it plays in reading and the appropriate way to measure it. We are even less certain when we attempt to concur on what are universal and orthography-specific building blocks, and the way in which these building blocks emerge from the "bottom-up" or from the "top-down."

Issues in the development of orthographic knowledge in L2 learners. In the area of reading in L_2 there is a tendency to import and apply in a wholesale fashion L_1 reading models. This practice is understandable given the dearth of L_2 reading models. At the same time such practice may lead to fundamental misconceptions and misinterpretation of crucial variables. In the context of discussing the development of orthographic knowledge as it is captured by performance on homophone and pseudohomophone tasks it may be fruitful to examine critically the assumptions listed with regard to L_1 learners and the extent to which these assumptions are valid in studying orthographic processes among L_2 learners.

To illustrate, children learning to read in their L_1 already have a good command of their oral language. When they begin to learn to read they use their rich repertoire of oral skills to facilitate word decoding and comprehension processes (Goodman,1989; Stanovich, 1993). They may know what a "boar" is even though they may not be aware yet of the fact that the particular spelling of /bor/ will depend on meaning. The L_1 learner comes to the learning task with accurate phonological representations of "boar" and "bore," and has to learn that the spelling of /bor/ (animal) is different from and more complex than /bor/ (send to sleep). In L1 researchers can assume that the more frequently a word is encountered in oral language and in print, the more familiar it becomes. Therefore, it is likely that the spelling of "bore" will be acquired before the spelling of "boar."

Learning to read and spell in L_2 may be fundamentally different—in many L_2 learning contexts (e.g., immigrant children, immersion programs, English for Special Purposes [ESP]) learners develop their oral and reading skills simultaneously, and therefore they cannot rely on high oral proficiency to facilitate the development of reading and spelling. One cannot reliably assume, therefore, that L_2 learners have had sufficient exposure to frequent words in the L_2 to make them familiar with those words. The L_2 learners are less likely to know the meaning of "knead" (unless one is a chéf enrolled in an ESP course). More importantly, a learner may find the meaning of "knead" by consulting a dictionary, be able to recognize the word on sight, spell it correctly and understand texts in which this word appears, but articulate it as /knīd/ (instead of /nid/). It is clear then that for such a learner "knead-need" are not homophonous.

Moreover, the second language includes some phonemes which do not exist in the L_1 and which cannot be pronounced accurately by the L_2 learner. Consider, for example, the subtle phonological differences in French among "de" (the indefinite article, singular), "des" (the indefinite article, plural), "dès" (since) and "deux" (two). Normally developing French L_1 learners can already pronounce these words accurately, though they need to learn how to spell each, and some elements, such as the silent consonant in "deux" may be problematic. However, to the uninitiated L_2 learner these words sound like homophones. In other words, items which are non-homophonous for L_1 learners may be perceived as homophonous by L_2 learners, and L_2 learners may learn to compensate for this problem by relying on higher level syntactic and semantic information sources.

To summarize, non-homophonous words may be perceived by L_2 learners as homophonous, and homophonous items may be represented phonologically as non-homophonous. L_2 researchers cannot take tasks developed for L_1 learners and apply them to L_2 learners in a hole-sail (or is it whole-sale...) fashion. The above discussion also suggests that the rate of acquisition of orthographic knowledge in a second language may vary as a function of negative transfer of phonological information from the L_1, and the inflectional complexity of the L_2. Inaccurate spelling may reflect trivial articulatory errors or inaccurate orthographic knowledge. Accurate spelling may be the result of a different strategy from the one used by L_1 learners. Researchers have to devise measurement tools that minimize such confounds.

SOME METHODOLOGICAL PRECAUTIONS

Many of the studies discussed in the chapters in this volume measured orthographic knowledge with choice tasks consisting of discrete lexical items. Three judgment-based task types recur: forced-choice, multiple-choice and yes-no. In the homophone choice task (see for example Assink & Kattenberg, chapter 3, this volume; Olson et al, chapter 1, this volume; Wagner & Barker, 1992; Stanovich et al, 1992) subjects are to select from an array of simultaneously presented printed words the homophone which is appropriate in a given context. For example, they hear the sentence "which is a fruit?" and have to choose between "pair" and "pear." In the pseudohomophone forced-choice or multiple-choice judgment task subjects see two simultaneously presented words, one of which is spelled correctly (e.g., "rain") but the other is an identical pseudohomophone (e.g., "rane"). The subjects' task is to judge which is the correct spelling (see for example, Olson et al, this volume; Stanovich et al., 1992; Wagner & Barker, 1992.) In the yes-no test paradigm subjects may hear a single lexical item and then see a written version of it. Their task is to judge whether or not it is spelled correctly (e.g., Manis, Szezulki, Holt & Graves, 1990).

The chapter by Olson et al (chapter 1, this volume) highlights some methodological pitfalls that need to be carefully considered with regard to the tasks surveyed above. One problem source concerns contamination of orthographic knowledge with linguistic and cognitive factors. For example, homophones can be challenging and confusing when individuals perceive them as homophones. Yet, as argued in the previous section, some L_1 children and L_2 learners may perceive more homophones than exist because of underdeveloped phonological representation. Another confounding factor mentioned earlier concerns the assumption that lexical items are familiar to the participants. A third confounding factor has to do with the confounding of metalinguistic development with what reading researchers refer to as orthographic knowledge. Specifically, when English speaking children hear the sentence "which is a number?" and then are to select between "ate" and "eight," or when Chinese children are asked in a forced-choice task to judge which of two characters means the same as a previously learned word (Jackson et al., chapter 2, this volume) the task becomes highly demanding as it requires the ability to separate meaning from graphic information.

Another methodological challenge faces researchers who use slightly different procedures to operationalize the same construct. For example, Olson et al. (chapter 1, this volume) and Manis et al. (1990) reached incompatible conclusions when they compared the orthographic knowledge of older reading disabled (RD) individuals with that of younger, normally achieving controls. Olson et al., who tested orthographic knowledge in reading and spelling with multiple-choice decision tasks, found the performance of the RD to be superior to that of the normal controls. Manis et al., on the other hand, who used a yes-no decision task found that the younger normals outperformed their RD older counterparts. Two interpretations of this discrepancy are likely. The interpretation favored by Olson et al. is that the finding that the orthographic knowledge of older RD is superior to that of their younger, reading-level matched counterparts is valid, and that a response bias in the Manis study was confounded with the "true" orthographic knowledge possessed by older RD children. Alternatively it is possible that, notwithstanding the influence of response bias, deciding whether a given spelling is correct (the procedure used by Manis et al.) is cognitively a demanding recall task. By comparison, multiple-choice or forced-choice tasks (the procedures used by Olson et al.) are less demanding recognition tasks, in which the crucial sub-lexical elements manipulated may become fairly salient, especially because the lexical items are presented simultaneously (see discussion above).

The use of reading level match designs, and what they tell us about normally achieving and reading disabled individuals, raises some persistent questions. Olson et al. (chapter 1, this volume) report on a series of studies in which a reading-level match (RLM) design was used to compare the orthographic knowledge of young readers to that of older RD participants who were reading disabled (RD), and who were matched to their younger normal counterparts. The older RD outperformed their younger, normally achieving counterparts, leading the investigators to conclude that these RD children have better orthographic knowledge (see also Siegel et al., 1994, for similar results.) In the Siegel et al. study, subjects are asked "which is more like a word—filk or filv?" Performance on this task requires ignoring meaning and focusing on form. In the Olson et al., studies better performance entails a more developed ability to integrate sound, meaning and orthographic constraints. The possibility that these studies are vulnerable to the confounding factors mentioned above needs to be seriously considered. Namely, older individuals are older. By virtue of being older they have presumably had more exposure and systematic instructional intervention than the young normals. They may be able to handle with more ease the metalinguistic components of these tasks than the young normals.

The work of Bowers and her colleagues (chapter 5, this volume), Berninger and her colleagues (see Berninger, Cartwright, Yates et al., in press) and Wolf and her colleagues (chapter 4, this volume) has begun to address sublexical orthographic processes. In these yes-no paradigms subjects have to decide whether a letter cluster was present or absent in a previously presented word. For example, the word "clock" is shown for one second, and then a letter cluster such as "cl" or "co" appears. Berninger reports that this form of orthographic recognition memory is related to more proficient reading of non-words. She argues that skill in recognizing sub-word orthographic patterns can help identify nonwords as well as words. While it is reasonable to assume that orthographic knowledge entails the gradual automatic recognition of sublexical clusters, it should be pointed out that performance on this task is confounded with a number of underlying cognitive and linguistic factors. So, as orthographic coding tasks are modified to include permissible and nonpermissible letter sequences, which is an excellent way to investigate the relationship between orthographic structure and orthographic coding (see Wolf et al., chapter 4, this volume), it will be important to consider alternative interpretations of the effects of permissible and nonpermissible letter sequences. For example, some clusters are more easily pronounceable (e.g., cl, co) whereas others are less so (e.g., cx). Thus performance on this task may be intricately related not only to frequency ("cx" never occurs in English, while the others do) but also to the pronounceability of the clusters. Pronounceable clusters could be retained in working memory for a longer time than non-pronounceable clusters. Performance on yes-no paradigms may also be confounded with attention. For example, children may perform poorly because of underlying attentional problems (rather than orthographic coding problems) and the task as designed does not allow one to tease apart that confound. Also, underlying problems in short term memory, independent of orthographic coding per se, could depress performance on this kind of task.

The importance of carrying out task analysis and examining the task demands of divergent tasks that purport to measure the same theoretical construct has been also articulated by

Bruck (1992) in trying to reconcile contradictory results pertaining to the RD obtained by Rack (1985) and Bruck (1992). In particular, Bruck found that the RD were less accurate on phoneme counting and phoneme deletion tasks, whereas Rack found that older RD were quite good at performing the Seidenberg and Tanenhaus (1979) rhyming task. Bruck argues convincingly that phoneme counting and phoneme deletion tasks require both automatic activation of orthographic information in auditory word recognition and the deliberate and conscious use of that information to perform the demanding tasks of counting and deletion. In contrast, orthographic effects in the Seidenberg and Tanenhaus tasks may be based solely on automatic activation. Bruck suggests that perhaps normals and dyslexics differ in their ability to use *deliberately* orthographic information in taxing and resource demanding tasks but not in their ability to activate that information.

Carrying out task analysis and examining task demands of divergent tasks purporting to measure the same theoretical construct may also help to reconcile what may seem like incompatible definitions of orthographic knowledge and an abundance of tasks used to operationalize this plethora of definitions. It may be useful to distinguish among measures tapping primarily orthographic representations that we already have in our memory (e.g., knowing that the fruit /per/ is spelt "pear"), and those assessing on-line processing required to activate orthographic representation. The latter is achieved by researchers in continuous recognition studies such as the one used by Berninger et al (chapter 8). Tasks that tap each of these use the same term "orthographic knowledge"; yet one set seems to focus primarily on products, whereas the other seems to focus primarily on process.

ORTHOGRAPHIC KNOWLEDGE AND VISUAL PROCESSING

The main thrust of our discussion so far has been on confounding factors stemming from linguistic, metalinguistic and cognitive factors. However, an examination of a wide range of research suggests that visual processing might also be intricately implicated in orthographic processing, and that there is a need to re-examine the widely held belief that visual processing deficits are not related to reading disabilities. For example, Corcos and Willows (1993) review studies, involving adults and children of varying ages and reading-skill levels, that attempt to avoid confounding orthographic processing with that of phonological and morphological information. They conclude that a strong relationship exists between the acquisition of orthographic knowledge and visual familiarity. Another review, by Willows, Kruk and Corcos (1993), provides further support for the need to consider the contribution of visual processes to word recognition and to the ways in which visual processes in early and late stages of visual processing interact with various linguistic processes. Additional support for the need to consider the contribution of visual processing is provided by Lovegrove and Williams (1993) who review psychophysical and physiological investigations and show that many reading disabled individuals are deficient in transient visual processing; it seems that the transient system of the reading disabled is less efficient, and that temporal aspects of transient system functioning can be affected by spatial frequency characteristics of text. Another perspective on the potential involvement of visual processing in word recognition processes comes from Seymour and Evans (1993) who examined the connection between visual processes and dyslexia, and argue that the visual deficit in dyslexia resides in a visual orthographic processor. They propose that reading difficulties in dyslexia can occur at several different stages: in early visual processing, in either a visual (object) processor or a visual (orthographic) processor which is exclusive to processing print, or in the central reading processes that incorporate higher cognitive and language aspects.

This body of research evidence suggests that beyond the issues dealt with by the authors in these chapters, the interface between visual processing and orthographic knowledge forms another dimension. Thus we have come full circle: We began our commentary by arguing that the line between phonological and orthographic processing is fuzzy. In many of the measures discussed in this book orthographic knowledge is tapped by examining similar sounding items that have different visual forms (homophones and pseudohomophones), and by contrasting abilities to process the sounds in words with the visual form of words. In future research, it is important to consider the extent to which there may be an essential visual component in orthographic knowledge that distinguishes it from phonological knowledge.

NOTE

1. In Hebrew there is also a relatively high number of homographs—identically spelled words that are pronounced differently. Texts written for fluent readers appear without vowels. This characteristic yields a special class of homographs in which the consonants are identical but the pronunciation and meaning differ (e.g., "s.p.r." pronounced as /siper/ [he told] and "s.p.r." pronounced as /sefer/ [book]). Another group of homographs includes words of identical spelling, varying in the stressed syllable and in meaning (e.g.,"k.m.h." pronounced /kamah (wheat) and "k.m.h." pronounced /kamah/ (she got up). Further discussion of related problems is beyond the scope of this commentary.

REFERENCES

Assink, E., & Kattenberg, G. (1994). Higher-order linguistic influences on development of orthographic knowledge: Illustrations from spelling problems in Dutch and assessment tools. In V.W. Berninger (Ed.), *The varieties of orthographic knowledge I: Theoretical and developmental issues* (pp. 111-136). Dordrecht, The Netherlands: Kluwer Academic Press.

Barron, R. (1994). The sound-to-spelling connection: Orthographic activation in auditory word recognition and its implications for the acquisition of phonological awareness and literacy skills. In V.W. Berninger (Ed.), *The varieties of orthographic knowledge I: Theoretical and developmental issues* (pp. 219-242). Dordrecht, The Netherlands: Kluwer Academic Press.

Berman, R. (1978). *Modern Hebrew structure.* Tel Aviv: University Publishing Projects, Ltd.

Berninger, V., & Abbott, R. (1994). Multiple orthographic and phonological codes in literacy acquisition: An evolving research program. In V.W. Berninger (Ed.), *The varieties of orthographic knowledge I: Theoretical and developmental issues* (pp. 277-317). Dordrecht, The Netherlands: Kluwer Academic Press.

Berninger, V.W., Cartwright, A.C., Yates, C.M., Swanson, H.L., & Abbott, R.D. (in press). Developmental skills related to writing and reading acquisition in the intermediate grades: Shared and unique functional systems. *Reading and Writing: An Interdisciplinary Journal.*

Bialystok, E., & Ryan, E.B. (1985). A metacognitive framework for the development of first and second language skills. In D.L. Forrest-Pressley, G.E. MacKinnon, & T.G. Waller (Eds.), *Metacognition, cognition, and human performance* (pp. 207-245). Orlando, Florida: Academic Press.

Bowers, P., Golden, J., Kennedy, A., & Young, A. (1994). Limits upon orthographic knowledge due to processes indexed by naming speed. In V.W. Berninger (Ed.), *The varieties of orthographic knowledge I: Theoretical and developmental issues* (pp. 173-218). Dordrecht, The Netherlands: Kluwer Academic Press.

Bowers, P.G., & Wolf, M. (1993). Theoretical links among naming speed, precise timing mechanisms and orthographic skill in dyslexia. *Reading and Writing: An Interdisciplinary Journal*, 5, 69-85.

Bruck, M. (1992). Persistence of dyslexics' phonological awareness deficits. *Developmental Psychology*, 28, 874-886.

Corcos, E., & Willows, D.M. (1993). The processing of orthographic information. In D.M. Willows, R.S. Kruk, & E. Corcos (Eds.), *Visual processes in reading and reading disabilities* (pp. 163-190). Hillsdale, NJ: Erlbaum.

Cunningham, A.E., & Stanovich, K.E. (1990). Assessing print exposure and orthographic processing skill in children: A quick measure of reading experience. *Journal of Educational Psychology*, 82, 733-740.

Ehri, L.C. (1993). How English orthography influences phonological knowledge as children learn to read and spell. In R.J. Scholes (Ed.), *Literacy and language analysis* (pp. 21-43). Hillsdale, NJ: Erlbaum.

Frost, R., Katz, L., & Bentin, S. (1987). Strategies for visual word recognition and orthographic depth. *Journal of Experimental Psychology: Human Perception and Performance*, 13, 104-115.

Geva, E. (March, 1994). *Universal and orthography-specific component processes in the development of basic reading skills in bilingual children*. Symposium presentation, Association of American Applied Linguistics (AAAL). Baltimore, MD.

Geva, E., & Share, D. (1994). *Orthographic and morphosyntactic factors in the development of orthographic awareness of Hebrew among second language learners*. In preparation. Ontario Institute for Studies in Education.

Geva, E., Wade-Woolley, L., & Shany, M. (1993). The concurrent development of spelling and decoding in different orthographies. *Journal of Reading Behavior, 25*(4), 383-406.

Goodman, K. (1989). Whole-language research: Foundations and development. *Elementary School Journal, 90*, 207-221.

Jackson, N., Lu, W-H, & Ju, D. (1994). Reading Chinese and reading English: Similarities, differences, and second-language learning. In V. W. Berninger (Ed.), *The varieties of orthographic knowledge I: Theoretical and developmental issues* (pp. 73-109). Dordrecht, The Netherlands: Kluwer Academic Publishers.

Katz, L., & Frost, R. (1992). The reading process is different for different orthographies: The orthographic depth hypothesis. In R. Frost & L. Katz (Eds.), *Orthography, phonology, morphology, and meaning*. Amsterdam, The Netherlands: Elsevier.

Lovegrove, W.J., & Williams, M.C. (1993). Visual temporal processing deficits in specific reading disability. In D.M. Willows, R.S. Kruk, & E. Corcos (Eds.), *Visual processes in reading and reading disabilities* (pp. 311-330). Hillsdale, NJ: Erlbaum.

Lu, W. H., & Jackson, N.E. (1993). *Children's developing metalinguistic awareness of properties of Chinese characters*. Paper presented at the biennial meeting of The Society for Research in Child Development, New Orleans.

Manis, F.R., Szezulki, P.A., Holt, L.K., & Graves, K. (1990). Variation in component word recognition and spelling skills among dyslexic children and normal readers. In T. Carr & B.A. Levy (Eds.), *Reading and its development: Component skills approaches* (pp. 207-259). New York: Academic Press.

Olson, R., Forsberg, H., & Wise, B. (1994). Genes, environment, and the development of orthographic skills. In V. W. Berninger (Ed.), *The varieties of orthographic knowledge I: Theoretical and developmental issues* (pp. 27-71). Dordrecht, The Netherlands: Kluwer Academic Publishers.

Rack, J.P. (1985). Orthographic and phonetic coding in developmental dyslexia. *British Journal of Psychology, 76*, 325-340.

Seidenberg, M.S., & Tanenhaus, M.K. (1979). Orthographic effects of rhyme monitoring. *Journal of Experimental Psychology, 5*, 546-554.

Seymour, P.H.K., & Evans, H.M. (1993). The visual (orthographic) processor and developmental dyslexia. In D.M. Willows, R.S. Kruk, & E. Corcos (Eds.), *Visual processes in reading and reading disabilities* (pp. 347-376). Hillsdale, NJ: Erlbaum.

Siegel, L.S., Share, D., & Geva, E., (1994). *The development of orthographic skills in normal and disabled readers.* Unpublished manuscript. Ontario Institute for Studies in Education.

Stage, S.A., & Wagner, R.K. (1992). Development of young children's phonological and orthographic knowledge as revealed by their spellings. *Developmental Psychology, 28,* 287-296.

Stanovich, K.E. (1993). Romance and reality. *The Reading Teacher, 47*(4), 280-291.

Stanovich, K.E., & West, R.F. (1989). Exposure to print and orthographic processing. *Reading Research Quarterly,* 24, 402-433.

Stanovich, K.E., West, R.F., & Cunningham, A.E. (1992). Beyond phonological processes: Print exposure and orthographic processing. In S.A. Brady & D. Shankweiler (Eds.), *Phonological processes in literacy* (pp. 219-235). Hillsdale, NJ: Erlbaum.

Treiman, R., Goswami, U., & Bruck, M. (1990). Not all nonwords are alike: Implications for reading development and theory. *Memory & Cognition,* 18, 359-367.

Turvey, M.T., Feldman, L.B., & Lukatela, G. (1984). The Serbo-Croatian orthography constrains the reader to a phonologically analytic strategy. In L. Henderson (Ed.), *Orthographies and reading* (pp. 81-89). London: Erlbaum.

Venezky, R.I. (1970). *The structure of English orthography.* The Hague: Mouton.

Wagner, R., & Barker, T. (1994). The development of orthographic processing ability. In V. W. Berninger (Ed.), *The varieties of orthographic knowledge I: Theoretical and developmental issues* (pp. 243-275). Dordrecht, The Netherlands: Kluwer Academic Publishers.

Willows, D.M., Kruk, R.S., & Corcos, E. (Eds.). (1993). Are there differences between disabled and normal readers in their processing of visual information? *Visual processes in reading and reading disabilities* (pp. 265-286). Hillsdale, NJ: Erlbaum.

Wolf, M., Pfeil, C., Lotz, R., & Biddle, K. (1994). Towards a more universal understanding of the developmental dyslexias: The contribution of orthographic factors. In V. W. Berninger (Ed.), *The varieties of orthographic knowledge I: Theoretical and developmental issues* (pp. 131-171). Dordrecht, The Netherlands: Kluwer Academic Publishers.

Address correspondence to:

Esther Geva
The Ontario Institute for Studies in Education
252 Bloor Street W
Toronto, Ontario M5S 1V6
CANADA

NEUROPSYCHOLOGY AND COGNITION

The purpose of the Neuropsychology and Cognition series is to bring out volumes that promote understanding in topics relating brain and behavior. It is intended for use by both clinicians and research scientists in the fields of neuropsychology, cognitive psychology, psycholinguistics, speech and hearing, as well as education. Examples of topics to be covered in the series would relate to memory, language acquisition and breakdown, reading, attention, developing and aging brain. By addressing the theoretical, empirical, and applied aspects of brain-behavior relationships, this series will try to present the information in the fields of neuropsychology and cognition in a coherent manner.

Series Editor

R. Malatesha Joshi, *Oklahoma State University, U.S.A.*

Publications

1. P.G. Aaron: *Dyslexia and Hyperlexia.* 1989
   ISBN 1-55608-079-4; 1994, ISBN Pb 0-7923-3155-9
2. R.M. Joshi (ed.): *Written Language Disorders.* 1991 ISBN 0-7923-0902-2
3. A. Caramazza: *Issues in Reading, Writing and Speaking.* A Neuropsychological Perspective. 1991 ISBN 0-7923-0996-0
4. B.F. Pennington (ed.): *Reading Disablities.* Genetic and Neurological Influences. 1991 ISBN 0-7923-1606-1
5. N.H. Hadley: *Elective Mutism.* A Handbook for Educators, Counsellors and Health Care Professionals. 1994 ISBN 0-7923-2418-8
6. W.C. Watt (ed.): *Writing Systems and Cognition.* Perspectives from Psychology, Physiology, Linguistics, and Semiotics. 1994 ISBN 0-7923-2592-3
7. I. Taylor and D.R. Olson (eds.), *Scripts and Literacy*: Reading and Learning to Read Alphabets, Syllabaries and Characters. 1994 ISBN 0-7923-2912-0
8. V.W. Berninger (ed.): *The Varieties of Orthographic Knowledge.* I: Theoretical and Developmental Issues. 1994 ISBN 0-7923-3080-3

KLUWER ACADEMIC PUBLISHERS – DORDRECHT / BOSTON / LONDON

GPSR Compliance

The European Union's (EU) General Product Safety Regulation (GPSR) is a set of rules that requires consumer products to be safe and our obligations to ensure this.

If you have any concerns about our products, you can contact us on ProductSafety@springernature.com

In case Publisher is established outside the EU, the EU authorized representative is:

Springer Nature Customer Service Center GmbH
Europaplatz 3
69115 Heidelberg, Germany

Batch number: 10816038

Printed by Printforce, the Netherlands